HYPNAGOGIA

HYPNAGOGIA

*The unique state of consciousness
between wakefulness and sleep*

Andreas Mavromatis

Routledge & Kegan Paul
London and New York

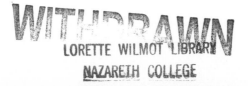

First published in 1987 by
Routledge & Kegan Paul Ltd
11 New Fetter Lane, London EC4P 4EE

Published in the USA by
Routledge & Kegan Paul Inc.
in association with Methuen Inc.
29 West 35th Street, New York, NY 10001

Set in Sabon, 10 on 12pt
by Columns of Reading
and printed in Great Britain
by Thetford Press Ltd,
Thetford, Norfolk

Library of Congress Cataloging in Publication Data

Mavromatis, Andreas.
Hypnagogia : the unique state of consciousness
between wakefulness and sleep.

Bibliography: p.
Includes index.
1. Hypnagogia. I. Title.
QP425.M38 1986   154.3   86-6592

British Library CIP Data also available

ISBN 0-7102-0282-2

To dream and altogether not to dream. This synthesis is the operation of genius. . . .

NOVALIS

I turned my chair to the fire and dozed. Again the atoms were gambolling before my eyes . . . all twining and twisting in snakelike motion. Look! What was that? One of the snakes had seized hold of its own tail, and the form wormed mockingly before my eyes. As if by a flash of lightning I awoke; and this time also I spent the rest of the night working out the consequences of the hypothesis.

KEKULÉ

One phenomenon is certain and I can vouch for its absolute certainty: the sudden and immediate appearance of a solution at the very moment of sudden awakening . . . a solution long searched for appeared to me at once without the slightest instant of reflection on my part . . . and in quite a different direction from any of those which I had previously tried to follow.

HADAMARD

I woke with a start and witnessed, as from a seat in a theater, three acts which brought to life an epoch and characters about which I had no documentary information and which I regarded moreover as forbidding.

COCTEAU

I am aware of these 'fancies' only when I am on the very brink of sleep, with the consciousness that I am so. . . . In these fancies – let me now term them psychal impressions – there is really nothing even approximate in character to impressions ordinarily received. It is as if the five senses were supplanted by five myriad others alien to mortality.

POE

In order to acquire continuity of consciousness, unaffected by lapses into unconscious states, you must hold yourself at the junction of all the states, which constitutes the links between sleeping, dreaming, and waking: the halfsleep or Fourth State.

FROM A TENTH-CENTURY TANTRIC TEXT

Contents

Acknowledgments

Thanks are due to a number of individuals and establishments without whose generous assistance this work would never have reached its present form. First, I should like to extend my thanks to the Social Science Research Council of Great Britain for awarding me a grant that enabled me to carry out the initial research, and to Brunel University for being instrumental in my receiving this grant. I should also like to thank the staff of Brunel University Inter-Library Loans section for their helpfulness, and in particular Ms Lorna Barnes for her tireless efforts in tracing and obtaining material from obscure and remote sources in this country and abroad. Special thanks are due to Dr John T.E. Richardson for his advice and encouragement throughout the initial research, to John Rowan for his constructive criticism, and to my editor David Stonestreet for his patience.

I am deeply grateful to the following for spending generously so much of their time and energy in translating for me hundreds of pages of very important material not available publicly in English: Adie Fishman, Heather Cox, Anne Vasseur, Annabelle Theodore, Liz Neville, Richard Pelling, Janice Selkirk, Jane Conway, Nigel Cooper, Ursula Riniker, Gabriele Simons and David Sladen. For the typing I would like to thank Jane Dawson, Isobel King and Sheila Rogers but mostly Jennie Dawson who took extra care in pointing out my occasional contortions of the English language – whatever is retained of this misuse is, of course, entirely my responsibility. For the illustrations I am particularly indebted to Chris H. Savvides, Tony Remali, Robert Stephenson, David Holt, and Michael Sandle. The list of investigators and experients to whose reports I owe so much is too long to mention here: tribute to them is hopefully paid throughout the text, appendices, references, and bibliography. Finally, I would like to thank all those friends and relatives who offered me moral and other support, not least my mother for calling out to the firemen in her pidgin English to save the typescript of the book when a fire raged through the house at the last stages of the writing of this work.

Figures: Chris H. Savvides **2.4, 2.5, 2.7, 2.9, 2.10, 3.1, 3.4, 4.1(a), 4.2(a,b,c,d), 4.5, 6.1.** Tony Remali **2.2, 2.11(b), 2.17, 2.18, 3.2, 4.4, 7.2(b,c), 8.3, 8.4.** Robert Stephenson **2.3, 2.6, 2.15, 2.16, 3.6, 8.8(a,b).** David Holt **2.19, 2.20.** Nick Constantas **4.1(b).** William Blake (by kind permission of the Trustees of the Tate Gallery, London) **2.11** *Satan in his Original Glory,* **4.3** *The River of Life,* **8.9(a)** *The Ghost of a Flea,* **8.9(b)** *The Man Who Taught Blake Painting in his Dreams.* Richard Doyle (by kind permission of the Trustees of the Victoria and Albert Museum, London) **2.14** from a fantasy sketchbook. From D. Milner and E. Smart *The Loom of Creation,* London: Spearman, 1975 (by kind permission of the publishers: C.W. Daniel Co. Ltd, Saffron Walden, Essex) **5.1(a,b,c), 8.5(a).** From S. Muldoon and H. Carrington *The Projection of the Astral Body,* London: Rider, 1965 (by kind permission of the publishers) **6.2(a,b,c).** The Bettmann Archive, Inc. **7.2(a).** Michael Sandle (courtesy of the artist) **8.1(a).** By kind permission of the Trustees of the Dickens House Museum, London **8.2.** Courtesy Dr Thelma Moss, Neuropsychiatric Institute, University of California, Los Angeles **8.5(b).** Salvador Dali (permission through DACS) **8.6** *Dream Caused by the Flight of a Bee Around a Pomegranate One Second Before Waking Up* (Thyssen-Bornemisza Collection, Lugano), **8.7** *Metamorphosis of Narcissus* (Tate Gallery, London). After M.J. Horowitz *Image Formation and Cognition,* New York: Appleton-Century-Crofts, 1978 (by permission of the publishers) **10.1(a,b).** UPI photos, New York **10.2.** After A. Besant and C.W. Leadbeater *Thought-forms,* Wheaton, Ill.: Theosophical Publishing House, 1975 **11.3.**

Preface

This is an exploratory book, and it is so in a number of ways not the least of which springs from the fact that its subject matter is much like a well-trodden and yet unmapped territory.

When I first began my investigations in this area I was struck by four important observations. To begin with, although a great deal of research had been done on sleep and dreams, there was hardly any organized work on the psychophysical states a person goes through immediately prior to sleep onset and at the time of awaking, otherwise known as hypnagogic-hypnopompic or presleep and postsleep periods. Psychologists spoke of this 'little-cultivated area' and complained that 'investigators worked in ignorance of one another's efforts'. Indeed, much of the original work is still unfortunately available only in obscure journals and other publications, and often in a language other than English. A great deal of this had to be translated specifically for the present work. Thus, one part of this exploration has been to carry out an exhaustive research of the literature, bringing together varied material from disparate sources and organizing it in what I believe to be a comprehensive and, I hope, comprehensible conceptual framework.

Many of the reports I collected from existing studies, and some of those I recorded in my own experiments over the last seven years, at first sight appeared to contradict one another in several respects. For example, some strongly indicated that the experiences were clearly hallucinatory, others emphasized that the person concerned was fully awake at the time and aware of the 'unreality' of the phenomena, and others still pointed out that the person was drowsing or that he even fell asleep for a few minutes. The vividness of the phenomena, the sense of modality involved, and the reported quality of thought also varied. Similarly, the conclusions drawn by investigators did not always agree with one another. This led me to a further, but parallel, exploration, namely to a systematic analysis of the person's attentional and cognitive-experiential states during these periods – which in its turn raised fundamental questions concerning the nature and definitions of wakefulness, sleep, and dreaming, and to which questions I addressed myself in gradual awareness of the fact that my answers would be controversial. In this, I found that personal experience was both necessary and invaluable.

A third exploration was prompted by the observation that although hypnagogic phenomena appeared to be related to a number of other states, processes, and experiences, on phenomenological and possibly aetiological grounds, no systematic studies along these lines had been undertaken. This task alone loomed enormous, and I cannot say with absolute confidence that I did it proper justice; in fact, in some important respects I only scratched the surface, but I hope that my efforts have been sufficiently consistent to present a reasonable and reasoned system around whose hub are coherently gathered these diverse phenomena, and suggestive enough to spur others on to further empirical and theoretical work.

My fourth kind of exploration constitutes an attempt to understand the functions of these experiences in a wider, evolutionary setting. Again, this has grown organically out of questions raised in the process of the research as a whole. It is at times speculative, and although great care has been taken to prevent such speculations from turning into flights of fancy, no doubt over-keen readers and specialists will be able to pick (small!) holes in some of my arguments, as I am sure they will in other parts of this work.

The book is also somewhat eclectic. In the first place, it is so because of the nature of the material and the sources from which it is collected. Second, it is also due to my own belief that the proper study of this area of experience should not be confined to narrow experimental procedures. In common with other modern thinkers, I hold that the future of psychology in general lies in the study of consciousness (and mind) and the development of 'state-specific sciences', and, as the reading of this book will reveal, the hypnagogic area contains all manner of what Tart has called 'discrete states of consciousness', and is for this reason a fertile ground for the application of such methods of investigation. Accordingly, I make no apologies for the use of material collected from outside the current mainstream psychology, such as that pertaining to occult, mystical, and spiritualist practices and 'parapsychological' studies, nor do I consider my inclusion of such sources as weakening the rigour of a scientific methodology. My approach is naturalistic and humanistic in the widest sense of these terms, which allows me to speak of, for example, psi, mystical, abnormal, creativity, and so-called paranormal phenomena and multilevel realities as *natural*, as common human experiences that one encounters frequently during the naturally occurring hypnagogic-hypnopompic periods.

Because of the breadth of the subject matter and the comprehensive nature of this work, certain themes – such as those dealing with logic, paralogic, certainty and conviction, reality sense and reality testing, loosening of ego boundaries – appear on more than one occasion and are treated from a number of angles, their meaning and significance becoming updated, expanded and elucidated as the investigation progresses. In all this, I tried to use the minimum of scientific jargon, and I hope that the meaning of those technical terms which are inevitably employed has been made sufficiently clear to ensure against hampering the understanding of the more general reader. On the other hand, in order to preserve maximum information content and assist the serious reader-investigator in furthering research in this area, I have made available detailed and extensive reference and bibliography sections. I have also considered it necessary to quote extensively from original sources for the purpose of familiarizing the reader with the richness and ramifications of the subject matter. In addition, I thought it appropriate to use drawings, sketches, and paintings both for purposes of illustration and in order to lighten the mood of this enterprise. It is very unfortunate that, due to printing costs, the commissioned drawings had to be made, and all illustrations reproduced, in black and white, while practically all visual hypnagogic reports speak of colourfulness.

In the general analysis of the various phenomena I have given precedence to the works and experiences of other investigators and experients upon whose reports and views I have frequently called. However, in critical and borderline cases, and on those occasions when finer analysis would be crucial in providing support for, or arguing against, central tenets of an important framework, I have tended to fall back, and reflect, on my own experiences. Whether this is the correct approach remains to be seen. The least I can say in this respect is that my close familiarity with the mental character of these phenomena has equipped me with a degree of insight. It has, for instance, enabled me to see with some considerable clarity the vast area of experience which lies between the Cartesian rational consciousness and the Freudian unconscious, and furnished me with more than an inkling concerning the unlimited epistemological possibilities and the range of possible ontological changes that exist therein.

Finally, and just in case any of my *theoretical* claims appear grandiose to some reader, let me reiterate McKellar's wise remark that 'those thought products which we call scientific theories are not wholly unlike those we call works of architecture', in which respect the edifice I have constructed here may be liked or disliked, agreed or disagreed upon, may enthuse or disappoint; hopefully, it will draw the attention of other 'architects' and generate reseaarch. As for my *practical* claims, any interested reader or investigator may test them for himself: this is an area of experience and observation not confined to the specialist but open, and naturally accessible, to every human being. To paraphrase Wittgenstein, all I have done is to gather driftwood and build a ladder which anyone may use to climb beyond.

Part I

Phenomenology

1 · *Introduction*

Background and incidence

Hypnagogic experiences are commonly defined as hallucinatory and quasi-hallucinatory events taking place in the intermediate state between wakefulness and sleep. The term 'hypnagogic' (from the Greek *hypnos* = sleep, and *agogeus* = conductor, leader) was introduced into the literature by Maury who used it with specific reference to the presleep or sleep onset phenomena.[1] Other terms suggested for these occurrences include 'presomnal or anthypnic sensations', 'visions of half-sleep', 'oneiragogic images', 'phantasmata', and 'faces in the dark'. Similar phenomena occurring at the other end of sleep are called 'hypnopompic',[2] that is, coming or leading out of sleep. The presleep period as a state or process has been variously designated as the 'hypnagogic state', 'borderland state', 'sleepening state', 'half-dream state', 'prae-dormitium', 'sleep onset', 'falling asleep', 'Einschlafen', 'endormissement', 'addormentamento'. Unfortunately, there is no single word in English equivalent to the Italian 'dormiveglia' (sleep-waking) which so succinctly describes both the 'hypnagogic' and the 'hypnopompic' states.

In general, there is a tendency among investigators in this area to employ the term 'hypnagogic' to refer to experiences occurring both at sleep onset and at the awakening side of sleep. Indeed, one early worker, Ellis,[3] protested against the introduction of the term hypnopompic into the literature and argued that it is 'pedantic' and 'unnecessary' to view the hypnagogic and hypnopompic as two separate states. Since there have not as yet been proposed strong phenomenological and physiological criteria for their distinction I shall continue in the same tradition and consider them as belonging in the same group of phenomena. I shall, furthermore, introduce the collective term *hypnagogia* to stand for the hypnagogic-hypnopompic state and all the phenomena and experiences encountered therein. However, the use of the two separate terms will be retained for the purpose of indicating the temporal occurrence of such phenomena.

Reference to hypnagogic experiences extends as far back as Aristotle, who remarked that anyone can convince himself of their occurrence 'if he attends to and tries to remember the affections we experience when sinking into

3

slumber', and that, in respect to the hypnopompic variety, a person can, 'in the moment of awakening, surprise the images which present themselves to him in sleep'.[4] In the third century AD, Iamblichus 'the divine', writing on 'god-sent' experiences and the conditions under which they take place, referred to 'a condition between sleeping and waking' and 'when sleep is leaving us, and we are beginning to awake' during which time and conditions 'voices are heard by us' and 'sometimes a bright and tranquil light shines forth'.[5] Leaning cites a number of writers in the sixteenth century who gave descriptions of their hypnagogic experiences.[6] In the seventeenth century Hobbes referred to his hypnagogic visions of 'images of lines and angles' as a 'kind of fancy' he could give 'no particular name' to,[7] and Cardano registered his displeasure when, as a child, his aunt interrupted his 'enjoying and looking intently upon' a 'festive' and 'wondrous' hypnagogic 'display' of 'various images as if they were bodies of air . . . . a collection of many things rushing together at the same time but not so that they were mixed up, rather, that they were hurrying by', and which included, besides such everyday things as people, animals, flowers, buildings and musical instruments, also 'winged creatures' and 'forms of bodies up to that day unseen by me'.[8] Both Leaning and Ellis[9] made reference to the descriptions of hypnagogic imagery recorded in 1600 by the astrologer Simon Forman in his autobiography. In the eighteenth century Emanuel Swedenborg reported his hypnagogic experiences, along with a method of inducing them, in a number of publications.[10] In the last century Poe spoke of them as

> a class of fancies, of exquisite delicacy, which are thoughts: they seem to me rather psychal than intellectual. They arise in the soul . . . only at its epochs of most intense tranquility . . . and at those mere points in time where the confines of the waking world blend with those of the world of dreams. I am aware of these 'fancies' only when I am on the very brink of sleep, with the consciousness that I am so.[11]

On the other hand, Mitchell noted that 'the borderland of sleep is haunted by hallucinations . . . voices . . . distressingly real visions seen during the prae-dormitium and at no other period'.[12]

Serious research into these phenomena began with Müller,[13] Baillarger,[14] and Maury.[1] Since then, there has developed a considerable, if fragmented, body of literature, with important reviews by Leaning,[6] by Schacter and by Mavromatis and Richardson.[15] With the advent of behaviourism, naturally interest in this area waned, especially in the English-speaking world. There was, however, still some important work carried on mainly in France and Germany and also on the part of clinical psychologists in the United States. More recently of course there has been a renewal of interest in mental imagery, and the last thirty or so years have seen a considerable growth of research into hypnagogic phenomena.

An early survey by Müller reported an occurrence of hypnagogic imagery of only 2 per cent in adults; similar results were also obtained by Galton. In

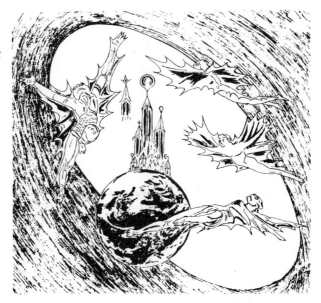

Figure 1.1 *Cardano:
'... bodies of air ...
winged creatures ...
forms of body up to that
day unseen by me.'*

her comprehensive survey Leaning found that the imagery occurs in about one-third of the adult population and to a much greater extent in children. McKellar and Simpson's[16] more recent calculations are in agreement with Leaning's findings. Lately, Owens,[17] Buck and Geers,[18] McKellar,[19] Richardson *et al.*,[20] and Richardson,[21] reported an incidence of 77 per cent, 72 per cent, 76 per cent, 75 per cent, and 74 per cent respectively. The real percentage may be even higher if we bear in mind 'false negatives' that 'seem to occur by a process of ignoring what one is not alerted to notice, as well as from emotional blockage'.[22] Indeed, it has been noted that people who never thought they had hypnagogic experiences come to realize that they have them frequently once they have been alerted to them.[23] Some workers have also drawn attention to cultural and social factors that prevent individuals from admitting that they have such experiences.[24] For instance, many people might deny having hypnagogic experiences because they are afraid that in doing so they would be admitting to having some kind of abnormal or pathological symptom.

Certain older reports that appear to argue in favour of a higher incidence of hypnagogic imagery among children have recently been challenged by the results of longitudinal studies of dreams in children carried out by Foulkes.[25] The de Manacéine[26] study, for instance, showed an incidence of 80 per cent in 6-year-old children and 40 per cent in 8-15-year-olds. The Partridge[27] survey on 826 children yielded the following incidences: 58 per cent in 13-16-year-olds, 59 per cent in 12-year-olds, 62 per cent in 11-year-olds, 65 per cent in 10-year-olds, 63 per cent in 9-year-olds, 60 per cent in 7-8-year-olds and 64 per cent in 6-year-olds. Foulkes, on the other hand, found that 61 per cent of the sleep interruptions of 9-10-year-olds yielded hypnagogic phenomena whereas with the interruptions of 3-4-year-olds the presence of hypnagogic imagery was only 18 per cent.

However, apart from the obvious fact that the more recent studies cited above show an overall higher incidence in adults, both the earlier investigations and the Foulkes study suffer from a methodological difficulty, namely the reliability of very young children to understand the instructions and/or have the capability to distinguish between hypnagogic and adjacent states and give accurate reports. In addition, the methods employed by these investigators differed widely from each other: Partridge used the survey method, and while Foulkes woke children from a clearly hypnagogic state, de Manacéine collected her data from hypnopompic awakenings only. Nonetheless, the Partridge study is the first to point out ebbs and flows in the occurrence of hypnagogic imagery: in the case of children there were found to be two peak periods, one around the age of 10 and the other stretching below the age of 6. Other researchers have also observed that hypnagogic experiences tend to occur in runs, appearing *en masse* for days or weeks, to disappear and re-appear later.[28] Leaning also noted that some people have hypnagogic experiences sporadically from early childhood whereas with others the experiences make their appearance for the first time in later life.

Again, although the earlier studies showed no statistically significant differences in incidence of hypnagogic imagery with regard to sex, the more recent ones by Owens, by McKellar,[29] by Richardson *et al.* and by Richardson[21] have shown that these experiences are more common in females. The Richardson *et al.* survey, carried out on 600 normal subjects between the ages of 20 and 80, has also shown a higher incidence among lower-class subjects and significantly lower incidence among subjects in their sixties and seventies. Unlike most other investigations of its kind which show a predilection for student subjects, the Richardson *et al.* study is a serious attempt to ensure that the sampling is representative of the general population in terms of social class, education, occupation and sex (300 males and 300 females). It is also one of a very few studies that surveyed the incidence of both hypnagogic *and* hypnopompic imagery, thus making it possible to observe that the same subjects tend to report both kinds of experience.

The evidence with regard to possible correlations between hypnagogic (sleep onset) experiences and physical and/or mental health is, at first sight, conflicting. While some investigators argue that hypnagogic phenomena occur when one is in good health and one's mind is calm,[30] others point emphatically to numerous cases of people whose hypnagogic experiences appeared for the first (and, sometimes, only) time, or became intensified, during poor health, severe general fatigue, fever, indigestion, nervous disturbance or shock.[31] Various writers hold that these phenomena are more liable to occur in nervous, impressionable, sensitive and thoughtful subjects of a reflective and perhaps anxious temperament.[32] McDougall considered hypnagogic experiences to be hallucinations occurring to sane and healthy people under 'more or less abnormal conditions'.[33] By contrast, de Manacéine noted that 'for these phenomena to attract attention a certain power of observation is required', from which she inferred that 'this is why they are chiefly found in intelligent persons'.[34] The soundness of the latter remark, however, has recently been disconfirmed by the results of the Richardson *et al.* study which showed no association of hypnagogic imagery with either verbal or nonverbal intelligence.

Nevertheless, both Leaning's and McKellar's investigations show that hypnagogic experiences are not statistically related to physical or mental ill-health. Moreover, a number of other studies argue that the occurrence of hypnagogic imagery not only is not suggestive of ill-health but that on the contrary, it is indicative of well-being and a balanced personality.[35]

Indeed, the fact that hypnagogic experiences tend to increase (or even appear for the first and only time) during ill-health in some people, (although they might decrease in others[6]), could be due to one or both of the following two factors: (1) the increase may be illusory, i.e. these people only noticed their hypnagogic experiences when they were forced, owing to their ill-health, to attend to their own internal states more than they would when in good health; it is also probable, as Galton suggests with reference to the appearance of faces, that although these might be present, 'the process of making the faces is so rapid in health that it is difficult to analyse it without the recollection of what took place more slowly when we were weakened by illness';[36] (2) there may be common factors (relaxation, turning inwards, etc.) attending both a case of fatigue or fever and a case of normal hypnagogia.

Similarly, the occurrence of a prolonged hypnopompic state has been related by some workers to physical and mental pathology.[37] De Manacéine makes reference to the medical literature to the effect that 'this half-waking state preceded the development of mental disease, of which it was, so to speak, the precursor', and that 'it is not found in persons whose conscious cerebral activity is highly developed'.[38] Her own investigations revealed that a prolongation of the hypnopompic state (from 15 seconds to 6 minutes; where it occurred for longer than 6 minutes she considered it 'wholly abnormal') tends to occur mostly in people whose work involves much exercise of the arms and feet (70 per cent) and who are stout, phlegmatic, and plethoric individuals: it very rarely occurs in nervous and sanguine persons.

De Manacéine made her observations on subjects who were awakened only after two and a half or three hours of 'quiet sleep'. The study was confined to observing people in the hypnopompic state, defined as a state that 'prevents them from gaining full consciousness, or from understanding where they are or what they have to do'. Her results showed a significant difference in incidence with respect to sex (men 35 per cent, women 20 per cent). The incidence by age was found to be 10 per cent in adults, 40 per cent in 7-14-year-olds, and 80 per cent in 3-7-year-olds. Working-class subjects showed an incidence of 25 per cent as opposed to 8 per cent in artists, merchants, military men and others, and 2 per cent in intellectuals. Children belonging to the working class displayed the longest hypnopompic state: between 5 and 6 minutes. The incidence in general was found to decrease between the ages of 25 and 40 and was again on the increase especially after 50.

This worker was the first to draw attention to cultural factors as influencing the incidence of the hypnopompic state by noting that out of 84 of her subjects exhibiting this state in a pronounced degree 27 were Finlanders. She considered this 'a national peculiarity' and went on to point out as a possible reason for this incidence 'the fact that amongst the natives of Finland it is nearly impossible to find a person of sanguine temperament'. She also noted 'a marked predisposition to a cataleptic condition of different muscular groups' in people who presented a long and profound hypnopompic state. Two of her subjects (sisters) who were 'remarkably predisposed' to the hypnopompic state since the ages of 7 and 8 developed chlorosis in their teens.

Some of de Manacéine's findings were not confirmed by the more recent Richardson *et al.* study which showed no significant difference in incidence between the sexes and a decrease in incidence in subjects in their sixties and seventies. Moreover, as with the sleep onset variety, the frequent occurrence of a lengthy hypnopompic state does not correlate statistically with physical or mental ill-health. For instance, as we shall see in chapter 4, Ouspensky made extensive use of this state in his studies on dreaming not only without any ill effects on his health but, on the contrary, with great psychological benefits.[39] Others make use of this state, and the catalepsy that sometimes occurs in it, for 'occult' purposes, again without ill effects (see chapter 6).

Hypnopompic experiences are less commonly reported than hypnagogic ones: only 21 per cent of McKellar's[40] subjects reported it, and although the Owens and Richardson *et al.* studies showed a much higher incidence – 51 per cent and 64 per cent – this is still lower than the hypnagogic reported in these studies, viz., 77 per cent and 75 per cent respectively.

Some observers noted that the imagery of their hypnagogic experiences appeared in a sense modality other than the one which predominated during their fully waking life.[41] However, this hypothesis which would argue, for instance, that poor visualizers should have more visual hypnagogic imagery than good visualizers has not been statistically confirmed. On the other hand, Leaning found that, of the 40 per cent of her mainly visual hypnagogist correspondents who provided her with information regarding their visualizing ability, nearly twice as many were considered good visualizers as compared to those who considered themselves bad visualizers. But, again, by themselves these results do not constitute a strong argument in favour of the proposition that visualizing ability contributes to, or correlates with, the occurrence of hypnagogic visions, mainly because (a) only 40 per cent of

Leaning's subjects provided the information under discussion, (b) there is no way of telling *why* these subjects provided this kind of information since they were not specifically asked to do so, i.e. there may be confounding motivational reasons especially because of the 'psychic' connotations of the survey, and (c) no standardized criteria were employed to define 'good' and 'bad' visualizers.

In respect to the relationship between waking imagery and hypnagogic imagery in general, Holt found a positive but insignificant correlation between the two.[42] As Holt himself, Starker,[43] and Schacter have pointed out, however, in future experiments a distinction needs to be drawn between volitional waking imagery and the more passive daydreaming type. This requirement acquires specific significance in the succeeding pages of this book both in defining the character of hypnagogia, one feature of which is passivity-receptivity, and in relating it to other states and experiences that share this particular dimension. Indeed, in view of evidence that hypnagogic imagery can be experienced with open eyes, that it does not necessarily lead to sleep, and that it can, to varying degrees of success, be controlled, or even deliberately formed, the passive-receptive aspect of hypnagogia acquires paramount importance both as a feature distinguishing this state from ordinary wakefulness and as a means of inducing and controlling it.

Various writers from diverse disciplines have made passing reference to the relationship of hypnagogia to a number of other states and experiences, but organized approaches to the problem of defining hypnagogia as a state of consciousness have concentrated mostly on differentiating it from, or relating it to, sleep, dreaming, and wakefulness.[44] There have been three main groups in this respect, two purely psychological and one concerned mainly with the physiological correlates of sleep onset. The latter is discussed in Appendix II.

Vihvelin[45] separated the two psychological approaches into the *internal* point of view represented by Burdach and Leroy, and the *external* point of view represented by Weygandt, Schultz, and Jaspers. The former view argues that an analysis of the phenomenon itself should show whether it is a hypnagogic experience or sleepdream, the latter view uses as criterion the subject's continued awareness of the external world. Vihvelin criticizes both viewpoints and offers his own according to which the subject in the hypnagogic state must retain both the consciousness of the situation, i.e. remain awake, and the ability to carry out voluntary movements. He further proposes that there are two stages in the process of falling asleep: '(1) the stage of *increasing fatigue*, which is characterized by the quantitative reduction of the conscious psychic processes; (2) the proper *hypnagogic* state or hypnagogium, the beginning of which is characterized by qualitative changes in the conscious psychic processes'. The end of the hypnagogic state is not sleep but a transitional state characterized by a vacillation between wakefulness and sleep, 'its chief distinctive mark being the interruption of the continuity of the state of wakefulness by constantly intruding dream-absences'. The disappearance of the consciousness of the situation marks the end of this transitional state and the beginning of the dream-consciousness. Thus Vihvelin anchors hypnagogia in the objective marks of the waking state (orientation, critical observation of phenomena, ability to make voluntary movements), emphatically maintaining that it is 'a state of consciousness utterly different from the dream-consciousness'.

But, Vihvelin's criteria for the use of the term 'hypnagogic state' are rather restrictive and not in line with evidence. On the theoretical side, he appears to ignore the common sense fact that the concept taken in its literal meaning stands for the whole transitional period preceding and leading into sleep; in which case Jaspers's definition of hypnagogic as the state encompassing all those events 'which appear in the period before falling asleep, from full wakefulness with closed eyes until the beginning of dreams'[46] would be more appropriate. (I would argue: with closed or *open* eyes until the beginning of *sleep*; see chapters 2 and 4). Further, since he does not tell us explicitly what he means by 'dream-consciousness' (except for the mark of 'the entire disappearance of the consciousness of situation'), and in view of the quantitative reduction of psychological processes and the introduction of qualitative changes in psychological processes, the latter being very similar if not identical to those reported as operating during dreaming, it is very difficult to sustain the view that hypnagogic experiences and dreams are two distinct geni as opposed to their being different species of the same genus (see chapter 4).

Furthermore, his stipulation that the hypnagogic state does not end with the disappearance of the consciousness of the situation (which mark, by the way, is not a sufficient condition, and in some cases, not even a necessary one, for the occurrence of dreams), but in an intermediate state of vacillation between wakefulness and sleep characterized by the intrusion of dream-absences, is simply arbitrary: if one lies down to sleep and is neither fully awake nor fully asleep, surely one is then in the presleep or sleep onset or hypnagogic state. A similar argument would be levelled against the prehypnagogic stage characterized by the quantitative reduction of psychic processes. In addition, Vihvelin's use of the term 'increasing fatigue' in respect to the first stage is a misleading generalization. It is true that there are many reports of 'fatigue' at this stage but this cannot be taken, by any means, to characterize all the cases. And in most of those reports that it occurs it is doubtful whether it is properly employed to convey the notion of tiredness as opposed to that of a feeling of deep relaxation and unwillingness to 'come out of it'. Both Leroy and Sartre,[47] for instance, talk of a deepening state of self-induced paralysis and autosuggestion. This observation would argue both against the use of the term 'fatigue' and Vihvelin's positing in the hypnagogic state a subject's constantly retaining the ability to make voluntary movements.

As opposed to Vihvelin's hypnagogium, numerous researchers have argued for a wider and more segmented or graded hypnagogia. The first investigators to point to the hypnagogic state as consisting of stages were Arnold-Forster[48] and Leaning who, on phenomenological grounds, suggested an early and a late hypnagogic stage. Davis *et al.*, using EEG indicators, divided the hypnagogic state into five stages (the fifth stage, in fact, belonging to sleep proper).[49] Liberson and Liberson attempted a four-stage classification.[50] Gastaut offered a three-stage division pointing out that in the third stage instead of hypnagogic hallucinations sometimes there may be some dreaming.[51] Under the term 'twilight states', Stoyva included, in terms of EEG patterns, stages which were mainly indexed by alpha rhythms, theta rhythms, and incipient Stage 2 'spindling' sleep.[52] Vogel, Foulkes and Trosman, viewing the hypnagogic state in terms of ego functions, divided it into three progressive stages: the intact ego stage, the destructuralized, and the restructuralized ego stage, or, as Trosman preferred, the early, middle, and late stages.[53] Oliver remarked that his own personal experience of the state showed that there are three stages: in the deepest stage he is unaware of his surroundings and his consciousness is filled with a dreamlike experience over which he has no control (this stage may, in fact, be subdivided into the stage in which he is totally unable to 'pull' himself back, and that in which he still retains the ability to re-establish contact with his surroundings), in the middle stage he is still unaware of his surroundings and cannot make verbal reports although he can review his imaginal experience, and in the lightest stage nearest to wakefulness he is aware of his surroundings and can report.[54]

It transpires then that theoretical considerations and empirical evidence support the viewing of a graded hypnagogic state as against Vihvelin's hypnagogium. Although it is clearly still too early to argue for very precise subdivisions and exact temporal patterns, it would be more in line with evidence and better facilitate research if efforts were made to tentatively group correlated phenomena, states of consciousness, and physiological observations, into three stages, viz. light, middle, deep, and then test and modify these groupings in the light of new evidence. The same grading, but in reverse order, i.e. deep, middle, light, would apply to the hypnopompic end of the state (see chapter 2 for hypnopompic gradations, and chapter 3 for suggested groupings and the identification of a hypnagogic syndrome).

The layout of this book

The book falls into three parts dealing respectively with the nature of hypnagogia, its relationship to other states and phenomena, and its function and evolutionary significance. More specifically, in the first part I examine the phenomenology of the state which I divide into two areas: the first area comprises somatosensory or perceptual and quasiperceptual phenomena (visual, auditory, etc.), and the second, cognitive-affective phenomena (quality of thought, mental attitude, etc.). In classifying the phenomena of the first area I make use of existing classificatory systems and suggest the employment of new ones. Concerning the cognitive-affective features of the state, not all of these are extensively examined in the first part. It seemed more appropriate to discuss some of them in greater detail in the second part in the process of comparing hypnagogia to other states and experiences.

Defining hypnagogia has been a difficult task. This is partly due to the transitional character of the state and the occurrence in it of cognitive modes and phenomena which are thought in general to be severally descriptive of – indeed, to characterize – other states of consciousness. Moreover, at the very introduction of the term 'hypnagogic', Maury clearly noted that the occurrence of these phenomena at sleep onset was not necessarily hypnagogic, i.e. they were not necessarily sleep-inducing! Thus, at the beginning of the book, a working definition of hypnagogia is offered which, however, is augmented as data about the state are presented and analysed, that is, an analysis of hypnagogia is begun in the first part and continued throughout the book.

In the second part, an examination of the phenomenological relationships of hypnagogia with a number of other states and experiences is carried out. Not all states and processes related to hypnagogia are examined to the same depth, particular attention being paid to dreams, schizophrenia, meditation, psi, and creativity. One of the striking findings in this part is the fact that some of these experiences are only distinguishable from hypnagogia by the subject's set of beliefs and the setting in which the experiences take place. Practically all of them contain a measure of hypnagogia, that is, they either begin with, or develop into, hypnagogic phenomena. Thus, hypnagogia is seen to be conducive to the production of these experiences, and vice versa, some of them develop into a hypnagogic state.

In the third part, I attempt three tasks. First, I try to show that the 'strange' phenomenology of hypnagogia and related states is correlated with activities of subcortical structures. Second, I argue that the core psychological phenomenon out of which springs the whole gamut of hypnagogic experiences is the loosening of the ego boundaries of the subject. This phenomenon, which is ontogenetically old and developmentally 'regressive', in that its tendency is to blur boundaries and fuse or multisociate concepts, entities, etc., strengthens, and is strengthened by, arguments supporting the involvement of subcortical structures. Third, I propose that hypnagogia constitutes the 'dream' component of life's triptych – 'dreaming', sleep, wakefulness – and that, due to its unique character of riding between wakefulness and sleep, facilitates the emergence into consciousness of material that might otherwise remain unconscious. It might, thus, also constitute the platform onto which is periodically raised the substratum of continuous but not always conscious mental activities taking place throughout life. As such, it opens great vistas of psychological exploration. Its introspective study may furnish the individual not only with the benefits of an integrated personality but also with the means of discovering new or little known modes of experiencing which will undoubtedly enrich him/her as a psychological entity.

Significantly, and as already alluded to in the Preface, in carrying out such introspections, one also becomes inevitably faced with ontological and epistemological questions whose discussion falls outside the scope of this book but whose mere raising in the mind of the reader will have gone a long way to justifying its writing.

2 · *Somatosensory phenomena*

Hypnagogic phenomena occur in all the sensory modalities, that is, there are visual, auditory, olfactory, gustatory and tactile experiences as well as somesthetic, kinesthetic, thermal and speech phenomena; and they range from the most vague and faintly perceptible to concrete hallucinations. Sometimes two or more sensory modalities are engaged in the same event, just as in waking life, while on other occasions only one sense is involved. These phenomena have been classified by a number of investigators along a variety of dimensions some of which are complementary to, or overlap with, one other whereas others traverse the whole field independently. In what follows I propose to list and examine hypnagogic experiences in terms of their occurrence in the various sensory modalities, indicate their main features, and discuss systems of classification. Since hypnagogic (sleep onset) phenomena are more widely reported than their hypnopompic variety, I shall devote more space to their presentation and discussion than to the phenomena of the hypnopompic state. Likewise, since by far the best researched hypnagogic phenomena are the visual kind, I shall spend more time examining them than any of the others. Indeed, the listing of the main features as well as the classification of these experiences in terms of content or some other, bipolar, dimension are primarily in reference to the visual sort.

Visual phenomena

The variety of visual hypnagogic phenomena appears to be endless: 'There are vignettes, charming, fantastic or comical. There are interiors, country-side and mountain scenery, seascapes, glorious snow scenes',[1] elaborate kaleidoscopic patterns, showers of flowers, lines of writing on a luminous ground,[2] and so on. Many subjects express their difficulty in trying to describe them with any precision. Collard, for example, writes:

> I have called them pictures, but that is a very inadequate description. At times it is a little like watching a succession of lovely forms on a

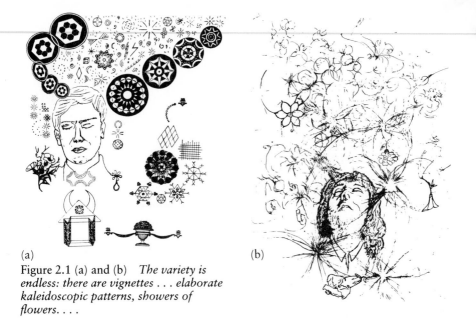

(a)

(b)

Figure 2.1 (a) and (b)   *The variety is endless: there are vignettes . . . elaborate kaleidoscopic patterns, showers of flowers. . . .*

cinematograph screen. It is a 3-D performance, and it is clear to me that I am observing them, not consciously creating them. Often they surprise and delight by their beauty and originality. . . . I have sometimes tried to portray them, but the most delicate technique, the clearest colours at an artist's command, fail to give the slightest idea of them.[1]

A great many reports begin with references to moving clouds of bright colours or mist and to 'little luminous wheels, little suns that whirl rapidly round, little bubbles of different colours that go up and down', 'luminous points and streaks, which shift and change in remarkable ways', 'thin threads of gold, silver, purple and emerald green, which seem to cross over or curl up in a thousand different symmetrical patterns, continuously vibrating, forming innumerable little circles, diamonds or other small regular shapes', and often developing into complicated structures, faces, scenes or landscapes.[3] Indeed, it may come as a surprise to the general reader to hear that when we close our eyes or stare into the darkness of a room we are hardly ever really confronted with total blackness but mostly with a range of visual phenomena the least structured of which are waves of pure colours, light-charged clouds, and dancing colour spots.[4] It is sometimes even claimed that 'a kaleidoscopic change of patterns and forms is continually going on.'[5] And the longer one stays away from actual light the brighter one's field of vision becomes. This phenomenon, known variously as ideoretinal light, luminous dust, entoptic light, or eigenlicht,[6] has been argued by a number of researchers to be the stuff out of which hypnagogic and sleepdream visions arise. James made a general principle of the eigenlicht by noting that 'any objective stimulus to be perceived must be strong enough to give a sensible increment of sensation over and above the ideoretinal light'.[7] And, although 'even in conditions of full daylight careful inspection will reveal luminous dust effects, an achromatic mottled atmospheric haze',[8] it is clear that the optimal conditions for observing ideoretinal phenomena are those of darkness or twilight during which James's increment is 'wholly or mostly absent'. In respect to hypnagogia, Hervey de Saint-Denys wrote:

> White smoke seems to blow across like a thick cloud driven by the wind. Flames burst out of it intermittently, so bright that they hurt my eyes. Soon they have absorbed the cloud; their brilliance is softened; they whirl and spiral, forming great plumes, black in the centre and red turning to orange towards their outer edge. After a moment they open out in the centre, now forming a thin golden ring, a sort of frame in the middle of which I think I see the portrait of one of my friends.[9]

The seeing of faces, as in the above quotation, is in fact one of the most common hypnagogic experiences. Such visions may be of people known or unknown, living or dead, stationary or in motion, single or in groups. Moreover, quite often these faces appear to express particular emotions, an observation that has led to their being referred to as 'the fleeting embodiments of some passion or some mood of the mind',[10] and which the following three reports clearly demonstrate:

> Two faces that stand out particularly in my memory were two jolly-looking middle-aged men in deep converse (profile to me). They suddenly became convulsed with laughter. I could almost hear them. One of them, a grey-haired man with grey moustache, opened his mouth so wide that I could see his teeth sideways, and his eyes went to slits with merriment.[11]

> Out of the whirl of uncouth figures to which I was accustomed, a big stout man, in a grey suit and Homburg hat, emerged, and came up (apparently) so close to me, staring pointedly at me, that I expected him to touch me. The movement and the figure were both so aggressive that I mentioned it to my family the next morning.[12]

An example from my own experiments (see page 19 and Note 17) reads:

> Portrait of an old man, about 70 (probably a farmer), standing in a countryside. The only background seen is the cloudy sky. The man is wearing a hat with warmers for his ears (like the sort worn by people living in very cold climates). He looks very relaxed and has a smile on his face. He is very pleased and contented with the life he has had in the past and continues to have now. He is smoking a pipe and continues to smile.

But even reports which deal specifically with 'faces in the dark' do not confine themselves to accounts of this type of visual content, i.e. faces, as can be seen from the following typical hypnagogic cases:

> For many years I have become accustomed to see multitudes of faces as I lie awake in bed, generally before falling asleep at night, after waking up in the morning, or if I should wake in the middle of the night. They seem to come up out of the darkness, as a mist, and rapidly develop into sharp delineation, assuming roundness, vividness, and living reality. Then they fade off only to give place to others, which succeed with surprising rapidity and in enormous multitude. Formerly the faces were wonderfully ugly. They were human, but resembling animals, yet such animals as have no fellows in the creation, diabolical-looking. . . . Latterly the faces have become exquisitely beautiful. Forms and features of faultless perfection now succeed each other in infinite variety and number.[13]

> At first, after lying quiet for a few minutes, with closed eyes, or, if in absolute darkness, with open eyes, there floats in front of me, and apparently a few feet away, a fleecy white and slightly luminous cloud. From this, sometimes gradually but generally with startling suddenness, the picture starts forth; the cloud rolling away from it, often to form a background, often disappearing entirely, . . . the colours are vivid and intense, the outlines and proportions absolutely life-like, and generally the illumination of the object is produced as if it were thrown by a limelight . . . they are like nothing I have ever seen in life or art. As a rule the expression [these faces] wear on their first appearance they retain unaltered during their brief stay; sometimes it changes, and extraordinary animation lights up every feature . . . the phantoms are not those of faces only, but of single figures, of groups of figures, of animals, landscapes, etc., all perfectly harmonious in their composition and colour, and generally brilliant in their illumination. Let me give one or two examples. Out of the fleecy cloud emerges an enormous book, closed, and held by two hands; the hands open the book, and the pages lying exposed are covered with curious written characters; then it disappears. Again the cloud rolls away, exposing the brilliant sunlit street of some Eastern city, but like none I have ever seen in pictures. The hard black shadows strike the ground and walls; the foreground is baked and arid, the distance bathed in a golden haze. Groups of people stand about – women veiled and men all clothed in white and bright colours. Then through the archway rushes a tumultuous mob of people, whose features, despite the numbers, are all painfully discernible. Those coming first bear all the impress of noble characteristics and are wonderfully attractive to look at; but as they file away, disappearing round a street corner, the succeeding ones are less pleasing; and the curious process of degradation goes on until there pours out of the archway a seething rabble such as a morbidly imaginative painter might draw escaping from hell.[14]

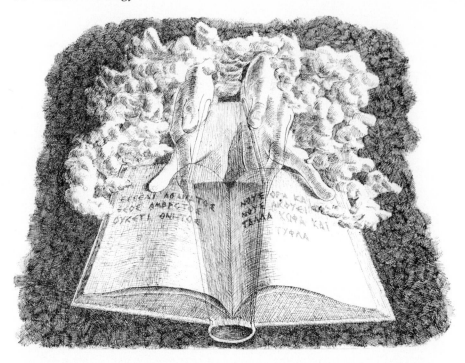

Figure 2.2 *'Out of the fleecy cloud emerges an enormous book held by two hands and covered with curious written characters. . . .'*

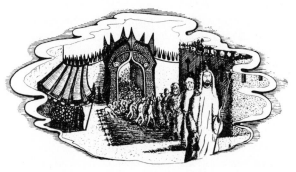

Figure 2.3 *At an Eastern city gate.*

Not only in the dark, but when I drowsily close my eyes in daylight, do I frequently see faces . . . ; but the faces that appear to me I have never seen in real life. Sometimes only the lower part of a face comes into view. At another time hands alone appear, looking most life-like. Nothing lasts more than two or three seconds, which is the more tantalizing because everything is perfect and beautiful, never ugly or grotesque. As in a cinematograph, often lovely scenery passes before me, such as a clear, rapidly-flowing river with its swirls and eddies, waving rushes on the bank. Then, for no reason, a perfectly-formed house may appear, such as I never could draw from memory. Again, I have the amusement of a street scene with all its busy traffic.

I had been reading a newspaper one afternoon recently, till my eyes closed drowsily. A charming Dutch peasant girl suddenly appeared, advancing towards me rapidly with smiling face and outstretched arms and palms held together. She wore a white cap, a blue dress, and a white apron which fluttered in the breeze. The vision was quite inexplicable as I have never been in Holland, nor had I been seeing Dutch pictures or thinking about Dutch maidens.[15]

A green hillock appears in the centre of my field of vision. Gradually I make out that it is a pile of leaves. They boil like an erupting volcano. The pile rapidly grows larger and wider, throwing off the moving parts. Red flowers sprout from the crater, forming an enormous bouquet. The movement stops. The picture appears very clear for a moment, and then disappears.[16]

The pictures I see generally appear at night before going to sleep, always in complete darkness, and I believe usually when I am rather tired. I can see them with my eyes open, but the colours are much less brilliant than when my eyes are shut. I am quite conscious at the time of the unreality of the scenes – indeed they seem to be very much like the constantly changing slides of a magic lantern, and I should say of the same size; when they disappear everything is black again. I see all kinds of things, generally in quick succession; never, however, blending into one another. I can never recall the same picture however much I try. I see landscapes, interiors and exteriors of houses, &c., and single objects, such as flowers, books, boots, feathers, pots, &c., &c., and sometimes figures – of which, however, I can never distinguish the faces. Once or twice I have seen a little scene enacted. I remember one distinctly. I saw a man in the dress of the last century riding down a lane. As he came forward, two men, also on horseback, rushed out on him from behind some trees and knocked him down. I longed to know the end of this little story, but it disappeared. I am never conscious that the things I see have any connection with what I have been thinking of, nor do I remember to have recognised a place I know amongst the many landscapes I see.[13]

In my own experiments[17] in which groups of subjects were guided, through a relaxation routine, to drift as close to falling asleep as possible (some did, in fact, fall asleep for short periods), the imagery in the collected reports is, on the whole, characterized by variety and apparent lack of associational links. Sometimes it is dramatic and highly original. Below are a few of these reports accompanied by drawings based on the subjects' own sketches:

I felt sleepy, then suddenly I saw a large green eye opening and closing. Also something very vague moving in the dark, like a train entering a tunnel or something similar, not very clear. Then, a landscape – outline of hills – very fluid – moving. A wolf's face grinning. Dark wood with pine trees and snow, a cold wet feeling of snow and dampness. The wolf walking in the wood. View of a tree from under the ground – seen as if I were lying under the tree looking up through its roots. 'Reflection' in a lake of old houses that did not exist! (Figure 2.4).

I had the feeling of looking down from the sky. I saw mountains and a waterfall. The act of sex! Swirling fog. Going down a well. I found myself in situations which appeared to be relevant to me – one was of a woman in a baby buggy – but when I came to they were senseless. I also found myself looking into a wooden port with a figure standing in a boat on the left hand side; dark water; large balustrade bridge looming up on the right from far bank; old large dirty streets and houses.

The impression of colour – bright greens and yellows – water falling into a cup or chalice – lines on a roof – movement of cross-shaped object. Hills, mountains or pyramids, a drinking glass on a shelf, a snail, the back of a person, three persons in a garden face on; also fish – I don't actually see it but I can smell it. Swirl of light. I had the sensation of heat, sweat, and a 'deep' feeling. (Figure 2.5)

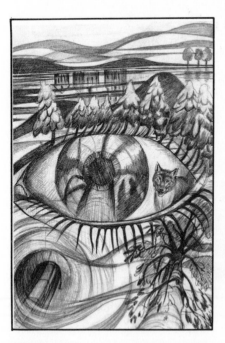

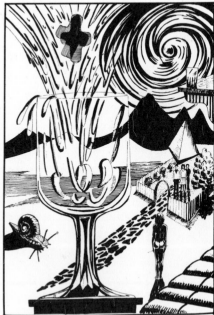

Figure 2.4   Figure 2.5

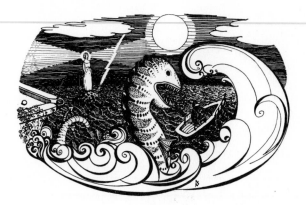

Figure 2.6

I saw a lot of blue, green, grey, white. Water. Combined pictures of water, and sun/moon. The colour red, then white, then swirling clouds of colours: an electric thunderstorm. Flashes of blue and white. Also impressions of a waterline with a diver drowning, fish swimming through green sea. A stormy sky. Something that looked like a lighthouse and/or a figure in Grecian-type dress standing on rocks. Lots of buildings from above. A fish tank. The corner of a billiard table. A ship being washed up on rocks, howling water, flashes of light, monster (serpent) coming out of water and attacking the boat, smaller boat in the wave washing towards rock, shipwreck. (Figure 2.6)

Brilliant rays of light. A great many geometric shapes. Something animate – could be human but animal-like with big teeth. Forest – lots of greenery and flowers. A dragon. Many interwoven snakes. Prehistoric creatures. Birds. All these were very vivid. Then other images that I've forgotten. A man walking a dog which changed into a policeman with police dog and then into a wolf and a soldier. Then I nodded off for a few minutes.

House with a tree and a plane flying above. There is a person sitting on a rocking chair. Spaceship travelling past the moon. Plane flying above New York city with St Paul's in the foreground. Felt a sense of foreboding. (Figure 2.7)

I had a very pleasant 'floating' sensation. I had lots of images of mansions, castles and houses. I heard the sound of wind whistling through trees and had a general feeling of calmness. Images of fire – connected with war maybe. I also saw a seaside but with a glass sheet in front of it where the shore would be; there was a big yellow sun in the background. Strange and beautiful buildings of coming ages – it *felt* as if I were looking into the future.

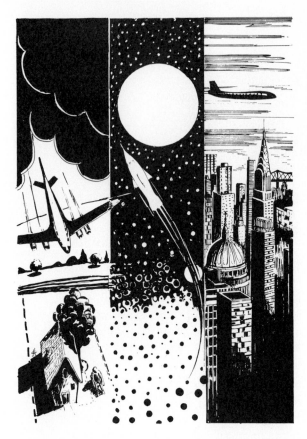

Figure 2.7

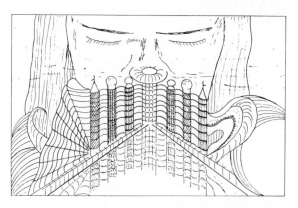

Figure 2.8 *'Strange and beautiful buildings of coming ages – it* felt *as if I were looking into the future.'*

Not infrequently, hypnagogic subjects find themselves 'drifting', 'flying' or 'floating' away from their bodies and their surroundings and into an 'imaginary' world in which, nonetheless, they feel a strong sense of reality. As one investigator reports:

With the appearance of scenery and interiors I acquire a new faculty –
that of travel. Though still aware that some aspect of myself remains in
the body, I go on exploring expeditions through houses, streets and
country lanes, or wander through the aisles of vast cathedrals. I meet
people on these journeys, but if they (or for that matter 'I') can be said to
be there at all, I am certainly invisible to them. I remember coming face
to face with a crowd of laughing children who, to my disappointment,
simply walked through me. At any rate, my sense of being present in
these scenes is so vivid that I have to remind myself that I can walk into
the houses unseen, and that I need not stop to open doors, but can pass
through them. . . . I once found myself, with an indescribable feeling of
happiness and freedom, walking down a corridor build of transparent,
iridescent planes set at angles to one another, rather as if I were inside a
prism, though the arrangement of planes was more complicated than
that; and although the effect was of glass or crystal there was nothing
solid about it. At the same time, without any effort of the imagination, I
was observing this thing from the outside.[1]

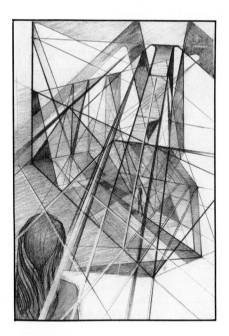

Figure 2.9 *'I found myself, with an
indescribable feeling of happiness and
freedom, walking down a corridor built
of transparent, iridescent planes set at
angles to one another.'*

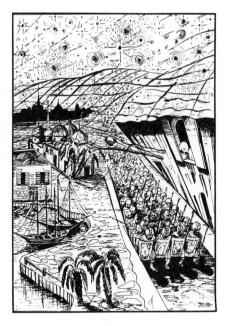

Figure 2.10 *Ouspensky's hypnagogic
experience in Istanbul.*

Ouspensky provides another example of this kind of experience:

> I am falling asleep. Golden dots, sparks and tiny stars appear and
> disappear before my eyes. These sparks and stars gradually merge into a
> golden net with diagonal meshes which moves slowly and regularly in
> rhythm with the beating of my heart, which I feel quite distinctly. The
> next moment the golden net is transformed into rows of brass helmets
> belonging to Roman soldiers marching along the street below. I hear
> their measured tread and watch them from the window of a high house
> in Galata, in Constantinople, in a narrow lane, one end of which leads to
> the old wharf and the Golden Horn with its ships and steamers and the
> minarets of Stamboul behind them. The Roman soldiers march on and
> on in close ranks along the lane. I hear their heavy measured tread, and
> see the sun shining on their helmets. Then suddenly I detach myself from
> the windowsill on which I am lying and in the same reclining position
> fly slowly over the lane, over the houses, and then over the Golden Horn
> in the direction of Stamboul. I smell the sea, feel the wind, the warm sun.
> This flying gives me a wonderfully pleasant sensation, and I cannot help
> opening my eyes.[18]

Indeed, some hypnagogic experiences are fairly lengthy, involved and
coherent dramas in which the subject himself participates. The best known
example of this kind is undoubtedly that recounted by Maury:

> I was slightly indisposed and was lying in my room; my mother was near
> my bed. I am dreaming of the Terror. I am present at scenes of massacre;
> I appear before the Revolutionary Tribunal; I see Robespierre, Marat,
> Fouquier-Tinville, all the most villainous figures of this terrible epoch; I
> argue with them; at last, after many events which I remember only
> vaguely, I am judged, condemned to death, taken in a cart, amidst an
> enormous crowd, to the Square of the Revolution; I ascend the scaffold;
> the executioner binds me to the fatal board, he pushes it, the knife falls; I
> feel my head being severed from my body; I awake seized by the most
> violent terror, and I feel on my neck the rod of my bed which had
> become suddenly detached and had fallen on my neck as would the knife
> of the guillotine. This happened in one instant, as my mother confirmed
> to me.[19]

The above are only a small sample of hypnagogic visions but they suffice
for the moment to demonstrate their variety and richness. Other examples
will be presented throughout the book for the purpose of illustrating specific
points and arguments. Before closing this section, however, it will be useful
to make a summary by classifying the phenomena in terms of content. To do
this I shall make use of Leaning's excellent classification, modifying it slightly
to accommodate some extra types. This classification, then, comprises the
following:

- *Formless* In this type belong waves of pure colours and light-charged clouds which in many cases appear to constitute the raw material out of which emerge more complex types.
- *Designs* A distinction can be drawn between the 'cloud-effect' or pure eigenlicht and 'phosphenes',[20] the latter being patterns and geometrical designs sometimes having the appearance of objects. They are often 'patterns of perfect symmetry and geometrical regularity', 'most beautiful decorative patterns, finials, curves, spirals, leaves, blossoms', 'like a thin gauzy pattern hung through the room'.[11]
- *Faces, figures, animals, objects* The seeing of faces is so widespread among the hypnagogic imagers that, as Leaning put it, it 'almost suggests that there is a special "face-seeing" propensity in the mind'. This propensity, however, is mostly observed in adults whereas 'in the children's census nearly twice as many speak of stars and colours as of people and faces'. Faces appear in a variety of ways but most often they seem to take shape out of a misty stuff, sometimes one face forming through another. On some occasions the faces are like 'drawings made with phosphorus on a dark wall at night' and on others 'a dim disc of light would suddenly appear and as suddenly brighten. There would be a whirling motion in the light which, with astonishing rapidity, develops into moving figures' that often come towards the subject.[12] Although the appearance of faces is sometimes fragmentary and 'flashed on and flashed out again suddenly', the process is usually one of gradual growth. The aesthetic quality of the faces ranges from 'transcendent beauty' to 'hideous and terrifying',[21] they may be weird faces that leer and grin horribly or strong, clearly defined, bearded, biblical ones.[22] They often appear to be looking at the individual in a very personal way, and sometimes they make remarks about him (see section on 'Auditory phenomena', page 33). In general they seem to represent particular moods or sentiments. Like the faces, figures appear in great variety, and so do animals and objects.
- *Nature scenes* The seeing of landscapes, seascapes, and gardens is usually accompanied by feelings of admiration and joy. Leaning found that landscapes form a large class of the visions of adults but do not figure at all in the children's census. Children tend to see more people, 'things', and animals than landscapes and scenes. Landscapes, like faces, usually have 'a cloud-accompaniment' in the shape of cloud formations which break and give a view of distant valleys or scenery in great brightness. More urbane landscapes are also reported in the form of outstanding buildings of unusual construction as well as of common streets and buildings. Other nature scenes include natural phenomena such as storms, flowing rivers, waterfalls and rain.
- *Scenes with people* As Leaning correctly remarked, 'if beauty character-izes the landscapes, life and movement in every variety are the chief features which distinguish the "scenes" from them.' A peculiar character-istic of the scenes is that they have neither beginning nor ending, they are

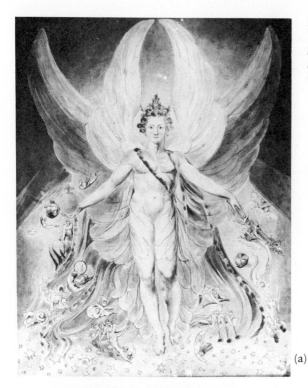

(a)

Figure 2.11 (a) and (b)
The aesthetic quality of the figures and faces ranges from 'transcendent beauty' to 'hideous and terrifying'.

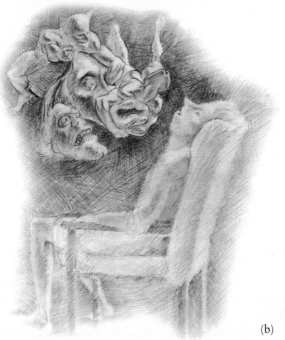

(b)

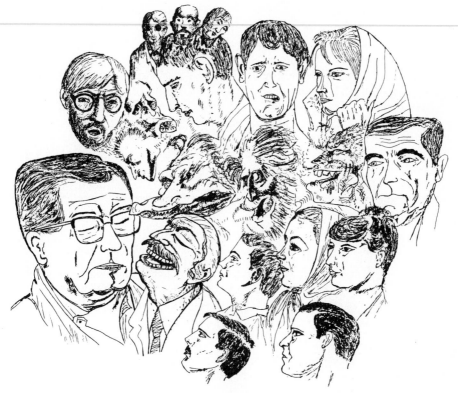

Figure 2.12 *Faces often appear to be looking at the individual in a personal way. In general, they seem to represent particular moods or sentiments.*

    something like trailers of a cinema film. They can be little dramas in exotic settings or ordinary street scenes.
- *Print and writing* This phenomenon, which has been reported by a number of subjects,[23] may occur in a variety of forms and languages including one's mother tongue, a foreign, ancient, or even an entirely imagined language.

The character of visual hypnagogic phenomena
Visual hypnagogic phenomena being of a great variety are, as we shall see at the end of this chapter, amenable to different types of classification. Thus, although the persistent appearance of certain features in the majority of reports may justifiably lead to their being considered as constituting the most prominent characteristics of the visual experiences in this state, it must be constantly borne in mind that the key feature is *variety*: for each *prominent characteristic* there is a range of less commonly reported ones. Also, as I briefly list and examine these main characters below, I would like to draw

attention to the fact that, since all perceptions, quasiperceptions and hallucinations involve a form of cognition, certain of these marks will be found to overlap with the 'more psychological' features of hypnagogia to be discussed separately in the next chapter.

Some of the most commonly reported features of hypnagogic phenomena are those of change, autonomy, and incoherence and absence of association. In general, the imagery appears and undergoes transformation before the eyes of the subject and in spite of any efforts he might make to preserve it unchanged: faces change expression, figures, animals, as well as inanimate objects, move, and events develop seemingly of their own accord. We are repeatedly told that these images are 'independent of any effort of imagination', they are 'not imagination at all, but entirely outside [the subject's] mental action'.[24] They are 'strikingly different from any deliberate visualization',[11] and appear to be seen 'in the eye' not the brain as is the case with visualization. They also 'differ from ordinary images of memory and fancy in being much more vivid, minute, detailed'. As Collard noted:

> I find by experiment that it is possible to hold a chosen thought-image in the mind, at the same time as, and quite independently of the visions. I am aware of consciously creating and controlling the thought-image, while the others appear automatic and objective.

Similarly, McKellar reports that some hypnagogic imagers are capable of carrying on a conversation while the imagery process continues. He offers a personal instance in which he was able to continue having visual hypnagogic images even during performance of such a complex act as manipulating the sound recorder on which he was recording his introspective reports.[25] Also, when one of his subjects was asked to inject into his hypnagogic imagery 'ordinary images', he reported that 'the hypnagogic sequence continued and the ordinary images did not blend with it'.[26]

However, although in the great majority of cases hypnagogic visions are characterized by autonomy, on occasion the subject is able to exert some control over their generation and subsequent transformation (see chapter 3).

On the whole, hypnagogic visions are brief in duration, changing speedily from one form into another. James, for instance, reported seeing 'a thousand different objects in ten minutes', and Müller referred to the 'rapidly changing forms'.[27] One of McKellar's subjects noted that his images changed 'at the rate of about one every three seconds'.[28] But occasionally we hear of the images becoming steady and lasting, passing slowly by and sometimes remaining.[29] Likewise, not all images or sequences of images are incoherent, although their associations in most cases are difficult to trace. As we shall see in later chapters, very often hypnagogic images are symbolic or metaphoric, and not infrequently autosymbolic, and therefore not always meaningless.

The angle from which hypnagogic visions are seen is sometimes very peculiar, like, for instance, seeing Humpty-Dumpty from the back, or seeing a stretch of tuft from an angle that would normally require one 'to lie very flat on the gravel walk, with one's face close to the turf',[11] or viewing the battlements of a castle from close quarters and from the outside as if one were floating in mid-air. On other occasions images 'are presented sideways or upside down', may constitute sections through earth, sea, or air, may be seen both from the inside and the outside simultaneously, may be seen 'through' as though one were able to view their far side in spite of their obviously opaque appearance.[30] Again, the behaviour of the imagery may be contrary to the known laws of perspective, as in the case of an image moving towards the subject without its becoming bigger (although it may become brighter).[31]

Another feature of hypnagogic visions is the manner in which they seem to be illuminated. On the whole, the light appears diffuse. Although the majority of images reported are in daylight with plenty of sunshine, even in night scenes one comes across this characteristic diffusion of light which renders them vividness and distinctness and appears rather to be internal to the seer, 'a penetrative quality in the seeing', as Leaning remarked. Again, most reports abound in expressions like 'strange luminosity', 'liquid fire', 'gorgeously coloured', 'endless variety of colours'. Müller, for instance, talks of highly illumined and coloured images.[32] Ladd reports: 'by far the purest, most brilliant, and most beautiful colours I have ever seen, and the most artistic combinations of such colours have appeared with closed eyes in a dark room'.[33] Collard writes:

> The colour is wonderful beyond anything I can describe, though
> occasionally they appear in black and white. I seem to see them as a rule
> in a clear, bright, crystal light; sometimes they are iridescent, as though
> seen through a rainbow.

Myers says that the 'subjective' hypnagogic images of his childhood 'were vividly and brightly, though unnaturally, lit. They might perhaps be described as being made of fire.'[34]

Most subjects keenly point out the externality, vividness, sharpness, and detail of hypnagogic visions. They are so sharp and detailed, as one subject put it in respect to faces, 'I could see the grain of the skin';[11] they possess 'a microscopic clearness of detail' and one can 'see *into* the material without its being made coarser as it would appear through a magnifying glass'. Another subject remarked that their 'clearness and solidity' is such, 'I have the impression that what I am seeing with my eyes shut must be before me.'[35] They are like a movie in 3D, and often 'as vivid as really "being there" as compared with looking at images'.[36] Even when subjects use the expression 'in the head' when referring to hypnagogic experiences, they either implicitly or explicitly assign some distance to the objects seen. Stead, for instance, writes:

> I saw all that without opening my eyes, nor did my eyes have anything to
> do with it. You see such things as these, as it were, with another sense

which is more inside your head than in your eyes. . . . The pictures . . . simply came as if I had been able to look through a glass at what was occurring somewhere else in the world.[37]

Greenwood, too, although he states that the hypnagogic images are in his head, places them five or six feet away.[38] Similarly, Alexander noted that 'they tend constantly to impinge upon "real" space'.[39] As one of Ardis and McKellar's subjects remarked, 'it seemed to be projected before me like a coloured film. . . It was quite unlike a mental image.'[40]

The 'sense of reality, of life-likeness' pointed out by many subjects in reference to their hypnagogic imagery often expands into 'feelings of *heightened reality*'.[40] It is interesting to note in this respect that Freud, among others, referred to hypnagogic visions as 'hallucinations' and not merely as images.[41]

The following example from Stead illustrates the autonomy, changeability, and lifelikeness of hypnagogic visions:

> There was no light in the room, and it was perfectly dark; I had my eyes shut also. But notwithstanding the darkness, I was suddenly conscious of looking at a scene of singular beauty. It was as if I saw a living miniature about the size of a magic lantern slide. . . . It was a seaside piece. The moon was shining upon the water, which rippled slowly on to the beach. . . . It was so beautiful that I remember thinking that if it continued I should be so interested in looking at it that I should never go to sleep. I was wide awake, and at the same time that I saw the scene I distinctly heard the dripping of the rain outside the window. Then suddenly, without any apparent object or reason, the scene changed. The moonlit sea vanished, and in its place I was looking right into the interior of a reading-room. . . . I remember seeing one reader . . . hold up a magazine or book in his hand and laugh. It was not a picture . . . it was there. The scene was just as if you were looking through an opera glass; you saw the play of the muscles, the gleaming of the eye, every movement of the unknown persons in the unnamed place into which you were gazing.[42]

In the above excerpt Stead refers to the hypnagogic vision as a 'living miniature'. Indeed, the majority of these visions appear to be experienced as miniatures. But although small, the images are not felt to be seen at a great distance; in fact, they are never located farther than a few feet from the eyes, and in some cases, as we saw earlier, are thought to be 'within' the eye itself. Not only micropsias but also megalopsias have been noted as occurring in the hypnagogic state, e.g. 'one subject reported seeing people known to him who "always grow bigger and bigger until I cannot picture them, or fade away to a single point".[43] Polyopsias, too, are sometimes reported, such as 'Rupert Bear with an elephant sitting in a toy tank going up and down hills . . . a whole string of bears and elephants one behind the other like a string of sausages'.[44]

Figure 2.13   *Example of polyopsia.*

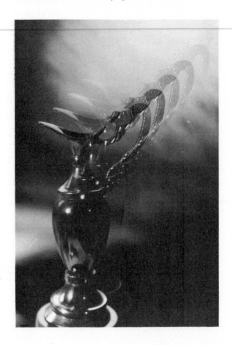

Another, common, feature of hypnagogia is that of synesthesia.[45] This comprises phenomena in which sensations in one modality call forth sensory impressions belonging to another. Hollingworth, for example, reported that, as he became drowsy while attending a concert, the three finishing blasts of the musical piece turned into 'the movements of some huge bug which came sailing from behind the wings, suddenly alighting on the stage, first on the two hind feet, then bringing down the middle pair, and finally the two front feet with the final blast'.[46]

A number of workers have noted that attending to one's hypnagogic visions increases the latter's duration and frequency.[47] It has also been observed that, contrary to their definition, these images do not always lead to sleep,[48] and, although in the main they are experienced with closed eyes, they are also seen with the eyes open.[49]

In general, hypnagogic visions are pleasant and even humorous. Indeed, whole comic scenes are often enacted in a hypnagogic state with or without the direct participation of the imager and, not infrequently, in the form of Disneylike cartoons, e.g. 'a cartoon sabre-toothed tiger tiptoes on hind legs up to some unseen victim, paws held up near face ... suddenly a striped tiger's arm comes around from behind and covers the sabre-toothed tiger's eyes.' Even otherwise macabre visions may appear amusing, as in the case of a person who saw 'a family of skulls in a car driving along', and, added, 'I could see the expression on their faces [sic]. I could tell it was a friendly family. They were all skeletons ... no, it wasn't at all frightening. On the

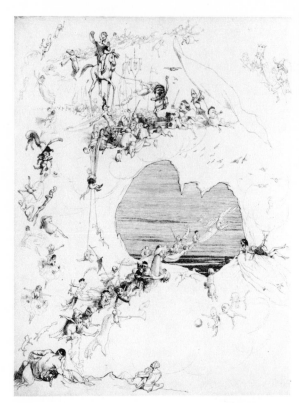

Figure 2.14 *Whole comic scenes are often enacted in a hypnagogic state. In such scenes, the characters may float through various layers of the same landscape.*

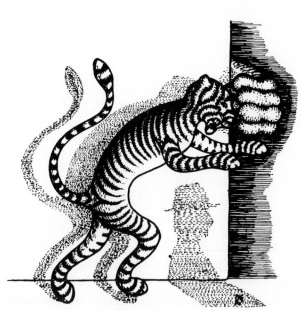

Figure 2.15 *Frequently, Disney-like cartoon episodes are experienced in this state.*

Figure 2.16 *A family of friendly skeletons driving along.*

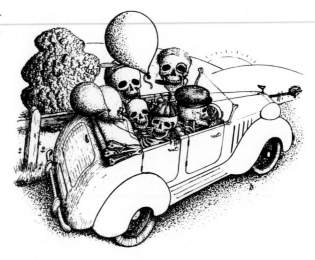

whole it was rather jolly.'[50] However, hypnagogic visions may sometimes be frightening, in which case they cause the subject to return to the full waking state.

Auditory phenomena

In describing their visual hypnagogic experiences many subjects refer to images of people making mouth movements like those of speech but, just as in a silent movie, no sound is heard; the same is said of animals, cars, seawaves, etc. Occasionally, appropriate sounds accompany the movements of figures or objects; for instance, one subject reports:

> There was quite a company of people about me, young women I believe, who looked towards me and passed on. One of them spoke. I heard the voice distinctly, soft and clear. It said '*He isn't asleep*'. . . . I am certain I am not confusing this with a dream.[11]

Fox reports the following personal experiences:

> Sometimes, just before falling asleep, I would see through my closed eyelids a number of small misty-blue or mauve vibrating circles . . . somewhat resembling a mass of frog's eggs, and only just on the border line of visibility. At first these circles would be empty, but soon a tiny grinning face, with piercing steel-blue eyes, would appear in each circle, and I would hear a chorus of mocking voices saying very rapidly, as though in tune with the vibration, 'That is it, you see! That is it, you see!' . . . [On other occasions] the light of the gas-flame grew dim and that mysterious pale-golden light from nowhere suffused the room. I

would hear strange noises, crackling and snapping noises, while little shafts of blue flame, like miniature lightning, darted from the corners of the room. And then came the apparition: a man with a grotesquely horrible face, a wolf with eyes of fire, a lion, a huge serpent, a great black bear standing erect so that it reached the ceiling.[51]

More often, voices of people out of view are heard, and less frequently music. One subject, recounting a hypnagogic experience in which she saw the bows of a ship at sea, says:

She cut through the water, making little waves that broke into foam . . . when quite clearly and *authoritatively* a voice spoke on my right a little behind my pillows: 'There's no occasion to warn her. We've got one ship off already'. It was the voice of a working man of the better class.[11]

Lady Berkeley wrote of hearing 'bells' and 'splendid organ music':

I not infrequently hear bells (or something like bells) mostly at night, and have often got out of bed, opened all windows, etc., to ascertain whether they really were ringing, only to be met by complete silence outside. . . . On returning to bed, putting balls of wax in the ears and shutting all sounds out with pillows, I hear again these grand organ-like vibrations, which then often end by rocking me to sleep (so to speak). In the same way I have at times heard musical harmonies which I was able (if I hurried) to play, and then write down.[11]

Some people when falling asleep hear crashing noises, bangs and explosions sometimes localized within the skull.[52] A usual auditory experience is the hearing of one's name being called,[53] another is the hearing of a doorbell ringing. Often the sounds are meaningless, or so they seem. Sometimes they are neologisms, e.g. 'Lacertina Wein', 'they are exposed to verbally interlection', 'or squawns of medication allow me to ungather', 'anzeema',[54] or strange remarks apparently heard in one's own voice such as 'I wanted to pull seven but I pulled nine instead',[55] irrelevant sentences containing unrecognizable names like 'Bill Hambra – Ju (sic) know him',[56] pompous nonsense often characterized by unintellectual wit, e.g. 'Buy stocks in the fixed stars. It is remarkably stable', 'he is as good as cake double', 'a leading clerk is a great thing in my profession, as well as a Sabine footertootro'.[57] Archer reports that often as he dozed off while reading he found himself substituting hypnagogically the last line of a poem or continuing with an extra line, or even composing an entirely new couplet quite meaningfully.[58] Maury spoke of 'sudden reproductions of sounds or notes which had struck the mind without its knowledge'.[59] Sometimes quotes, references to spoken conversation, and remarks directed to oneself are reported, some of which are apparently part of the visual scene while others seem to be unrelated to it. Arnold-Forster reports hypnagogic experiences in which a certain sentence, apparently unrelated to her thoughts of that moment, would come through, followed almost immediately by a visual translation of its contents, e.g. the sentence 'newly fledged birds on a tree – all grey' gave rise to its visual equivalent.[60] On other occasions, hypnagogic auditory experiences may be meaningful responses to one's thoughts of the moment or somehow related to one's thoughts prior to the experience.[61] Froeschels noted that mostly statements made in one's auditory imagery are egocentric, i.e. they are not directed to anybody.[62]

Leaning remarked that 'the impression conveyed is that there is something about them [i.e. auditory images] which corresponds to the colour, perspective, etc., of the visual images, and probably with sufficient data we might find every point paralleled'. Oliver's impression from his own experiences is that 'auditory images resemble the visual imagery in that they often appear at first to be meaningless, but if their symbolic connections can be determined, a meaning can be deduced'.[63]

In a recent investigation carried out by McKellar on a group of 400 New Zealand University students, auditory imagery was found to be less common than the visual.[64] The results were: *Visual*: (male) 48 per cent, (female) 61 per cent, *Auditory*: (male) 31 per cent, (female) 38 per cent. Foulkes and Vogel also found that 'hypnagogic experiences are primarily visual in character'.[65] The results of these investigations disconfirm McKellar and Simpson's earlier conclusion that auditory hypnagogic experiences predominate.

Olfactory and gustatory phenomena

Hypnagogic smells vary from 'a horrible stench' to the smell of a rose that 'smelt much nicer than ever a real rose could smell',[66] and they are often, but not always, accompanied by an appropriate visual image.[67] Some hypnagogic smells are so realistic that, for instance, people may get out of bed to make sure that they have not left the oven on or that there really isn't a gas leakage somewhere in the house. Maury and Leaning also reported gustatory images.

Somesthetic, kinesthetic, tactile, and thermal phenomena

In this group belong experiences called by Mitchell[68] 'primary sensory stuff', e.g. 'a feeling of rending', 'a shock like that which a sudden arrest of motion causes', 'a bolt driven through the head', an 'upward surge of indescribable nature', 'an electric sort of feeling', 'skin sensations as of an electric shock'. Both Mitchell and Roger[69] speak of the 'numbness, or swelling mounting rapidly from the extremities or the epigastrium to the head whereupon the shock occurs'. One may be given the description of the head swelling like a balloon till it bursts with an explosion.[70]

Tactile sensations include 'a sense of cold water poured over the head', the feeling that one is being touched, 'a feeling of "hot" flow down one or both legs' or from one arm to the other, a pain shooting from neck to fingertps, buzzing in the head, a sudden spasm.[71]

Feelings of bodily distortion or 'body image disturbances' include the enlargement or shrinkage of parts of the body, the disappearance of parts of the body, the blurring of bodily outlines or parts of it, 'mouth distortions', weightlessness.[72] Sartre notes that 'one's body is but vaguely felt, and even more vaguely, the contact with the bed sheets and mattress. The spatial position of the body is but poorly localized. Orientation is confused. The perception of time is uncertain.'[73]

Another phenomenon, that of myoclonic jerking, may vary from mere twitches to violent spasms which tend to appear *en masse* for nights or weeks and then disappear for a period to reappear again.[74] This phenomenon seems to be statistically very common, occurring sporadically to more than 80 per cent of the normal population.[75]

Another interesting phenomenon in this group is the experience of falling which is 'more uniformly associated with a bodily jerk than are the other varieties of bodily shock'.[76] Quite often the fall forms part of a hypnagogic 'dream' in which the subject, for instance, finds himself falling off a cliff to escape a ferocious beast, or off a toppling ladder, missing a foothold while climbing steps or tumbling down the stairs at his home.[77] In such cases the subsequent waking may be the result of the subject's alarmed attempt to arrest the fall, or the outcome of the imaginal impact. Thirty-three among 134 persons Oswald questioned said that falling was the commonest of their types of sensory experience accompanying a jerk. Harriman reported the falling phenomena as occurring in 27 out of his 44 subjects (61 per cent), and McKellar found that 144 out of his 182 subjects (79 per cent) had falling experiences.[78] It is possible, McKellar suggests, that this phenomenon, so obviously related to muscular tension and relaxation, is a universal one. Grouping all the above experiences together he reported that they occurred to 21 per cent of his male and 35 per cent of his female 400 New Zealand university student subjects.[79]

The hypnopompic variety

We are all familiar with the feeling of disorientation we occasionally experience on awaking, or the feeling of having awoken in strange surroundings. Some people even have visual illusions in this state, as in the case of the man who, on seeing someone squatting by the wall in his room, 'jumped out of bed, caught the intruder by the throat, and found he was a dirty linen bag, with the neck tied.'[80] When Myers coined the term 'hypnopompic', however, he defined it as 'pictures consisting generally in the persistence of some dream-image into the first moments of waking'.[81]

On emerging from sleep a person sometimes opens his eyes to find that a

Figure 2.17 *Caught the intruder (dirty linen bag) by the throat.*

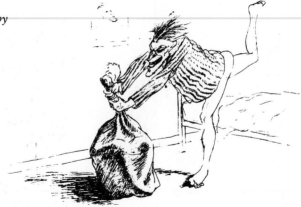

dream he has been having continues, and that having shifted his attention to an object in the real world of his room the dream imagery is somewhat interrupted but resumes its full strength as his attention is removed from the immediate surroundings. The following is one such an experience reported by the philosopher Spinoza:

> One morning, as I woke out of a very heavy dream (it being already day) the images which had come before me in my dream remained before my eyes as lively as if they had been the very things, and especially that of a scurvy black Brazilian, whom I have never seen before. This image vanished for the most part when, in order to divert myself with somewhat else, I cast my eyes on a book or any other thing; but so soon as I removed my eyes from their object without looking with attention anywhere the image of this same negro appeared as lively as before and that again and again, until it vanished even to the head.[82]

Another subject reports:

> Once I had a most vivid dream about a man whom I knew well. On suddenly waking, I saw him, in the light of early morning, standing at my bedside in the very attitude of the dream. I looked at him for a second or two, and then putting my foot out, I kicked at him; as my foot reached him, he vanished.[83]

Two more episodes of this kind come from de Manacéine.[84] In the first, she dreamt of seeing an image of Christ, crowned with thorns:

> The face of Jesus was admirably reproduced, and full of sweet and profound sadness; but suddenly the expression began to change, and in my dream I was so astonished that a mere painted image could thus change its physiognomy that I awoke, and yet still continued to see the divine face before me with an expression of sadness on it, slowly

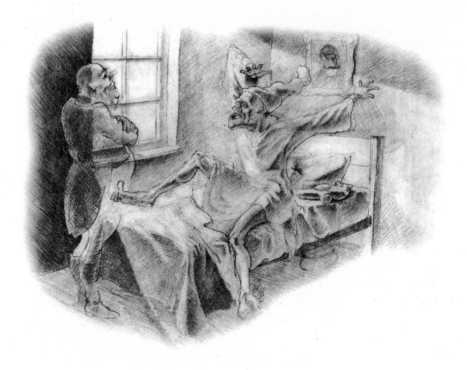

Figure 2.18   *'I kicked at him but as my foot reached him he vanished.'*

changing into a mild and joyous smile which at last completely effaced its earlier melancholy. In this case awakening took place in the morning when it was quite light.

In the second dream, she found herself sitting in an easychair in her study when someone came into the house bringing to her the Russian flag:

> The appearance of the national flag in my house surprised me so much that I awoke, and on opening my eyes still saw it before me with the three national colours, the eagle, and the two golden tassels, while the staff was slightly bent towards me. . . . It was still night, and the bedroom was in absolute darkness.

McKellar points out two groups of phenomena in this state: hypnopompic speech and hypnopompic imagery. As an example of the former group he offers the case of a young woman who woke up to find herself murmuring 'put the pink pyjamas in the salad', an utterance interestingly pointed out for its likeness to schizophrenic speech. When not expressed in overt speech, McKellar notes, hypnopompic thoughts are retained and expressed subvocally. In the second group belong phenomena of an anticipatory character such as 'watching' oneself getting up and beginning the events of the day but 'knowing' that one is still in bed.[85] McKellar explains this character of the hypnopompic state by ascribing to it 'the function of protecting the sleeper from the harsh realities of getting up in the morning'. It is doubtful, however, whether this feature is indeed protective since such anticipatory experiences just as often have the opposite effect of waking up the sleeper, as in the case of one of McKellar's subjects who, having dreamt of toasting bread, 'awoke quite quickly to smell toast burning' and got up to check whether the oven had been left on. Myers reported a woman he once knew whose dream images would continue 'for a short period after she awoke and had, for example, to pick her way through a mass of crabs on the carpet to the light to switch it on in order to reassure herself that they were not really there. On such occasions she would sometimes continue to see the images in the full light.'[34]

Sometimes, visual hypnopompic images appear in colours complementary to those seen in the dream.[86]

On the auditory side, we occasionally come across reports of people who, having woken, continue to hear dream music which fills them with 'exquisite peaceful joy'.

In contrast to the above, various workers have presented data that argue for a variety of hypnopompic experiences which are not continuations of dreams.[87] Some of these phenomena commence as the subject begins to wake while others occur after he has woken. McNish, for instance, noted that one may wake and see visions of people in his room which one takes for real and thus resort to shouting and calling for help.[88] Kanner proposed that children's nightmares transpire during such semi-waking states.[89] On the other hand, many of these experiences are far from being frightening. As one subject reported:

> I have often, when waking in the middle of the night, found the room apparently blazing with light, heard loud music, generally of a band and seen a number of men and women, generally dancing or in rapid motion.[90]

Two other cases read as follows:

> When in bed I see in the wall a round window through which I not only see but hear all sorts of things. One morning I saw hundreds of bluebottles and could hear them buzzing. Another morning I saw a farmyard with a shippen and two large green doors. At the left was a brown and white cow, on the right a black and white one. The brown one was mooing and it jumped over the door. As it jumped, the door opened and inside were stalls with four more cows.

> Some time ago I awoke early one morning. I was amazed that very suddenly a picture appeared. In it I saw Christ toiling up a hill, wearing

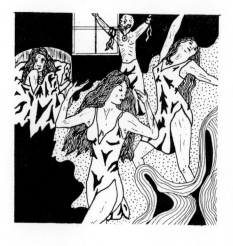

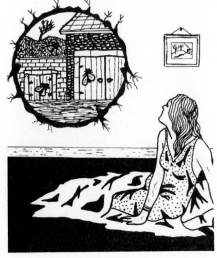

Figure 2.19 *'I have often woken in the middle of the night to see people dancing. . . . '*

Figure 2.20 *'When in bed I see in the wall a round window through which I not only see but hear all sorts of things.'*

a loose white garment, a crown of thorns on his head and the cross upon his back. He was accompanied by a powerfully-built, dark-skinned man, and behind was a long line of people.[91]

Another interesting example is one reported by McKellar in which an elderly woman woke in the middle of the night to find her room 'full of angels'. On other occasions, 'strange, symbolic figures' may appear 'with explanations of their meaning on scrolls or shields'.[92]

Here also belong what may be called 'warning' and 'problem solving' cases. In the former, the subject wakes to see the vision or hear the voice of a person (known or unknown to him, dead or alive) which warns him of some impending danger or 'informs' him of an important event such as the death of a close friend or relative; sometimes the warning may consist of no more than a feeling or sense of imminent danger or death, and on other occasions, while no actual information is passed, the very awakening of the subject may lead to the prevention of some personal disaster (see chapter 6). In other cases, on waking, the subject is confronted with the solution of a difficult problem (see chapter 8).

An interesting case of linking dreaming with wakefulness in the hypnopompic state, but hardly ever mentioned in the literature, is that of Descartes who, having become aware of dreaming while asleep, began to interpret his dream and continued to do so after waking and opening his eyes – he also reported frequently seeing 'sparks scattered about the room' as he opened his eyes on coming out of sleep.[93]

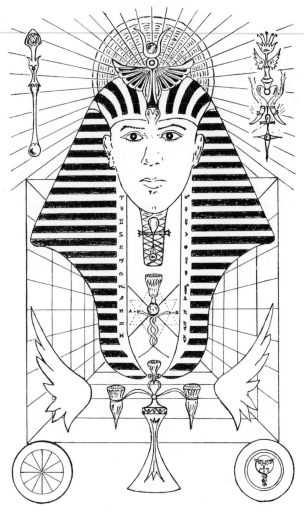

Awakenings of subjects from various stages of sleep have shown that there is a 'carry over' effect from particular sleep stages into the waking state.[94] Interestingly, awakenings from the REM stage yielded more 'dreamlike' responses than awakenings from other stages. Although this latter finding does not support in particular the view that hypnopompic experiences are always continuations of dreams, it does, however, point out that they transpire in a climate of 'dreaminess'.

As with the sleep onset kind, hypnopompic experiences (which are not continuations of dreams) may involve any of the sense modalities: hypnopompic sounds and voices (hearing knocks on the door or one's name being called) are not at all unusual in this state; haptic hallucinations and smells are also reported.[95]

Speech phenomena

Hypnagogic-hypnopompic speech phenomena are, on the whole, apparently nonsensical or irrelevant statements or responses the subject makes as he falls asleep or wakes up. An example of the hypnopompic kind has already been given above, viz. 'put the pink pyjamas in the salad'. Another one, which I shall have occasion to refer to again (chapter 7), is that reported by Mintz as having occurred to a Russian woman.[96] In the process of waking up one morning the subject asked her husband to 'set the towel on fire' (or 'light the towel': the Russian admits of both meanings). Similar phenomena are also encountered on the hypnagogic end of the state. For instance, Maury reported that while drowsing during a lecture he responded to a question by the lecturer with the irrelevant sentence, 'There is no tobacco in this place.'[97] Hollingworth offers a number of examples of his own, e.g. '(H's wife) Let's hurry and get there by ten o'clock. (H) That's easy. I could get there by a nickel to ten . . . [the time was 9.50].' '[H's wife] How curious the moon looks behind the clouds! (H) Yes, just like a thin place in the sky.'[46] Other examples are given in later chapters.

Classifications

In a way, the manner in which data have been presented so far constitutes a number of classificatory systems. One such system, for instance, is the grouping of hypnagogic phenomena according to sensory modality, another is the distinction between experiences during which consciousness of the situation is retained and those which constitute dreams or full hallucinations; on the hypnopompic side, a distinction is readily drawn between dream continuations and postsleep experiences. A third can be derived by grouping the phenomena in terms of intensity of character and/or number of features. A fourth, already pointed out and made use of, is that of classifying the experiences in terms of content. In Part Two we shall see that there are many hypnagogic phenomena whose particular set and setting may cause them to be classified and referred to as other than hypnagogic, e.g. as dreams, phenomena of meditation, psi experiences, psychotic mentation, acts of creation, and so on.

In this section I shall concern myself with the examination of some fairly well-known classifications which, as already noted at the beginning of the chapter, are mainly dealing with visual phenomena and in particular with the sleep onset variety. However, it must be borne in mind that whatever is said of these rather specific classifications in the process of examining them is also applicable (with certain obvious qualifications) to the visual experiences of the hypnopompic state and the auditory phenomena of hypnagogia as a whole. To a certain extent some of my remarks will also apply to the experiences of the other sensory modalities, although care needs to be exercised here since not only is extensive research lacking but also there are important differences between what have come to be called distant receptors, viz. visual and auditory modalities, and the other senses – or, more properly put, important differences are *thought* to exist between them, for, as we shall see in later chapters, in hypnagogia whatever is 'seen', 'heard' or otherwise 'perceived' is also 'felt' kinesthetically, thus pointing to a common unifying denominator of the senses.

Now, as distinct from Leaning's classification by *content*, other writers have attempted to classify visual hypnagogic experiences along various *bipolar* dimensions, such as: *external or objective – internal or subjective* (Jaspers),[98] *hallucinatory – quasihallucinatory* (Schultz),[99] *distinct – shadowy* (Leonhard),[98] *visions of somatic connections – visions of psychic connections* (Vihvelin),[100] *perseverative – impersonal* (McKellar),[101] *objective – subjective* (Myers),[102] *meaningless*, i.e. formless, geometric forms – *meaningful*, i.e. single objects, integrated scenes (Richardson).[103] Leroy also distinguished between *the visions which are reproductions of recently seen objects*, and *the stereotypical terrifying visions of children*.

External or objective vs. internal or subjective

Jaspers's classification has been criticized[104] on the grounds that the criterion of space is insufficient for determining the substance of some visual hallucinatory phenomena, and that, in the case of hypnagogic visions, this is often connected with considerable difficulty. Personally, I find that the criticism is as general and vague as is the employment of the concepts of internal and external, subjective and objective. There are, certainly, cases where one can use the concept 'internal' to mean subjective and, likewise, 'external' to mean objective, but in the case of hypnagogic visions the exchangeability or assimilation of these terms may lead to a great deal of confusion. As we have seen, hypnagogic subjects tend to place their visions 'in front' of them. There is no doubt that these are 'subjective' in the sense that they are only experienced by the subject, but they are clearly not 'internal' in the same way that thoughts, intentions, desires, or even reminiscences are. Moreover, since hypnagogic visions can also be experienced with open eyes and are then more clearly located 'externally', it will be very confusing to identify the 'external' with the 'objective' since the experience is still 'subjective' in the sense that it is experienced only by the subject.

Hallucinatory vs. quasihallucinatory, and distinct vs. shadowy

Schultz's classification, although based partly on pathological cases, may be useful in that it suggests the employment of a cognitive dimension, that is, hypnagogic visions may be distinguished along a continuum of involvement and absorption. (This approach is discussed in more detail in subsequent chapters.) Likewise, Leonhard's distinction between vivid and shadowy visions may be related to particular physiological or psychological conditions of the subject, that is, such conditions as physical or mental fatigue or degree of absorption or relaxation may be found to correlate with the vividness of hypnagogic imagery and its acquiring hallucinatory qualities. On the other hand, vividness may turn out to be a useful indicator of certain personality variables (e.g. good visualizers vs. poor visualizers, relaxed vs. tense personalities).

Meaningful vs. meaningless

In contrast to Jaspers's, Schultz's, and Leonhard's classifications which may, in fact, be placed on a common dimension and identified as functions of the subject's attentional state, Richardson's classification of visual hypnagogic phenomena in terms of meaningfulness-meaninglessness is not only arbitrary but also confusing. It is confusing in that, although his proposed dimension is in reference to content, the employment of the concept on which it is based is primarily dependent on the subject's mental state and/or past experiences, e.g. a triangle or a circle, which are meaningless in Richardson's terms, may convey important subjective meaning whereas an object or scene may not.

Perseverations and nightmares

Leroy's first group of phenomena, viz. visions which are reproductions of recently seen objects, is very similar to, if not identical with, that of Ward's 'recurrent sensations', F.W.H. Myers's 'cerebral after-images', Titchener's and Hanawalt's 'recurrent images' Warren's 'delayed after-sensations', Vihvelin's 'visions of memory-images', and McKellar's 'perseverative' images, and will be discussed later.[105] His second group, that of the stereotypical terrifying visions of children, although arbitrary, may suggest lines of research and classification along a number of dimensions, including that of the statistical incidence of pleasant as opposed to terrifying hypnagogic visions in childhood.

Visions of somatic connections

Vihvelin's data on hypnagogic visions were collected from the self-observations of three subjects over a period of two years. From the data of these subjects Vihvelin selected only 'those . . . whose characteristic features are connected with the subject, i.e. traceable to the personality of the observer', excluding those 'phantastic' phenomena which, as far as he could ascertain, did not have any 'especially established connection with the subject', i.e. they could not be found to have had a somatic or psychological connection with the subject's past experiences.

Vihvelin subsumed under 'visions of somatic connections' the following two main groups of hypnagogic visions: (a) visions of memory images, and (b) synesthetic visions. In the first group he includes (i) hypnagogic visions of objects on which the subject had concentrated intensely during the day; (ii) hypnagogic visions which are linked to earlier memory-images but not to an intensive previous sensory stimulus; (iii) hypnagogic visions that are called forth in an associative and reflex way, as in the case of seeing a car crash during the day and then later in the evening having the hypnagogic vision of a crashed car actually seen years earlier; (iv) hypnagogic visions which are called forth associatively by other sense modalities, e.g. auditory, thermal, tactile, as in the case of hearing the roar of a motorcar, having the hynagogic vision of a wheel revolving synchronously with the motorcar noise, and being able to trace the vision of the revolving wheel back to a definite perception.

The second group deals with phenomena in which a sensation in a sensory modality other than the visual gives rise to an original visual sensation in the shape of a hypnagogic vision, and in which one can determine with evidence that the peculiar features of the provoking stimulus are reflected in the figures of the vision, as in the case of having a hypnagogic vision of a slightly cupped left hand and then becoming physically aware of one's left hand being pressed under his head as he is resting on the bed. Hypnagogic visions belonging to this kind are, as one of Vihvelin's subjects emphasized, entirely different in their characteristics from other hypnagogic phenomena: they are fragmentary, silhouette-like and immovable, with opaque, greyish-white, blurred contours, and one always notices them first and only later the stimulus that gave rise to them. These experiences Vihvelin calls 'primary synesthetic hypnagogic visions' and distinguishes them from hypnagogic visions that are synesthetically caused but complemented by associatively kindred memory-images. He suggests that synesthetic hypnagogic visions may be projections of parts of our body schema resulting from corresponding physiological changes.

Visions of psychic connections

In contrast to hypnagogic visions of somatic connections which are considered devoid of psychological content, the hypnagogic visions of psychic connections are such that their appearance 'can be traced back to a certain definite actual mental content, and . . . a psychologically comprehensible connection can be established between subject and hypnagogic vision'. The contents of the earlier psychic experience may be abstract or concrete and the resulting hypnagogic vision may be direct and indirect: the direct one is that in which the mental contents 'seem to transform themselves immediately into corresponding images, and which the subject can perceive with hallucinatory distinctness';[106] the indirect visions are those that occur at a more or less prolonged period of time after the original psychic experience. In this latter case the vision may begin as a memory image and 'then the part of the vision springs up in which the contents previously experienced by the subject (e.g. as a train of thought either concrete or abstract) are given in a visualised form.' In this fashion, earlier mental contents reappear in the shape of a hypnagogic vision. There are 'faithful visualizations' in which 'the representation of the object is given as an image of it', and 'altered visualizations' in which 'the mental contents tending to a visualization, are given as images associatively related to the primary mental contents'. As an example of altered visualization, Vihvelin cites Kollarits's experience as the latter struggled with eyes shut one evening against falling asleep; combined with this struggle was an effort to find a possible connection between cyclophrenia and schizophrenia. (See also the discussion of 'autosymbolic' phenomena in the next chapter, page 56.) As he grew sleepier and sleepier, Kollarits reports,

> I could observe that there were leaps and bounds in the association of my ideas. . . ; suddenly the thinking process ceased entirely and instead a plain appeared before my eyes, I felt as if I were looking from above on a blackboard, upon which two lines intersecting vertically become visible – the system of co-ordinates, and this geometrical system had a horizontal wavy line: the sinus-line, and a vertical one: the tangent-line, distinctive from each other along both lines – as if they were railway tracks – two small freight waggons were running. One of them was going from left to right on the sinus-line, the other from the top to the bottom along the tangent-line. They had no label whatever but I know that the first one corresponded to manic-depressive psychosis, the second (along the tangent-line) to schizophrenia, and that their movement ahead meant the course of both these diseases.

As opposed to the above kind of hypnagogic vision, Vihvelin continues, in which the actual mental contents must be interpreted as primary components, and the corresponding hypnagogic vision as secondary, we often find cases where the reverse seems to apply, that is, a primary somatically caused vision acquires its contents and 'psychic connection' only in a secondary manner, by means of a superimposition of the subject's actual mental contents. For instance, one of his subjects reported that as he sat during a train journey with his elbows resting on his knees and his face in his hands feeling very drowsy but unable to sleep, he had the hypnagogic vision of a fragmented human face that was smiling ironically: 'seeing this malicious mimicry', the subject reports, 'I at once recognised the railway guard (by the awareness accompanying the vision). . . . Connection: an hour ago I had an altercation with the guard, and had felt vexed at the injustice of that official.'

Vihvelin concludes that

> owing to the frequent presence of the accompanying awareness of significance and to the reshaping of the contents in a 'symbolic' way, the visions of psychic connections can – from the inner point of view – be compared to dreams, but on the other hand – from the viewpoint of formal peculiarities (elementariness and fragmentariness of the figures) – they are similar to visions of somatic connections. . . . [however], these hypnagogic visions have not been perceived in dream consciousness, but in the hypnagogic state, and . . . the observer regards these unexpectedly appearing phenomena with a feeling of strangeness and criticism.

He also draws a distinction between hypnagogic visions appearing in 'internal space' and those taking place in 'external space'.

Vihvelin's classification, although detailed, is nevertheless incomplete due to the limits imposed on it by the investigator himself. In the first place, he discarded all those reports that were 'phantastic', i.e. that could not be related to the subject's past experiences. The puzzling question here is: If we cannot relate a present experience to a past one does it mean that *there was not* one to relate to or that we simply *do not remember* one? To opt for the first alternative is arbitrary. As we shall see, there is evidence that these visions are very common and their occurrence may reveal a very important psychic component of human nature. Second, Vihvelin restricted his definition of the hypnagogic state by introducing the stipulation that the subject must not lose his consciousness of the situation during the experience, thus excluding beforehand hypnagogic dreams (see chapters 3 and 4). In respect to the distinction he draws between hypnagogic visions taking place in internal space and those occurring in external space, since he does not provide any clarifications as to what he means by these terms there is not much one can say about them.

Objective vs. subjective

Myers distinguishes between objective and subjective hypnagogic images. The first group is made up of (a) postcognitive images, that is, hypnagogic images that could be related to 'past perceptive experiences of the observer', (b) precognitive images 'being the core of future perceptive experiences of the observer', and (c) unidentified images, that is, hypnagogic images that cannot be placed in either of the previous two categories. The postcognitive kind clearly includes all of Vihvelin's hypnagogic visions of 'somatic connections' and could easily be extended to include his visions of psychic connections. The precognitive kind belongs in a class of its own, very difficult to justify in a classificatory system since at the time of its occurrence it can only be classed together with the unidentified kind (this latter being one of the kinds excluded from Vihvelin's classification). Its presence may, however, be justified if it is placed in a different dimension, namely, that of the awareness of significance accompanying a vision, which is discussed in the next chapter. The unidentified imagery of a hypnagogic vision, Myers argues, may, in fact, belong to either the precognitive or the postcognitive kind, but its past or future actual occurrence is so far removed in time that at the time of the experience it cannot be seen as belonging to either. Another possible explanation Myers offers for the occurrence of the unidentified imagery is that it may belong to another mind, viz. it may be a thought in somebody else's mind which is being picked up by the hypnagogic subject (see chapter 6).

Myers's second group, that of subjective hypnagogic images, refers to nightmarish experiences wherein one sees ugly and frightening objects or faces.[107] He calls these phenomena subjective to distinguish them from those in the previous group which can be related to events in the external world. This group may, in fact, be classed as a member of McKellar's 'impersonal' kind to be discussed next.

Perseverative vs. impersonal

McKellar distinguishes between 'perseverative' and 'impersonal' hypnagogic images. The former are 'those whose content can easily be explained in terms of past experiences, particularly those of the day before'. For instance, one may have hypnagogic images of plants and flowers if one happened to have spent one's day in a garden:

> Recently I did a mixed weeding. That night I had a veritable hypnagogic botany lesson on the weeds of a New Zealand Garden. They were all there, docks, dandelions, convolvulus roots, and several more which I could not name although I had been dealing sternly with them all afternoon. I had not myself consciously decided on this review of the afternoon's events, but – like the typical hypnagogic imager – I watched the performance with interest.[108]

Leroy also writes:

> When I was studying anatomy, I very frequently experienced a hypnagogic vision not rare among medical students. Lying in my bed with closed eyes I would see most vividly and with complete objectivity the preparation on which I had worked during the day: the resemblance seemed perfect, the impression of reality and, if I may say so, of intense *life* which emanated from it was perhaps even deeper than I experienced when facing the real object.[109]

Leaning, writing of 'cases in which some scene, or some object has engaged concentrated attention during the day, and an absolute reproduction takes place spontaneously against the background of darkness', lists Flournoy's 'visions', Hobbes's geometric figures, and Müller's microscopic preparations as examples of this phenomenon. Titchener referred to these experiences as

> *recurrent images*, those troublesome and haunting images to which most of us are subject at times: the tunes that run in our head and that we cannot get rid of, the rows of figures that obsess us after a long morning of calculation, the bright disk that keeps cropping up after we have spent several hours at the microscope.[110]

Dallenbach noted that having travelled all day, when he lay down in the evening 'the movement of the car was retained in kinesthetic imagery and was transferred in perception to the bed upon which I lay'; he also reported

> visual after-images of movement which were projected upon the field of my closed eyes or, with open eyes, within the darkness of the bed-room. The movement was toward me, a positive duplication of the perceptions

aroused from watching the roadway. During the entire time of driving I kept my eyes fixedly upon the road directly ahead of the car. . . . Stimulation was constant and of long duration; it was also intense, particularly during the last half of the trip which was made under the illumination of strong headlight.[111]

Hanawalt, reporting on the hypnagogic images of blackberries he had one evening as he retired and closed his eyes after a day out picking the fruit, writes:

> The images greatly impressed me for they were neither after-images in the usual sense nor were they memory images. The images were positive and appeared to be located in the eyes rather than projected. They were very vivid; they could be *seen* not just imagined as in the case of memory images. In this respect they were like the usual after-images. Introspectively they appeared to be retinal phenomena. . . . My wife and I both saw idealized images; . . . In place of the almost prohibitive brier patch, the berries hung upon open shoots; . . . in our images not an imperfect berry appeared.[112]

Comparing 'recurrent images' with Jaensch's[113] eidetic images, Hanawalt notes that

> according to Jaensch, the eidetic images can be seen after a brief stimulation. Recurrent images, contrariwise, occur only after long and intense stimulation. Again, such evidence as we have seems to indicate that recurrent images are located in the retina; eidetic images are projected into the environment. Recurrent images tend to occur with eyes closed or in very dim light; eidetic images can be seen with eyes open in broad daylight.

However, this polarization between eidetic images and recurrent images is not quite justified. Nor is Richardson's subsuming of recurrent images under the heading of after images. Richardson argues that 'though the circumstances in which these visual recurrent images appear might lead to them being called hypnagogic images the antecedent conditions of prolonged and intense retinal stimulation makes them a distinctive phenomenon and in this respect more like the after-image'.[114]

But, to begin with, recurrent images do not occur only after long and intense stimulation: an attentive glance may suffice, as both Maury[115] and Vihvelin noted. One of Vihvelin's subjects, for instance, reporting on the hypnagogic vision of 'a heap of electrocardiograms' he had one evening, writes:

> In that evening, before leaving the laboratory and before turning out the laboratory lamp, I threw an attentive glance on my working table, where the heap of the electrocardiograms was seen. This was the last relatively

intense optical perception I had that evening. The image of the vision corresponded exactly to the earlier perception.

Second, the locating of recurrent images in the retina or 'in the eye' as opposed to their being projected into the environment is rather confusing and misleading. What is meant by 'located in the retina'? Describing his own hypnagogic images, Hanawalt says that 'they could be *seen* not just imagined as in the case of memory images. In this respect they were like the usual after-images.' But if we 'see' something surely this something must be placed in front of us. This is not only logically necessary but experientially discoverable: even in the case of the usual after-image this is projected in front of us.[116] In fact, Hanawalt closes his paper leaving the argument open to the possibility 'of breaking up the eidetic image into two types: recurrent images and visualizations'. (See chapter 9 on 'eidetic imagery'.)

Similarly, Richardson argues that recurrent images are not perfect counterparts of original sensations or perceptions but 'idealized images'. He notes that

> In one study of eidetic imagery it was found that an 'idealized image' of a leaf resulted when a series of seven different shaped leaves had been previously presented one at a time. Such reports are similar to the results of experiments on composite photography (Galton 1883) where, for example, the heads of four or five women may be photographed in the same position on the one negative producing an idealized woman.[117]

He continues his argument pointing out that in stereoscopic experiments in which different full-face photographs are presented to each eye the result is often a fusion of the two which is typically experienced as more attractive than either face when seen alone.

Be that as it may, the fact remains that not all 'recurrent images' are 'idealized' ones, and that, as the evidence indicates, some are 'absolute reproductions' of original sensations or perceptions.[118]

In contrast to the 'perseverative' hypnagogic visions which are characterized by the recognizability of their imagery contents, the contents of the 'impersonal' type 'cannot easily be located in the imager's personal experience. Moreover, the images, by virtue of their originality, often seem strange and foreign to the personality of their author.'[119] Indeed, the majority of Leaning's correspondents (61 per cent) declared that they were unable to recognize objects and people in their hypnagogic images; a further 5 per cent could only very rarely recognize them, and 14 per cent could recognize only parts of their images. The rest (20 per cent) stated that their images were 'usually, or often recognized'.

A fourfold classification

In view of the evidence presented above, McKellar's two categories of hypnagogic phenomena, the 'perseverative' and the 'impersonal', are clearly too general. To begin with, the 'perseverative' type includes at least two groups of phenomena that warrant more attention and which, with wider research and more detailed analysis, may be seen to form two subclasses of the same category or even two entirely separate classes. The evidence so far, then, suggests that the perseveration of images is of at least the following two kinds: (a) images which, in Leaning's words, are 'absolute reproductions' of objects seen during the day (or sometime in the past), and (b) images which are not exact reproductions of their originals in the sense that they are not seen exactly from the same angle, and may exhibit added characteristics which, although they may belong to the nature of the object, were not actually present in the perception; moreover, this latter case may give rise, by some form of association, to experiences of similar objects. Of course, since images are not restricted to the visual modality, perceptual experiences in other parts of the sensorium may give rise to images in their respective modalities. For instance, listening to or performing Beethoven's music for long hours may not only, or necessarily, result in an accurate hypnagogic reproduction of the performance but may also, or instead, lead to auditory hypnagogic images of Beethovenesque compositions; similarly, as a result of travelling by car all day, one may have kinesthetic hypnagogic experiences of accelerating, swerving, etc., which do not literally correspond to actual experiences that took place during the course of the travelling. Returning to the first subclass, one may also notice that it contains perceptual details which are not within the normal memory capacity of the individual and which, for that reason alone, may surprise the subject as they make their appearance in the hypnagogic reproduction.

It seems to me, then, that in the 'perseverative' type we are dealing with two groups of phenomena, the first having a great deal in common with 'traditional' eidetic imagery, while in the second a certain amount of memory and 'imagination' are implicated. Concerning the 'impersonal' type, in this category we may have even more subdivisions, but suffice it to point out at this stage that the contents of this type are not all fantastic and unrecognizable although the majority of them might appear to be so at first sight.[120]

Thus, McKellar's twofold classification might be more accurately replaced by a fourfold one, namely: (a) reproductive, (b) perseverative, (c) familiar, (d) unfamiliar. The first class will comprise 'absolute reproductions' of perceptual experiences (this will include (i) and (ii) of Vihvelin's 'visions of memory-images'): the second will be made up of perseverations, that is, of images that persist in a 'reverberative' and 'echoic' manner implying a certain degree of departure from the exact original and allowing for the introduction of a restricted play of imagination (this will include Hanawalt's visions of 'idealized' objects); the third class will contain images of immediately or easily recognizable objects (this may include (iii) and (iv) of Vihvelin's 'visions of memory-images'); the fourth class will consist of entirely phantastic images of (α) plausible and (β) implausible objects, that is, of things, faces etc., whose appearance (shape, construction, etc.) is plausible but outside the subject's conscious memory – indeed, they may never have been encountered in waking life – and of things, faces, and so on, whose appearance (shape, construction, behaviour, etc.) is implausible (flying monsters, angels, devils, and so on). In subclass (α) we may include Myers's 'unidentified' images.

Naturally, this fourfold system does not exclude combinations of categories – on the contrary, some hypnagogic experiences will fall into one combination or another; for instance, the experience of a hypnagogic reproduction of a childhood event will be classified as a reproductive familiar hypnagogic experience. Moreover, the same event might, retrospectively, be viewed as reproductive unfamiliar if the subject does not recognize it as a childhood event at the time but does so subsequently (perhaps as a result of visiting the location of the event or seeing a photograph of the location or through some other vital clue or through hypnosis). This latter case would, I think, fruitfully suggest that at least some hypnagogic images might be traceable to distant or subliminal perceptions.

Other, and possibly more useful, dimensions of classification will be suggested in the succeeding chapters. Clearly, at this stage of research into hypnagogia, the greater the amount of data presented and the greater the number of angles from which they are viewed or classified the wider and more fruitful the field of research will be rendered to subsequent investigators.

3 · Cognitive and affective characteristics

In this chapter I shall delineate and discuss the salient psychological features of hypnagogia, offer an analysis of the attentional state of a person when involved in the induction, prolongation and control of hypnagogic imagery, and identify a hypnagogic syndrome. The term 'psychological' is being used advisedly here since all the phenomena described or referred to in the main body of this book are, in the last analysis, psychological. But, whereas in the previous chapter attention was primarily paid to the phenomena themselves, and in particular to their *perceptual* character, in the present chapter we shall be looking into the *mental state* of the hypnagogist (more accurately, into his *psychophysical* state).

Suggestibility-receptivity

Suggestibility appears to be one of the most prevalent features of hypnagogia. This is to be understood not only as the subject's susceptibility to accept suggestions by an external agency, e.g. an experimenter, but also as the subject's readiness to accept, incorporate and elaborate perceptual (both exteroceptive and proprioceptive) and imaginal data, as well as 'freely' associate and elaborate concepts and ideas, that is, as the subject's autosuggestibility.

A number of workers have noted the readiness with which external stimuli tend to become incorporated in hypnagogic mentation and have drawn attention to the possibility of their being causally involved in the genesis of hypnagogic experiences.[1] Hollingworth remarked that hypnagogia possesses 'the tendency to magnify simply sensory impressions',[2] and Arnold-Forster noted that 'when we are nearest to sleep the senses become abnormally acute'.[3] Davis *et al.* were the first to observe through EEG an increase of responsiveness to sound as the subject moved from wakefulness to drowsiness.[4] More recent research has confirmed these observations.[5] For instance, Ornitz *et al.*[6] found that averaged evoked responses to 60-decibel clicks (ambient noise 30 decibels) clustered in their largest amplitudes around sleep onset, viz. during the 10-minute period immediately preceding and following the first sleep spindle, that is, during the deeper hypnagogic state. These investigators conclude that 'there would seem to be either a special facilitatory influence or a decrease in inhibitory influence associated with the transition from wakefulness to sleep', and point to other supporting evidence provided by de Lisi and by Oswald[7] in respect to the occurrence of sudden bodily jerks at sleep onset as indicators of facilitation or decrease in inhibition.

Jastrow spoke of hypnagogia as 'that state upon the verge of sleep in which the mind seems peculiarly open to suggestion', McDowell wrote that 'the impressions that are introduced at such a time tend to operate with abnormally great effect', and Arnold-Forster referred to the 'special receptiveness of the mind to suggestion and communication in the borderland state'.[8] Similar views are held by numerous other investigators.[9]

The autosuggestibility of the subject in hypnagogia was dramatically pointed out by Sartre who proposed that hypnagogic catalepsy is 'a condition which may be described as paralysis by autosuggestion ... distantly related to hysterical pythiatism and to certain frenzies of influence'.[10] No less dramatic, and just as important and interesting, is the discovery by many hypnagogists that they can influence, or even generate, their imagery by mere suggestion. For example, Alexander reports: 'an image appears, and I say to myself curiously "that resembles a frog (an alligator, or what not)." Forthwith the image transforms itself into a frog.'[11] One of Leaning's correspondents reports that, having been awoken in the middle of the night by the barking of a dog, he resolved 'to be calm, quite calm, and lay passive'. Presently, he continues,

> I saw the big trunk of a tree, with mossy roots, at the foot of the trees even several small indistinct white objects. I wasn't sure what they were – 'Mushrooms, perhaps?' I thought – and they clearly became mushrooms! Then they shifted again – and 'No' I thought 'they are not mushrooms, they're PLAYING CARDS'. And in a trice they became playing cards. I saw the black and red pips on them; then all gone. This was becoming interesting and I waited for the next picture. It came as a bank of dense plants, clumps like very large forget-me-not plants – nothing else, only the leaves. I thought 'Now can I get these plants *to blossom*.' I had no sooner formed the wish than I saw flowering stems and buds pushing out from among the leaves; they grew by degree, and unfolded. I was so thrilled I hardly dared to breathe. .... Most certainly I was not asleep. My mentality was most keenly awake and absorbed in this quite new development. 'If another comes,' I said to myself, 'I'll try to get something alive.'. ... There came a sort of confusion and shaking in the darkness – indistinct bunches that *moved* – then I saw hanging down several legs and feet of game birds, the claws and scales on the legs lifelike; below them rose the head and forepart of a little animal that looked like a rat, its head was turned over, and the mouth open. I saw the pink tongue and lips. Then all vanished.[12] (Figure 3.1)

Figure 3.1 *To the suggestible and receptive mind of the hypnagogist, perceived images can be modified to fit the concept of what he thinks he is experiencing, and ideas and desires may give rise to appropriate imagery which unfolds before him most lifelike.*

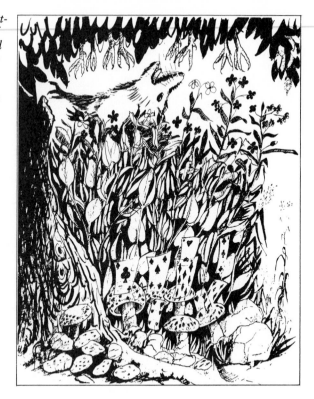

Indeed sometimes the 'suggestions' and the resultant image are so quickly and subtly formed that one may seriously wonder whether the hypnagogist is not engaged in an act of 'knowing' rather than 'suggesting'. That is, there are at least some cases in which the subject may not so much suggest as know what the image is going to be before the latter appears.[13] (Interestingly, this almost incidental observation may have far-reaching epistemological implications in its indicating how simplistic, and possibly false, is the view of clearly distinguishing between knowledge and autosuggestion in the wider context of wakefulness.)

Budzynski claims that in the hypnagogic state subjects 'are super-suggestible and capable of learning certain things more efficiently and painlessly than during the day, when logical and analytical faculties are in control'. He reports that by means of an electromyograph subjects are trained to reduce tension in forehead muscles through biofeedback and thus decrease cortical and autonomic arousal as well. Once they have learned to put themselves in this relaxed state, which is characterized by theta EEG activity, they are further 'trained to maintain the theta pattern indefinitely with a device called Twilight Learner'. He maintains that because in this state the constricting influence of logical thinking is laxed or absent, subjects can be helped to break down mental blocks, prejudices, biases, resistances, bad habits, headaches, anxieties, and learn new material, such as languages, easier and quicker. He offers as evidence some of his own work and his colleagues', and cites other instances from eastern Europe, in particular the Russian tutorial method known as 'hypnopedia' which uses repetition of material over several days or weeks.[14] Budzynski's own findings appear to support the hypothesis put forward by earlier workers[15] that sleep onset is the most effective period for 'sleep' learning.[16]

In her hypnopompic experiments, in which she woke her subjects after two or three hours of night sleep and made various suggestions to them while they were still in this half-awakened state, de Manacéine found that a considerable number of them transformed or incorporated the suggestion into the imagery of an ensuing dream.[17]

Awareness of significance and affective response

Another important feature of hypnagogia, and one which is often overlooked, is the accompanying awareness of significance which seems to equip the subject with an understanding of his imagery. As we shall see in later chapters, its occurrence in hypnagogia may be a congruent accompaniment of creativity, have mystical overtones, or be clearly psychotic. Although this feature is reported by Vihvelin[18] as a character of a particular type of hypnagogic vision, careful examination of reports in the literature shows it to be a more commonly occurring feature of hypnagogia in general. It is a defining characteristic of the 'autosymbolic' phenomenon first reported by Silberer[19] and subsequently by other workers. My own observations suggest that its appearance and the particular form it takes depend on the mental set of the subject both prior to and during hypnagogia itself.

Silberer observed that when the following two conditions were present, (a) drowsiness, and (b) an effort to think, an autosymbolic phenomenon made its appearance, that is, 'a hallucinatory experience which puts forth "autosymbolically", as it were, an adequate symbol for what is thought (or felt) at a given instant'. All autosymbolic hypnagogic phenomena, according to Silberer, are the result of the above-mentioned two conditions, the former being a passive condition not subject to will, the latter an active one controllable by the will, and 'it is the struggle of these two antagonistic elements that elicits . . . the "autosymbolic" phenomenon'.[20] He distinguishes three types of the phenomenon, noting that often a hypnagogic experience may be a mixture of two or all three. The first type, which he calls 'Material (content) phenomenon', consists of 'autosymbolic representations of thought contents, that is, of content dealt with in a thought process', such as ideas, groups of ideas, and judgments. For instance:

> In a state of drowsiness I contemplate an abstract topic such as the
> nature of transsubjectively (for all people) valid judgements. . . . The

content of my thought presents itself to me immediately in the form of a perceptual (for an instant apparently real) picture: I see a big circle (or transparent sphere) in the air with people around it whose heads reach into the circle. . . . In the next instant I realise that it is a dream-picture; the thought that gave rise to it, which I had forgotten for a moment, now comes back and I recognize the experience as an 'autosymbolic' phenomenon.

Another example offered by Silberer is the following: 'My thought is: I am to improve a halting passage in an essay. *Symbol*: I see myself planing a piece of wood.'

The second type of autosymbolic phenomenon, which Silberer calls 'Functional (effort) phenomenon', represents the condition of the subject experiencing the phenomenon or the effectiveness of his consciousness, that is, it has to do with the mode of functioning of the subject's consciousness and not with the content of his thought. Example:

I am thinking about something. Pursuing a subsidiary consideration, I depart from my original theme. When I attempt to return to it, an autosymbolic phenomenon occurs. *Symbol*: I am out mountain climbing. The mountains near me conceal the farther ones from which I came and to which I want to return.

The third type he calls 'Somatic phenomenon' and it reflects 'somatic conditions of any kind: external or internal sensations, such as pressure, tension, temperature, external pain and position sensations . . .', chemical, optical, and other stimulations. Thus the somatic phenomenon may arise from various physiological sources, such as pressure of a blanket, itching, rheumatic pains, palpitations, smells, apnoea, a breeze touching one's cheek, and so on. For instance: 'I take a deep breath, my chest expands. *Symbol*: With the help of someone, I lift a table high.' Another example:

My blanket rests so heavily on one of my toes that it makes me nervous. *Symbol*: The top of a decorated canopied carriage scrapes against the branches of trees. A lady hits her hat against the top of her compartment. *Symbol-source*: I had attended a flower parade that day. The high decorations of the carriage often reached to the branches of the trees.

The 'somatic phenomena' are somewhat different from the other two kinds in that the 'effort to think' is not relevant in their genesis, and 'in the struggle against drowsiness the "will" is replaced by sensations or feelings': all that is needed for the production of these latter phenomena is that one should resist falling asleep when very drowsy, but at the same time must not force oneself into full wakefulness. Silberer noted that the material for the symbols in these phenomena is taken (as in the example of the flower parade above) mostly from recent experiences. It should be noted, for later reference, that in all three kinds of autosymbolic phenomena the interpretation of the symbol is given during the phenomenon itself, that is, Silberer *knows* what the imagery conveys to him either while having the experience or as the imagery fades away but he is still in hypnagogia.

Besides Kollarits's example in the previous chapter, which is clearly an autosymbolic (material) phenomenon, in the next chapter we shall see a number of 'somatic' and other autosymbolic experiences reported by Ouspensky as examples of his studies on dreams during hypnagogia. Vihvelin has also presented numerous reports of his subjects in which there is clearly an accompanying awareness of the significance of the symbolism in the vision. For instance:

> A vision of one's empty shoes appears, seen from above. According to the accompanying awareness, this is to signify that one must put them on and go out. *Connection*: shortly before the mental content was present that one will have to go out soon.

Slight reports that if, while in hypnagogia, some problem presents its solution or a memory is recovered after some effort, a person may have the image of a bridge over which he seems to have crossed and looks back feeling that he has crossed after difficulty but he is relieved by the fact that the crossing is completed.[21] Leroy offers a number of autosymbolic phenomena that include personal experiences and reports by subjects.[22] Rapaport, reporting on his attempt to remain awake in hypnagogia, describes the sudden emergence of the image of two waves which he was trying to bring together and of the vision of someone who was frantically trying to get to a door which was slowly closing.[23] A remark by Maury suggests that he, too, was probably aware of this phenomenon. He writes, 'As soon as the mind stops on an idea, a corresponding hypnagogic hallucination produces itself, if the eyes close.'[24] Importantly, Maury's observation points out the possibility of having autosymbolic experiences, which are not 'somatic phenomena', in the absence of a struggle between trying to think and the desire to fall asleep. This, it will be argued later, may point to hypnagogia's having its own

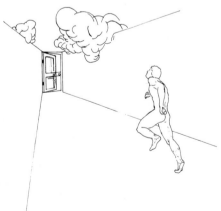

Figure 3.2 *An attempt to remain awake in hypnagogia often results in the sudden emergence of an autosymbolic phenomenon, such as the vision of someone trying to get to a door which is slowly closing – the phenomenon being an adequate symbol of the person's current mental state.*

'cognitive function' which is distinct from that of the waking, 'logical', thinking.

Two of my own hypnagogic experiences may be included here. The first belongs to the 'material phenomenon' type whereas the second is mainly 'functional' but with an added 'intuition' to it. Lying in bed with eyes shut, half asleep, I am thinking of the difficulties of trying to remain awake in hypnagogia. I have the picture of a man (I feel, myself) rolling a stone bigger than myself up a small conically shaped hill and trying to place it on its tip. The idea behind it is that if I achieve this I will then be able to have a clear view all round. But every time I roll the big stone to the top I only succeed in getting a glimpse of the surroundings before the stone begins to roll over to another side of the cone. It never exactly rolls off my hands completely, but I have to go along with it until I manage to stop it rolling away and then start all over again, this time from another side of the cone. In fact, I never manage to get it to the tip but sort of get to just below it and then keep going round the tip trying to stop it from rolling away. As I reflect on this imagery while the experience is coming to its end I realize that the whole vision is a representation in picture form of my thoughts about the difficulties of maintaining waking awareness during hypnagogia. The second experience begins with my thinking about a particular weakness in my behaviour and of how I could best conceal it. Suddenly, I have the hypnagogic vision of myself squatting on the ground in front of a hole (about 15 × 15 cm) which I am trying to fill up with earth. As I am doing this I realize that in order to fill up the hole I am, in fact, making another hole next to it as I dig to get the earth I need to fill up the first hole. Then, just as suddenly, I have a flash of understanding in which I see that there is no way of really covering up any weakness and that no matter how much I gloss over it the fact remains that I myself know about it.

An interesting observation made by Silberer, and emphasized by Slight, is that symbols appearing in hypnagogia are not static and universal but particular ones which carry specific meanings for the individual concerned. Moreover, what makes the symbols what they are is not only, or always, the significance they normally have for the individual but often the significance they have or acquire at the time of their appearance or very soon after while the person is still in hypnagogia. The interpretation obtained in this state, according to Slight, 'has that note of reality and surety which a true and real self-knowledge alone can give.' In this respect, hypnagogia appears to be a most appropriate state in which to carry out interpretation of symbols.

It must be noted, however, that awareness of the significance of the symbolism is not always present, and in the majority of cases imagery remains a puzzle until one begins to pay attention to it and enters into a form of 'conversation' with it. The difficulty here lies in the degree of willingness on the part of the subject to enter into this form of 'associating' or 'talking to oneself'. As Jung pointed out in respect to allowing one's unconscious to emerge, this 'becomes possible only when the ego acknowledges the existence of a partner to the discussion.'[25] Furthermore, van Dusen notes that the process of balancing oneself between waking and sleeping requires the ability 'to relax enough to continue to observe the hypnogogic without blocking it by an excess of ego. *Very clearly it is the antithesis of ego.* Where ego is absent, it can appear.'[26] And when this happens, the autosymbolic nature of hypnagogia becomes obvious. 'When one first runs into the hypnogogic,' van Dusen further notes, 'it seems to be just a lot of random firings of the brain, bits of images and phrases. . . . Upon closer examination it appears rather clearly autosymbolic.' This autosymbolic feature may stretch all the way from the eigenlicht to the deepest layers of hypnagogia. The seeing of geometric patterns, for instance, may represent the analytical mind of the subject. 'My own fern-leaf designs,' van Dusen remarks, 'seem to go with a very peaceful languid state, the feeling suggested by ferns growing in shaded areas.' The same applies to the phenomena of the auditory modality: peculiar combinations of sounds or strange names may also be autosymbolic. 'At the moment the name explodes in awareness,' the same author writes, 'it seems to represent the background feelings it came from by the arrangement of its sound qualities.' Towards the deeper end of hypnagogia, the 'conversation' method may elicit more meaningful responses. For instance:

> I once asked the hypnogogic whether or not I should change jobs and circumstances. . . . I saw a river that had worn down through a gorge for centuries and heard 'Wear down like a river'. I came out of it with a feeling of the great pleasure of knowing one place for centuries.

Van Dusen suggests that hypnagogia may consist of a hierarchy of levels roughly as follows:

> (a) random bits of images and phrases: (b) experiences that are pretty clearly autosymbolic or representative of one's state at the moment; (c) hypnogogic experiences that are instructive, including the possibility of questioning the process and learning from it; (d) hypnogogic experiences that break into trance-like periods of enlightenment.

In the depths of hypnagogia, he claims, the questioner and the answerer become one in a kind of satori or enlightenment.

One phenomenon in this state, van Dusen reports, which does not appear to have been noticed by anyone before is the following:

> when nearly asleep I find myself locked into some kind of logical relationship. There may be a fixed image and I go over the logic within its form repeatedly. I have the impression it is like a perfectly balanced, very complex, logical presentation. When I awaken it is difficult to remember though. I may come out with some very paradoxical statement. When, within it, all its logical relationships seem perfectly clear although complex and often paradoxical.

He attempts to explain this phenomenon as perhaps having to do with his

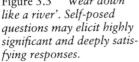

Figure 3.3 *'Wear down like a river'. Self-posed questions may elicit highly significant and deeply satisfying responses.*

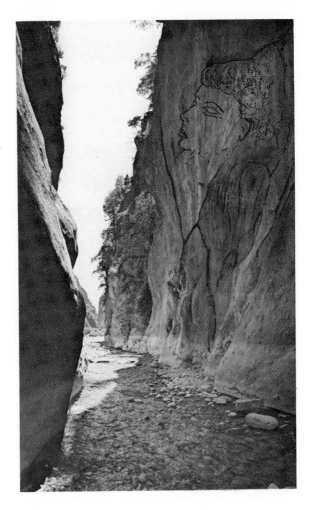

personal desire to see things in the world fit each other in a perfect comprehensive whole.

The same or very similar experience was also noted by Hollingworth who reported that he frequently recorded fantastic experiments and conclusions late at night which at the time of their conception 'seemed highly rational, strikingly original and wonderfully significant'. More specifically, Hollingworth noted that in hypnagogia 'an idea, plan or desire is . . . able to make unimpeded progress from stage to stage of its development with what seems at the time to be unerring logic', and that this state 'behaves much as do the familiar dream states in which cosmic riddles are solved and impossible mechanical devices evolved' (see chapters 7 and 8).

Hollingworth uses the term 'substitution' to describe phenomena encompassing synesthetic, autosymbolic, and 'transformational' events. He appears to consider synesthetic and autosymbolic phenomena as paraphrastic, that is, as reverberations or restatements in a sensory modality of thoughts or perceptual and imagery experiences taking place in another sensory modality. Under the term 'sensory substitution' he describes what I would call transformational and incorporative phenomena, such as those that occurred in the first example of his report in which the sound of waves washing against the sides of the ship in which he was travelling assumed the role of a foreign salesman, and those that occurred in his third example in which his tossings and turnings in bed became transformed into the combination numbers of his gym locker.

Relevant in the present discussion are Leaning's remarks in connection with the aesthetic quality of hypnagogic visions, and in particular of faces which range from 'transcendent beauty' to 'hideous and terrifying'. Leaning's explanation of the quality of these visions is that they might have 'some relation to the thought-tone of the persons seeing them, and may be a transcription in symbol of the unconscious morality and instinctive emotional reaction to life which lies under the surface of the conscious and the controlled'. She makes references, in this respect, to Müller's comparing notes with Goethe and noting that the differences in their respective visions were proper to their respective mental endowments. Greenwood spoke of his 'faces in the dark' as sometimes having 'a profoundly meaning, or appealing, or revealing look'.[27] Other hypnagogists may consider their visions to be omens (see chapter 6).

Interestingly, however, several investigators have noted that visual hypnagogic experiences are generally accompanied by lack, or considerable decrease, of affect, irrespective of their content or aesthetic quality.[28] Indeed, Foulkes and Vogel pointed out 'emotional flatness' as 'the primary affective characteristic of the hypnagogic period' and noted that 'even in the minority of hypnagogic reports which do contain indications of the presence of affect it is quite rare for this affect to be at all intense'. As one subject reports:

> Finally, one image presented itself. A frightful one that did not, however, truly frighten me. The distorted face of a man; wrinkled and lined by folds of flesh; his one eye was like a very old apple that has turned pale brown and shriveled. It stood out of his eye socket. I saw no other eye. This image lasted several seconds, it seemed, and I got a good look at this face; it was alive, the changeless grimace seemed alive somehow, and the head turned somewhat. As I say, I was aware that this was a hideous image, yet I was not afraid so much as curious to watch it to see what it might do.[29]

On the other hand, some workers have held that in hypnagogia there occurs a variety of emotions.[30] However, careful examination of reports shows that not only are strong emotions rare in this state but also that their occurrence is not conducive either to the induction or the prolongation of hypnagogia. For instance, hypnagogic nightmares in normal subjects bring the state to an end.

Figure 3.4 *A wrinkled and distorted face with a rotten apple for an eye: 'I was aware that this was a hideous image, yet I was not afraid so much as curious to watch it to see what it might do.'*

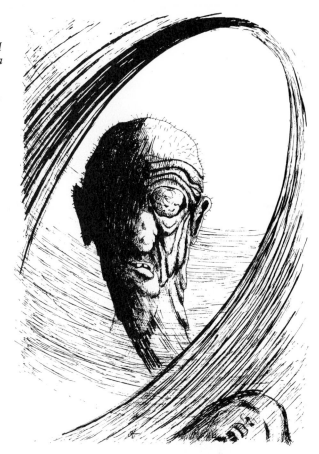

Similarly, strong emotions would prevent hypnagogia from occurring naturally in the first place. As distinct from this, most subjects report that they experience 'relaxed numbness' and 'curiosity', that they are 'much interested and entertained', 'surprised and interested', or merely 'disinterested'.

Changes in the quality of thought

Thinking in images, which dominates hypnagogic mentation, is thought to appear in the earliest stages of the cognitive development of children.[31] In this respect, practically all workers in the area have pointed out the 'regressive' character of hypnagogia. Hollingworth, for instance, remarked that 'in this state the condition of early childhood is reproduced', typified by examples of magic-childlike thinking. Analysing one of his hypnagogic experiences, Silberer wrote:

My abstract chain of thought was hampered; I was too tired to go on thinking in that form; the perceptual picture emerged as an 'easier' form of thought. It afforded an appreciable relief, comparable to the one experienced when sitting down after a strenuous walk. It appears to follow – as a corollary – that such 'picture thinking' requires less effort than the usual kind.

In agreement with Freud,[32] he posited that 'this is in many respects a primitive form of thinking'. As McKellar[33] points out, this view is highly compatible with the theory later developed by Rivers according to which dreaming is 'an expression of early modes of mental functioning which have been allowed to come into action owing to the removal of higher restraining influences derived from the experience of later life'. It is also compatible with Bergson's[34] theory of 'mental effort' in respect to perception, and Jung's[35] distinguishing between 'directed thinking' and 'dream or phantasy thinking'. According to Jung, the former type of thinking is 'troublesome and exhausting' whereas the latter 'does not tire us; it quickly leads us away from reality into phantasies'. James referred to the latter as 'merely associative' thinking and wrote:

> Our thought consists for the great part of a series of images, one of which produces the other; *a sort of passive dream state of which the higher animals are also capable.* This sort of thinking leads, nevertheless, to reasonable conclusions of a practical as well as a theoretical nature. As a rule, the links of this sort of irresponsible thinking, which are accidentally bound together, are empirically concrete things, not abstractions.[36]

McKellar refers to hypnagogic mentation as 'autistic',[37] that is, thinking dominated by inner fantasy life, and Oswald uses the term 'dereistic'[38] to convey the disregard of, or divorce from, reality apparent in this kind of mentation. These two Bleulerian terms are very similar to Piaget's 'egocentric' employed in the description of mentation encountered in early childhood, dreams, and half-sleep states.[39]

Like the above workers, Rapaport also noted that as he slipped into hypnagogia he began to lose reflective self-consciousness together with the ability to exert effort and think logically, while at the same time his visual imagery increased in frequency and vividness.[40] Similarly, Singer found that effortful thinking was difficult to carry out and that 'reminiscing proved to be the easiest task'.[41] Proust spoke of the presence of a 'form of reasoning totally contradicting the laws of logic and the evidence of the present',[42] and Forbes observed that in this state 'one may simultaneously visualize a familiar landmark and recall a recent "wise-crack" and perhaps some third impression'.[43] Often, items of experience, which clearly belong to different and unrelated frames of reference, may fuse to give rise to novel, if strange, combinations.

Figure 3.5 *The complexity of awareness in hypnagogia: One may simultaneously visualize a familiar landmark, recall a 'wisecrack', and have a third impression. Such events may unfold autonomously and in apparent independence of each other, and thus give credence to the notion that the human psyche consists of 'layers' or 'streams of experience' which can exist separately and in parallel to one another. (See chapter 7 et seq.).*

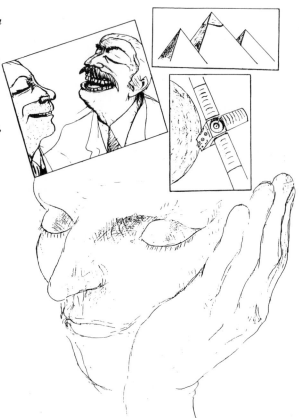

Hollingworth remarked that here 'the essential thing is the release of all intellectual inhibition' and that 'formal, practical and conceptual constraints being removed, resemblances of a sensory and ordinarily unnoticed kind ... become predominant'. He noted the following as typical occurrences in hypnagogia: unusual verbal combinations, absurd juxtapositions, bizarre analogies, attention to irrelevant details, naive confusion of related concepts. The last of these was stressed by Froeschels who pointed out that *similarity* between two or more items may turn into *sameness* or identity[44] (see chapters 7 and 8).

Leroy cited a case in which both the element of suggestibility and the tendency to turn similarity into sameness were clearly present. His subject reported that at first he saw the image of a carpet being shaken from a window. As he watched this it seemed to him that the carpet looked like a tooth, whereupon the carpet turned into a molar tooth with two roots protruding from its base which represented – played the part of – the legs of the person shaking the carpet from the window![45] Such imagery, as we shall see later (chapter 8), is made constructive use of by surrealist painters.

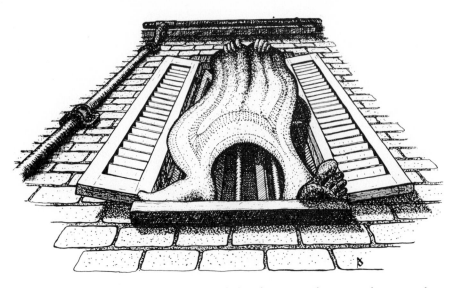

Figure 3.6 *The carpet, which was being shaken from a window, turned into a molar tooth whose roots turned into the legs of the person who was shaking the carpet!*

Now, hypnagogic mentation as a whole appears to be related to a mode of experiencing that functions at a lower level of energy requirement than the active, waking kind of mentation. Furthermore, and in agreement with Silberer's observation above, the mere functioning in the former seems to be connected with a gaining in energy rather than expending. In my own studies in which subjects were asked to sit in a relaxing position, close their eyes and turn their attention inwards watching receptively for whatever imagery might emerge, practically all subjects reported feeling 'refreshed' and 'invigorated' at the end of each experiment. To a certain extent this was to be expected since relaxation formed an integral introductory part of every experiment. But it was soon noted that reports of 'refreshment' and 'invigoration' were both more forthcoming and more emphatic from those subjects who also reported as having experienced a considerable amount of imagery as opposed to those who reported very little or none. Moreover, my studies also suggest that, given the initial relaxation and psychological withdrawal, emerging hypnagogic imagery (and the accompanying mentation) may deepen the former and thus initiate a self-perpetuating cycle of ever deepening relaxation and imaginal experiences. This seems to be in agreement with Leroy's and Sartre's seeing hypnagogia as a deepening state of self-induced paralysis. The 'refreshing' and 'invigorating' features may, in fact, be functions of the hypnagogic components of 'passive volition' and 'absorption' to be discussed below. In which case the term 'regressive' is rather misleadingly employed here if it is to be understood *merely* as 'a primitive form of thinking'.

Thus, although, when viewed in ontogenetic terms, hypnagogic mentation may indeed be called 'regressive' – using the term in its usual psychoanalytic definition of referring to a channel of expression belonging to an earlier phase of development[46] – it is arguable whether the term, with its pejorative connotations, is justifiably employed in those cases where hypnagogic mentation appears in the absence of tiredness either spontaneously or when deliberately induced, in a presleep setting or in psi experiments, religious prophesying, or in any other setting in which it is intentionally produced (see, for example, chapters 5 and 6). As Tappeiner rightly points out, the word 'regressive' 'is a somewhat biased term which does not take note of more recent studies which interpret the return to "primary process thinking" as neither regressive nor progressive but in terms of organismic intention'.[47]

By 'recent studies' Tappeiner is mainly referring to Deikman's paper on 'Biomodal consciousness' in which it is proposed that human beings function primarily in two modes: '(1) the receptive mode oriented toward the intake of the environment, and (2) the action mode oriented toward manipulation of the environment'.[48] In the action mode, Deikman explains,

> the striate muscle system and the sympathetic nervous system are the dominant physiological agencies. The EEG shows beta waves and baseline muscle tension is increased. The principal psychological manifestations of this state are focal attention, object-based logic, heightened boundary perception, and the dominance of formal characteristics over the sensory; shapes and meanings have a preference over colours and textures. The action mode is a state of striving.

By contrast, in the receptive mode,

> the sensory-perceptual system is the dominant agency rather than the muscle system, and parasympathetic functions tend to be more prominent. The EEG tends toward alpha waves and baseline muscle tension is decreased. Other attributes of the receptive mode are diffuse attending, paralogical thought processes, decreased boundary perception, and the dominance of the sensory over the formal. . . . This mode would appear to originate and function maximally in the infant state.

The point being made here, and one which will be argued throughout the book, is that hypnagogic mentation is a function of the employment of the receptive mode, and as such, it is not so much regressive as much as an expression of a specific 'functional orientation' of the human nature.

Fascinated attention

The attitude of openness and sensitivity to physical stimuli in hypnagogia is paralleled, as we saw earlier, by openness and sensitivity on a psychological level. Indeed, this latter feature, along with that of 'psychological incorporability', will be seen later to constitute essential elements of the important phenomenon of *loosening of ego boundaries* (LEBs) which, lying as it does at the root of all hypnagogic experiences, may hold the key to hypnagogic mentation, and its presence may help to explain mentation in other psychological states. Depending on the prevailing cultural and psychological setting, it may take on names such as 'role-playing', 'adaptability', or 'egolessness'. Significantly, behind these latter terms there appear to lie the important hypnotic factors of 'absorption' and 'fascination'[49] whose presence is believed to result in an altered sense of reality and imperviousness to distracting events,[50] and it is of importance that the same or similar terms have been employed by a number of writers to describe the psychological states of meditation, expanded awareness, aesthetic, mystical and peak experiences;[51] it is also of interest to note that Aristotle in his *Poetics* used the term 'psychagogia' (ψυχαγωγία = soul-leading, soul-guiding) to describe the state of the spectator in the theatre whose mind is 'enthralled', 'entranced', 'absorbed', 'transported'.[52]

In such a state of 'fascination', in which the representational system is fully engaged, a person 'cannot . . . maintain salient qualifying "meta-cognitions", that is, thoughts *about* the primary representation, such as "this is only my imagination" or "this is not really happening".'[50] This, in fact, is a characteristic of an advanced hypnagogic state wherein the subject becomes completely absorbed in imaginal activities, that is, he becomes 'fascinated' and loses his ability for reality testing. Similarly, Sartre states that 'hypnagogic phenomena are not "contemplated by consciousness": *they belong to consciousness*', 'we do not contemplate the hypnagogic image but are fascinated by it'.[53] He further explains that

> what happens here is similar to certain psychoses which possess a
> simple and also a delirious form. Hypnagogic images belong to the
> delirious form. I am still able to reflect, that is, to become conscious of
> being conscious. But to maintain the integrity of this primary
> consciousness it is necessary that the reflexive consciousness be in turn
> charmed, that it does not place before itself the acts of primary
> consciousness in order to observe them and describe them.

It should also be added that the activities of primary consciousness are here accompanied by 'primary logic' as it is encountered in the receptive mode. But before we move further on this line of argument there are certain points brought out by Sartre that need clarification.

First, Sartre uses the term 'fascination' in a derogatory manner to mean 'deterioration of consciousness', that is, the charming of secondary consciousness and the maintenance of the integrity of the primary consciousness are considered 'regressive': they are a following into 'bondage'. Second, the 'charmed' and 'fascinated' attributes are in reference to the dimension of attention as it is understood to operate in the normal waking state. He proposes that when consciousness is 'fascinated' it is not centred in the manner of attention because 'all phenomena of attention have a motor basis (convergence, accommodation, contraction of the visual field, etc.)', and 'these different movements are for the time being impossible: to produce them we must emerge from the condition of paralysis in which we find ourselves, in which case we return to the wakeful state'. To pay attention to something, he continues, means assigning it spatial localization. In this way, 'there results a sort of objectification of the subject in relation to the object (be it a sensation or a thought)':

> In falling asleep the motor basis of attention is weak. From it there results a different type of presence for the object. It is there but without externality; we cannot observe it, that is, build hypotheses and control them. What is lacking is precisely a contemplative power of conscious-ness, a certain way of keeping oneself at a distance from one's images, from one's own thoughts, thus permitting them their own logical development. . . .

Now, Sartre's approach to the subject raises a number of problems not least of which is that resulting from his apparent equation of the notion of attention with that of contemplation. It is of great importance to clarify these notions if we are to avoid conceptual muddle and better advance our understanding of hypnagogia. Contemplation is clearly an attitude of placing a spatial and/or temporal distance between oneself and objects, the latter being anything that is not considered to be part of the 'self'; it can also be the placing of a distance between the 'assumed' psychophysical self (i.e. one's physical body, instincts, emotions, intentions, thoughts, etc.), which is thus considered to be the object, and an occult or metaphysical self with which one identifies. (Here we are not concerned with the common-view distinction between 'active life' and 'contemplative life' since this is only a distinction between external and internal *activity*.) In contemplating, one obviously directs one's attention to the object of contemplation somehow dividing it between the object and self-awareness. But this is not all that should be understood by attention. Deikman pertinently distinguishes between 'focal attention', which is the component of the active mode, and 'diffuse attention', a component of the receptive mode. And although it might be argued that in 'diffuse attention' the object is not 'centred' in the generally understood sense of focal centring, we must be careful to observe that it *is* 'centred' in the sense that one is absorbed in it. As Tellegen and Atkinson have also noted, 'absorbed attention is highly "centred" (in a roughly Piagetian sense).'[50] Now, attention in hypnagogia is both *diffuse and absorbed*: it is so because of the subject's general state of relaxation which alone is often sufficient to elicit hypnagogic imagery whose very nature is characterized by the subject's absorption in it. Indeed, it is the manipulation of these two features, diffusion and absorption of attention, that, as we shall see later, may facilitate a state of double-consciousness and complete or partial dissociation.

Ellis's reference to Ribot's distinction between *voluntary attention* and *spontaneous attention* may further clarify the present discussion especially since it introduces the notion of *will* as the defining characteristic of the terms.[54] As Ellis explains, the former type of attention 'is accompanied by some feeling of effort. It always acts on the muscles and by the muscles.' This, being precisely the definition given by Sartre to his concept of attention, indicates how incorrect is the latter's view of the *singularity* of the notion. The concept of voluntary attention is highly compatible with Deikman's action mode as 'a state of striving' in which attention is 'intimately associated with the striate muscle effort of voluntary activity, particularly eye muscle activity'. By contrast, spontaneous attention is characterized by 'muscular weakness'.

In such a state of diffuse-and-spontaneous attention, the latter is drawn and absorbed by the ensuing imagery thus giving rise to a *subjectification of the object*, as opposed to Sartre's 'objectification of the subject'. This subject-object immediacy endows the imaginal environment with a sense of reality which is 'more vivid' and 'more real' than ordinary reality. In this state of fascination there is, indeed, a sense in which one's attention is 'caught', one is held captive: It is a state of self-hypnosis in which the separative, contemplative aspect of self is ostracized. It is of great relevance here that 'absorption' was found by Tellegen and Atkinson to be the factor most 'consistently associated with hypnotic susceptibility': it shows how in hypnagogia a person may gradually relinquish the attitude of contemplation and, by being absorbed in imaginal activities, become 'fascinated' (or, vice versa, one may become 'fascinated' by being absorbed in imaginal activities and thus relinquish the attitude of contemplation). Autosuggestibility and psychological incorporability or internalization of the environment (subjectification of the object) are thus attentional attributes of that aspect of receptivity which is operational in hypnagogia.

It can now be seen that Sartre's argument that the centring of consciousness in hypnagogia 'is not in the manner of attention' is refuted, unless it is qualified and restated as 'not in the manner of contemplative or reflective attention'. Also, the motor basis of attention considered by Sartre to be necessarily involved in the localization of thoughts and images may be entirely absent once the imaginal object is 'internalized' or 'subjectified', that is, one need not emerge from the condition of temporary hypnagogic 'paralysis' in order to be able to 'attend' to one's thoughts and images (see cases of spontaneous as well as induced hyypnagogic-hypnopompic catalepsy in chapter 6). Indeed, in many cases, the greater the feeling of physical paralysis the greater the freedom one experiences in observing and controlling one's imaginal world. But, although this clearly constitutes an advanced form of dissociation, let us not lose sight of the fact that hypnagogia is a graded state consisting of stages and that, therefore, the subject's attention is fascinated to varying degrees depending on his depth of relaxation and absorption. Thus, there is an abundance of evidence to show that once diffusion of attention and a certain degree of withdrawal from the environment have set in, a person may achieve a state of double-consciousness wherein he retains awareness of his situation while his attention is mainly absorbed in the observation or control of his imagery. And it must be constantly borne in mind that in hypnagogia such psychological attitudes as attention, concentration and observation are employed 'receptively' as opposed to being used 'actively'. The same is also the case with the notion of 'will'. These observations will become clearer in the following section.

The mode of induction, control, and prolongation of hypnagogic imagery

It was noted in chapter 2 that, although not very common, on occasion hypnagogists can generate and control or prolong their hypnagogic imagery. Also, many subjects are able to induce in themselves experimentally a hypnagogic state and prolong the hypnopompic kind. For example, Poe claimed to have had 'the capacity of inducing or compelling it'.[55] A correspondent to the *Journal of the Society for Psychical Research* stated that she had trained herself by cultivating her concentration 'when in the dark, to see the letters of the alphabet, one by one – a gold thread on a black ground': as a result she began to experience spontaneous hypnagogic visions of letters.[56] Burdach was able to make his terrifying hypnagogic faces disappear by concentrating his attention on architectural forms that produced kaleidoscopic figures.[57] In the same way, Myers reported that although unable to bring on consciously a desired image when he wished to do so, a similar one would appear, 'e.g. I wish to see a herbaceous border and I see a curtain patterned with floral designs.'[58] My own studies suggest that this is a common phenomenon. For instance, in trying to visualize a red rosebud some subjects saw an open pink rose, others a withering red rose, and yet others saw different flowers including a row of flowering plants on a windowsill. To Goethe, we are told, whenever he closed his eyes and thought of a rose, a rosette made its appearance continuously unfolding and bringing forth a succession of petals.[59] Similarly, Mitchell could call up visions before falling asleep but once they appeared he had no control over them.[60] Ladd stated that very frequently he could simply choose some simple schema such as would serve as a framework for a corresponding object, fixate it in idea with closed eyes and make it appear in the retinal field.[61] One of Galton's subjects could bring back to its 'starting point' the image of a crossbow that had undergone nearly a dozen changes, and could call up the image of a rosebud and make it open its petals.[62] Janet claimed that he could summon a hypnagogic image almost at will: 'all I need to do is to think about an object in semi-sleep for it to become a hypnagogic image.'[63] Maury reported summoning in a similar manner a portrait he saw in a gallery.[64] Herrick, although unable to generate any imagery, could, once it appeared, prolong it by paying close attention to it.[65] One of Oliver's subjects could shift his point of view of the object and look at it from different directions in space.[66] Some of McKellar's subjects

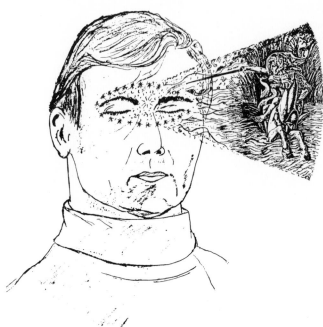

Figure 3.7 *Obtaining images by concentrating on the retinal light.*

not only could control their hypnagogic images but could even participate in ongoing hypnagogic stories.[67] Delage[63] and Warren[68] both reported that they were able to picture hypnagogic scenes voluntarily. The latter wrote:

> I obtain these visualizations by concentrating the attention on the retinal field endeavouring to form pictures out of what I see, and projecting them into a real scene. At first I see only the play of indefinite retinal light, which I weave into a picture with the help of imagination. Then all at once the picture becomes vividly real for an instant. I have never succeeded in prolonging these images. The effort to observe them attentively always throws them back into their former state: and often the attempt to control them voluntarily has the same result.

It is of importance to note that Warren's inability to control and prolong the appearance of his images is clearly due to the adopting of an inappropriate attentional attitude. In this respect, and in agreement with my discussion of attention in the previous section, Ardis and McKellar drew a distinction between *attention* and *scrutiny*, noting that the latter is not conducive to the flow of hypnagogic images.[69] Leroy also says that 'in order to prolong the phenomenon a certain "absence" of voluntary attention is necessary, as in the case of its generation'.[70] Sartre concurs that 'if they are to appear one must carefully avoid paying attention *to the images themselves*'. Myers remarked that concentration on the interpretation of the images interrupts their flow.[58] Indeed, the flow of images, Edmunds notes, is interrupted not only when active attention is paid to them 'but also in another fashion, namely, by starting to think about something. Merely readying the attention as if to think sufficed, even without formulating a problem.'[71] By contrast, those subjects who have claimed some control over their hypnagogic imagery speak of the employment of 'passive concentration', 'passive volition' and 'receptivity'. Sherwood, for instance, noted that 'the only successful attitude is one of quiet receptivity and interest ... unbidden, a vivid picture will glow into reality and remain as long as one can hold a purely receptive attitude'.[72] Similarly, Poe wrote that hypnagogic images 'arise in the soul ... only in its epochs of most intense tranquility'.[73] Edmunds's observation is very much to the point here:

> The experience afforded a critical test of one's ability to be aware through two channels simultaneously. Without losing the picture one could think lightly and descriptively about it: or could perhaps have described it aloud to another person. Alternatively music or even conversation could be listened to in a rather vague background fashion – but the moment definite attention was given to any of these, the picture vanished. This was a real object lesson on the difference between passive diffuse reception of incoming sense signals, and actively going out to meet them with focussed attention.[74]

In this state of diffuse double-consciousness a person may bring about changes to his hypnagogic imagery not so much by willing them as by 'suggesting' them. Leaning appears to be indicating a similar distinction when, in her discussion on the control of hypnagogic imagery, she says that 'a difficulty arises by the casual use of "willing" where one suspects *wishing* would be a more correct term'. More recently, McKellar, writing on the control of hypnagogic imagery some of his subjects reported, says:

> One subject – he has the imagery more or less nightly – defined his control in these terms. He told me that he sees a lot of landscapes. He said, 'The scene is going on of its own accord, but I can put something in it'. He gave an example: 'I can't say, "I'll have a square cloud", but I can say, "I'd like a different one, thanks". And a different one will come. I can't specify'. His gratitude and word of thanks towards his obligingly autonomous imagery system may be noted![75]

Figure 3.8 *In 'double' consciousness: having a hypnagogic experience while being aware of the immediate physical environment.*

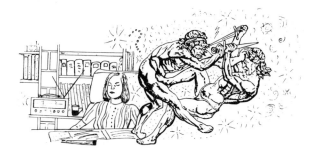

Similar experiences have been reported by other workers.[76]

Moreover, as can be seen from the examples given earlier in this section, 'suggestions' or 'wishes' can in fact be more specific and precise than in the above report. What is of paramount importance here, for the experimental induction and prolongation of hypnagogia as well as for the exercise of control over its imagery, is the subject's general attitude of receptivity. This is a psychophysical condition in which a person's body is behaving parasympathetically while on the psychological level the attitude is one of empathy, that is, one of taking-in, merging, internalizing (somewhat akin to digesting on the physiological side).

It would be instructive to remind outselves here of Foulkes *et al.*'s observation that those subjects whose hypnagogic imagery emerges easily and appears rich and profuse are persons with more relaxed and self-accepting personalities as opposed to hypnagogic non-dreamers who have rather restrictive and defensive personalities.[77] It is obvious that a person with a defensive personality most of the time would be using his sympathetic system and concentrating focally and separatively. This would clearly prohibit the emergence of hypnagogic imagery. What is apparently needed here is an attitude diametrically opposed to that of defence-alarm reaction which employs characteristically the sympathetic system.

The defence-alarm reaction is said to have had survival value in early man's history and has thus become strongly established in his genetic make-up[78] (although it may be argued that an opposite attitude put in an appearance probably earlier in man's history: see Part 3). Survival here implies '*fighting* for survival' in an environment which is inimical or believed to be so. By the same token one may say that the opposite psychophysical state of affairs would prevail when the environment is not thought to be threatening and in which the defence-alarm reaction becomes, therefore, obsolete. Such a state of affairs is precisely what is required for the induction and establishment of hypnagogia. In this respect, it has been noted that '"letting it" happen is the single most important factor in attaining the kind of altered states of consciousness associated with theta EEG feedback and hypnagogic imagery'.[79] What is also of importance is that this same state of affairs is in itself a *method* and a *justification*, a way of knowing as well as the legislator of the criteria of this knowledge and the judge of its status. Thus, the images and associations that arise in hypnagogia are the result of the employment of this method, the very employment of which conditions consciousness and confers a cognitive attitude – it employs a different logic from that used in the active mode. As Poe remarked in relation to the ecstasy he experienced during his hypnagogic visions, the viewing of the latter carried a conviction as to their source and nature which seemed a portion of the ecstasy itself.

Sometimes, while in this relaxed state, a fearful idea or image may rise into consciousness resulting in a switch to focal attention and active mode, thus terminating the state. This would not explain *why* hypnagogic nightmares occur but it would explain why hypnagogia cannot be maintained in the presence of fear or anxiety. However, having attained a state of deep physical and mental relaxation in hypnagogia, one can then engage in observational and manipulative activity *within the receptive mode*, that is, a person can observe and manipulate the imagery provided he continues to regard it as part of an environment of which he is himself an integral part, a part not in the sense of adding one unit to another to obtain a whole made up of two separate units but rather in a chemical or 'field' sense ('field' as in 'electromagnetic field'). This feeling of being chemico-electromagnetically related to one's imagery is exemplified in comments to the effect that one experiences oneself 'moving towards the object in the image',[80] or that 'the distance between the object and me changes slowly in such a way that I'm unable to say whether it is the object or me that is moving'.[81] This is in clear opposition to the differentiating 'I-It' attitude one adopts in manipulating objects in normal wakefulness. Here one is dealing not with an 'It' but with a 'Thou'.[82] The 'It' either disappears altogether, in which case one is 'fascinated' or falls asleep, or recedes into the background: in the latter case it merely represents the vaguely perceived physical environment including the investigator. Even the verbal report itself tends to become gradually more 'introverted', that is, while the subject describes what he is experiencing he has less and less the feeling of speaking to a physically present person, i.e. the investigator, and more and more a feeling of talking to the imagery itself or to oneself. As Bertini *et al.* noted, some subjects in their ganzfeld-hypnagogic experiment 'after a period of relatively controlled ideation, went over into what seemed like a trance-state' in which they appeared to be 'speaking from a dream, describing an ongoing dream experience'. Sometimes, this 'introverted' reporting may become so internalized that, again, the subject does not retain any memory of his report.[83]

In my own studies (see Appendix III) I found that it was not always easy for a subject to retain a clear memory of his hypnagogic imagery without constant rehearsal. The latter was carried out either at the end of a hypnagogic experience or punctuated it. In the former case, often a certain amount tended to be lost both quantitatively and qualitatively, that is, bits and pieces of hypnagogic imagery would be lost temporarily or irretrievably, as instanced by remarks like: 'There was something else I saw ... eh ... I forgot. ... I've lost it now ... eh ... oh, yes, there was this strange-looking object like a clock, and after that ... eh ... oh, it's ... oh, I can't remember it. But I'm sure there was something else.' I strongly suspect that this difficulty in remembering was due to the fascination and absorption experienced by subjects which prevented them from contemplating and rehearsing. The quality of imagery also suffered a loss in recall: although qualities such as colour, brightness, sharpness and detail, and accompanying feelings were often still there in an 'afterglow', if the subject were not asked to report his experiences immediately after they took place they would change qualitatively, due perhaps both to the fact that they were not hypnagogic any longer, that is, they had become memories, and to constant rehearsal which was found to be necessary in order to 'capture' and 'solidify' the fleetingness and changeability of the imagery. On the other hand, when rehearsal was carried out in the midst of the experience it had a halting effect on it, it interrupted its flow and often terminated it.

It was then decided to have the subjects report their imagery as it occurred.[84] This initially inhibited the flow of imagery because, as it was expected, when readying themselves to report the subjects inadvertently became more alert and analytical. With practice, however, some learned to retain their diffuse attention and receptivity while they reported verbally. Interestingly, when they learned the 'knack' of balancing themselves in this state, the flow of imagery, its brightness, vividness and 'reality' increased again. It was observed that subjects who achieved this degree of control of hypnagogic imagery, although relaxed, were not at all drowsy. On the contrary, these experiences, as noted earlier, had a refreshing and invigorating effect on the subjects who often remarked that after the experiments, which were carried out between the hours of 7.30 and 10.00 in the evening, they felt so full of energy that they could begin another day's work all over again. Personally, I found that this type of induced hypnagogia can be brought on at any time of the day and, obviously, does not lead into sleep unless the intention to observe and report is abandoned – or never formulated in the first place. In general, however, 'most mentally active people', as Edmunds observed, 'seldom achieve this state until they *are* nearly asleep', in which case they may decide to make use of this naturally occurring state and, having drifted as close to sleep as possible without entirely losing reality testing, i.e. without falling asleep, may briefly hold themselves in this delicate borderland and obtain hypnagogic imagery.

It can thus be said in summary that hypnagogic imagery may be observed and explored and that this can only be achieved by the subject's entering hypnagogia by means of physically and mentally relaxing,[85] turning his diffuse attention inwards, and remaining in this state *paying primary attention to the hypnagogic reality*. This constitutes a form of dissociation wherein a degree of automatism may be observed, that is, the subject 'transfers' his awareness to the hypnagogic reality while his sensorimotor systems, along with some kind of automatic consciousness, may operate almost independently, i.e. he may hear music, conversation, doors opening and closing, traffic, etc., all of which register as background events. Simultaneous verbal reporting can also take place so long as attention is not drawn towards an active search for words, conscious generation of grammatical structures, or intellectual concern for the expression of abstract ideas. On the other hand, once a strong rapport with the imagery has been established, a considerable increase of mental activity may take place without interrupting the state.

On the hypnopompic side, the procedure becomes one of either preventing oneself from waking fully or, having woken, remaining receptively in a 'dreamy' mood. The phenomena here, as we have seen in chapter 2, are of two kinds: continuations of sleepdreams, and postsleep experiences. The following is an example of the former kind:

> I woke so far as to know perfectly where I was, and to be aware of the passage of time; yet my dream went on parallel, as it were, to my waking consciousness – imaginary people continued to say and do things, quite uncontrolled by my will. Thus I was able, for an appreciable space of time – perhaps a minute, or even more – *to watch myself dreaming.*[86]

A number of examples of the latter kind are given in chapters 2, 4, 6 and 8.

The hypnagogic syndrome

Given the analysis carried out so far, we are now in a position to identify a *hypnagogic syndrome* which is characterized by the following features:

(1) Psychophysical relaxation
(2) Shift to 'passive volition' (marked by quantitative reduction of thought processes)
(3) Shift to parasympathetic predominance (accompanied by receptive mode shift)
(4) Reduction of exteroceptive and proprioceptive input
(5) Psychological withdrawal (marked by inwardly turned diffuse-absorbed attention and the appearance and increase of qualitative thought changes)
(6) Decreased arousal (marked by shift to high amplitude low frequency EEG rhythms – mostly theta)
(7) Need or intention to sleep and/or dream

This can also be instructively seen in the general context of the conditions for hallucinatory activity proposed by West and by Stoyva.[87] West's perceptual release theory of hallucinations postulates that a hallucination appears when the following two conditions prevail: impairment of effective sensory input, and a level of arousal sufficient to permit awareness. (Effective sensory input may be impaired, according to West, in three ways: (i) absolute decrease or depatterning, e.g. sensory deprivation, (ii) input overload or 'jamming the circuits', e.g. high excitement, manic ecstasy, and (iii) decreased psychological contact with the environment through the unusual exercise of dissociative mechanisms, e.g. by 'concentrating' on an object or an image.) With stress on the induction of twilight states, Stoyva adds three more postulates to those of West: reduction of internal or proprioceptive input, shift to a condition of 'passive volition', and shift from sympathetic to parasympathetic predominance.

It is worth noting, in respect to West's postulates, that hypnagogia can be induced by a combination of depatterning and decreased psychological contact with the environment (see chapters 5 and 6, and section on sensory deprivation in chapter 9). But there is a crucial difference between hypnagogia and West's conditions for hallucination, namely that in the former there is nothing 'unusual': it is a natural phenomenon occurring spontaneously to all of us. Moreover, since hypnagogia is a transitional state, not all of the above features and postulates are to be found in the same degree throughout the whole of the state. Thus, full hallucinations are only encountered in the deep stage of hypnagogia, whereas the experiences of the light and middle stages are quasihallucinatory. This has the important implication that the subject in hypnagogia may, as we have already seen, observe the unfurling of his own hallucinations in full knowledge of the nature of their character – which, however, does not necessarily imply that they are dismissed as 'unreal', nor that any criteria for reality testing normally applicable to the 'physical' world need be applied here: indeed, they might be inappropriate. In this state there is often the realization or insight that the so-called 'reality' of the physical world is only one of a number of realities which coexist,[88] and that awareness of one reality or the other is merely a matter of altering one's state of consciousness. It might even be argued that the stages of hypnagogia constitute discrete states of consciousness in their own right, each addressing itself to a different reality.[89]

To the extent that hypnagogia is a transitional state in which the features of the syndrome are applicable by degrees – which is another way of saying that hypnagogia consists of stages – we may attempt to identify hypnagogic experiences by stage. (The following is only an indication, not an exhaustive classification.) Thus, at the deep end we have full hallucinations such as hypnagogic dreams characterized by ego involvement and total psychological withdrawal from the environment. In the middle-to-deep stage, when the physical component is totally relaxed but a certain degree of mental 'activity' is present, autosymbolic phenomena make their appearance. In the light-to-middle hypnagogia, when physical relaxation is considerable but mentally there is an awareness of external reality, body schema distortions and floating or drifting are reported. Davis *et al.*, for example, noted this experience in their subjects while the latter were in alpha EEG: the alpha rhythm was practically always interrupted by a depression prior to the drifting or floating experience.[90] Flashes of light and colour spots and clouds seem to belong to the light stage and appear as the subject begins to relax and withdraw at sleep onset or as he begins to awake at the hypnopompic end. Vividness, luminosity and intensity of colour are also dimensions that increase in accordance with the depth of the state. A hypnagogic report recorded by Horowitz is very much to the point here as it shows clearly the hypnagogic progression:

> Customarily as I drift off to sleep I find a succession of visual
> experiences. When I close my eyes I see darkness but then it lightens to

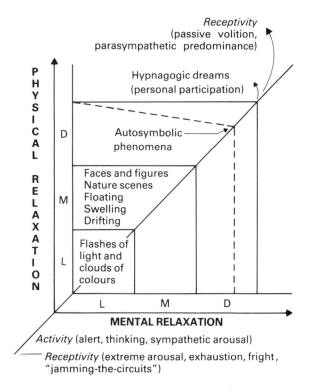

Figure 3.9 *The stages of hypnagogia, and a tentative identification by stage of some of the most common hypnagogic phenomena (L = light stage; M = middle stage; D = deep stage).*

gray. Next I see colored lights and sometimes very complex geometric forms that dance, rotate, or sparkle about. Soon a succession of images of people and scenes parade before me. I find these quite interesting and often go to sleep watching them. At times, however, I get vivid hallucinations which may frighten me awake. For instance, once all of a sudden I saw a spider on my pillow; another time a crab. They were ugly and scary and caused me to start up in bed thinking they were real.[91]

In the great majority of spontaneous hypnopompic cases the direction of the values of the hypnagogic syndromic features is, naturally, reversed, as one gradually returns to wakefulness; there are, however, many occasions when a person may not awake fully but only sufficiently as to be aware of the fact that he is not asleep, and remain in a *dreamy* state for some time observing the phenomena unfolding therein. In the latter case, and especially if the person actually returns to sleep, however briefly, the hypnagogic syndrome as outlined above is fully operative. In fact, we now know that sleep itself is not a homogeneous, continuous and uninterrupted affair, but a multiphase conglomerate kind of state punctuated by partial or complete, if brief, awakenings during which 'conscious' dreaming may take place. The presence of the syndrome is also clearly obvious when the halfawakened person sets out deliberately to remain in, or re-enter, hypnagogia for the express purpose of experimenting (see chapters 4 and 6).

Finally, the usefulness of identifying a syndrome and its gradual application by stage can be seen in at least two very important respects at this juncture. First, it helps us resolve contradictions in statements made by one and the same author regarding hypnagogia, as well as in statements made by different writers concerning the same state. For example, on one occasion Archer states that hypnagogic images are as real to him as any dream experience, and are symptoms of a cessation of full consciousness, and yet on other occasions he says that he 'was perfectly conscious throughout, and was consciously studying the phenomena' and that the latter are 'waking dreams' or 'dream-activity proceeding under the observation of the waking mind'.[92] Likewise, we have seen both investigators and hypnagogists variously argue that hypnagogic phenomena are experienced in wakefulness, drowsiness (or semisleep), and in short periods of what is clearly sleep. Such apparent contradictions are resolved when viewed in the perspective of the syndrome and its by-stage presence. Second, a brief glance at the syndrome will show that, if, while hypnagogia is in progress, the 'need or intention to sleep' diminishes or disappears totally (either spontaneously or experimentally) while the other symptoms remain unaffected, hypnagogic experiences become indistinguishable from phenomena which are usually allocated to other states. This, as we shall see in Part Two, places hypnagogia in a very significant position in terms of its making available to any individual a wide range of often inaccessible, hard to get to or, in the main, unconscious phenomena. Moreover, as we shall also see, the 'need or intention to *dream*', in the absence of a 'need or intention to *sleep*', literally turns hypnagogia into a state of wakeful dreaming.

Summary and conclusions of Part One

In this first part of the book an examination of the occurrence and nature of hypnagogic phenomena was carried out in which the latter were found to be quite common in incidence. They were also found to be of a great variety occurring in all the sensory modalities and involving motor-kinesthetic and speech mechanisms.

The best researched hypnagogic phenomena are those of the visual modality. On the whole, these are characterized by externality, autonomy, clarity of detail, brevity of duration, vividness of colour, by the diffused quality and 'internality' of their illumination, and the sense of reality they impart in the subject. Although usually minute in size, they also appear in gigantic proportions. They differ from ordinary images of memory and fancy in being much more vivid, sharp and detailed, and they do not blend with ordinary images when attempts to inject them with the latter are made. Their classification by content includes formless images (colour clouds and lights), designs, faces, figures, animate and inanimate objects, nature scenes, scenes with people, print and writing. Other, bipolar, dimensions of classification have been offered, most of which can be accommodated in a four-group arrangement comprising reproductive, perseverative, familiar, and unfamiliar visual hypnagogic phenomena.

Auditory hypnagogic phenomena include the hearing of crashing noises, one's name being called, a doorbell ringing, neologisms, irrelevant sentences containing unrecognizable names, pompous nonsense, quotations, references to spoken conversations, remarks directed to oneself, meaningful responses to one's thought of the moment. Less frequently, music is heard and poems are composed. As with the visual kind, auditory hypnagogic phenomena are characterized by externality, autonomy, and vividness.

Other hypnagogic phenomena include somesthetic, kinesthetic, tactile, thermal, gustatory, olfactory, and synesthetic experiences such as myoclonic jerks, falling, the feeling that one is being touched, numbness and swelling and other body schema disturbances, a sense of heat or cold coursing through the body, a variety of smells and tastes, and the seeing of a visual image in response to a sound.

Like the sleep onset phenomena, the hypnopompic variety of hypnagogia occurs in all the sensory modalities. This includes continuations of dreams, anticipatory experiences, and phenomena occurring after the subject has woken. 'Warning' and 'problem-solving' phenomena are also reported. Hypnopompic experiences are less commonly reported than sleep onset ones. An experience that occurs at both ends of the state is the speech phenomenon which consists of apparently nonsensical or irrelevant statements or responses made by the subject.

On the cognitive-affective level, hypnagogia is characterized by receptivity and susceptibility to suggestions (paralleled on the physiological level by a sensitivity to external and internal stimuli), readiness to incorporate external and internal stimuli into hypnagogic mentation, and the frequent presence in it of an awareness of significance which seems to equip the subject with an understanding of the occurring symbolism and which is the defining characteristic of the autosymbolic phenomenon. Many workers have also pointed out the regressive character of hypnagogic mentation and the decline of affect concomitant with the increase in hallucinatory experience. As I have argued, however, the word 'regressive', as applied to this state, is a rather biased term carrying pejorative connotations. It is, thus, suggested that it is more appropriate to view it as a feature of the receptive mode which is another way of engaging the world distinct from the active, analytic, mode. Indeed, hypnagogia as a whole appears to transpire in the receptive mode, characterized on the physiological level by parasympathetic predominance and on the psychological side by a loosening of ego boundaries (LEBs) typified by openness, sensitivity, internalization-subjectification of the physical and mental environment (empathy), and diffuse-absorbed attention. These same features are also pointed out as the conditions for the induction, prolongation, and control of hypnagogic imagery. Specifically, in this respect, it is suggested that a 'conversational' attitude towards one's hypnagogic imagery both increases the latter's occurrence and renders it amenable to control.

A hypnagogic syndrome is also identified, based on the conditions present in spontaneously occurring hypnagogia. Since hypnagogia is a progressive state consisting of stages which stretch from mere relaxation to hypnagogic dreaming, the symptom-conditions of the syndrome can be seen as applying by degrees. This, in turn, enables us to identify hypnagogic experiences by stage. Moreover, the stress placed on the analysis of the conditions conducive to the induction, prolongation, and control of hypnagogic imagery can now be more properly justified. To begin with, since the occurrence of hypnagogia necessitates the presence of psychophysical relaxation, the induction of hypnagogic imagery of necessity requires the subject to relax, i.e. let go physically and mentally, which alone might prove of great health value. Second, the method of prolonging the hypnagogic imagery both requires the subject to become accepting of his own mental processes and helps him gain insight into them, i.e. into his own mental nature. Third, the presence of the core phenomenon of LEBs renders the hypnagogist more accepting in general by virtue of its loosening of existing strictness. Fourth, acquiring control of, and participating in, his own hypnagogic imagery places the subject in a unique state of consciousness which is distinct from both wakefulness and sleep. Functioning in hypnagogia, a person may thus gain knowledge of aspects of his mental nature which, although ontogenetically old, are by no means obsolete, and which may in fact constitute fundamental underpinnings of all adult thought, in addition to holding their own ground as essential counterparts to the analytic, logical, active mode of experiencing.

Part II

Hypnagogia and its relationship to other states, processes, and experiences

Introduction

In this part of the book I shall further expand the examination of hypnagogia in the process of relating it to a number of psychological states and experiences. In carrying out this task I shall propose that the preceding observations and those to be made in this part concerning the character of hypnagogia will provide clues to the kind of 'realities' encountered in these states, processes, and experiences. Conversely, I shall avail myself of the existing data and theories concerning these latter to shed more light on hypnagogia.

Since hypnagogia is a natural state we all enter at least once daily (or nightly), phenomena encountered in *induced*, *abnormal* and *unusual* experiences, processes and states, which also occur in hypnagogia, will be considered hypnagogic in nature – the rationale being that if a phenomenon occurs naturally, as well as under abnormal or experimental conditions, it makes sense to consider it natural in essence rather than unnatural. Thus, for instance, the use of certain terms such as 'psychotic' and 'paralogical' mentation should not be taken as implying an abnormality when applied to hypnagogia: they are merely terms which arose within areas that have been studied earlier and more systematically than hypnagogia, and connote research orientations as well as indicate the kind of reality within which they were coined. As already pointed out, and will be further argued in this and the following part of the book, hypnagogic experiences transpire in a 'reality' different from that of ordinary wakefulness, and terms employed to describe them being coined in the latter are, therefore, invariably evaluative. Thus, when referring to hypnagogia such terms should be stripped of their connotations and taken merely as descriptive of phenomena.

4 · Dreams

In Part One I made reference to hypnagogic experiences sometimes turning into full-blown dreams. I shall now expand on this and, in what follows, discuss the phenomenological similarities between some hypnagogic experiences and sleepdreams, presenting data and arguments to support the view that the former can be comparable in all respects to the latter. In doing this, I shall also argue that there is a wide range of types of dream, some of which can be experienced in the absence of sleep, that in hypnagogia a person may observe his imagery turning into a full-blown dream without a break in consciousness, that hypnagogia is the most suitable state for understanding dreams and controlling them and that it offers the opportunity of experiencing simultaneously wakefulness and dreaming.

Hypnagogic experiences as dreams

Given the character of the hypnagogic syndrome, it is hardly surprising that opinions should differ concerning the relationship of hypnagogic phenomena to sleepdreams, that is, it is reasonable to expect that the gradual application of the syndrome in the naturally occurring hypnagogia should give rise to a variety of experiences not all of which could be classed as dreams. Thus, subjects and investigators whose experiences are primarily those of light hypnagogia argue that these phenomena 'are not dreams – they are "pure" images, following one another without, as a rule, any connecting link between them except, sometimes, an association of ideas'.[1] Moreover, hypnagogists who either spontaneously or as a result of training have had hypnagogic experiences in a state of double-consciousness in which although deeply involved in their imaginal activities are still aware of their physical surroundings may come to hold that 'these things are *not* dreams. . . . They have not the feel nor the appearance of dreams.'[2]

On the other hand, many workers have noted close connections between the two, and some have contended, with strong experiential evidence as we shall presently see, that at least certain hypnagogic experiences are indistinguishable from sleepdreams, or that the genus dream includes a species derived from hypnagogia. For instance, Purkinje called hypnagogic visions 'the elements of dreams'; for Gruithuisen they were 'the chaos of the dream'; for Baillarger 'anticipations of dreams'; for Maury they were the 'forerunners of dreams', 'the embryogeny of the dream';[3] Leroy proposed that dreams and hypnagogic visions had the same origin and that the latter constituted the elements of the former;[4] Arnold-Forster divided the phenomena of the hypnagogic or 'borderland state' into two major groups one of which 'embraces experiences which stand in so close a relationship to our dreams that no clearly defined boundary can be drawn between them'.[5] Archer, reporting on his own hypnagogic experiences, spoke of them as 'dreams and nothing else'.[6] Gastaut maintained that 'it is impossible to differentiate between hypnagogic dreaming and true dreaming'.[7] As one experimental subject reported, 'these things are practically dreams, but I am awake enough to catch them.'[8]

A mark that was thought by earlier researchers to be present in sleepdreams but not in hypnagogic experiences, and was therefore used as a distinguishing characteristic, was organization or internal coherence. Hypnagogic experiences were thus thought to be discrete bits and pieces, too fragmented to be called dreams. Further, various workers have argued that, unlike dreams and hallucinations, hypnagogic experiences, even when they present themselves as coherent stories, are like shows which the subject watches as a passive spectator.[9] Leroy, for one, concedes that they are sometimes complete dreams except for the subject's lack of participation.[10] They are, he says, 'hallucinations of a special kind, hallucinations that the subject watches, but which he does not mix in with his life', 'the images present themselves as spectacles of the reality in which one does not believe, but one contemplates it, in most cases, with curiosity and sometimes with a real pleasure', the subject 'waits without seeking to comprehend and without prejudging anything.' For instance, in a hypnagogic experience in which he saw a milk float doing its rounds, Leroy reports:

> I say to myself 'where is the car going?' without really wanting to
> know, and without attaching the least importance to this absurd
> question, since I know that these animated images are not real; I reply:
> 'It's going to the purchasers!' thinking at the same time that what I have
> just said is quite stupid, that these are the words of a 'drunkard'.

However, not all of the hypnagogic cases recorded by Leroy can be characterized as detached observations. One subject reported to him that on seeing the hypnagogic vision of a maggot being threaded on a fishing hook 'I feel my fingers working away', and another case he reports in the same work is unquestionably a dream, complete with personal participation and characteristic dream logic. Indeed, although on the whole Leroy wants to retain a distinction between hypnagogic visions as 'spectacles' and dreams as 'adventures', he appears to concede that the distinction is not always easy to adhere to since in some hypnagogic cases the images extend themselves into sleep without losing their character, whilst, on the other hand, certain characteristics of sleep, such as motor impotence, and of dreaming, such as the belief that one can move one's limbs in response to the contents of the vision (personal participation), appear also in hypnagogia. In respect to becoming involved in one's hypnagogic experiences, McKellar reports:

> I am still quite cross about one of my own hypnagogic images. In it I saw a group of people: as usual they were strangers. Then another stranger appeared, produced a handgun, and proceeded to shoot them down. Although the image was the product of some subsystem of my own mental life, I was very indignant. These people were doing nothing to hurt anybody: they were innocent victims of unprovoked aggression. . . . One does feel responsible. . . . ; at times the imager on return to wakefulness feels an obligation to doze off again and put things right in some previous hypnagogic episode.[11]

In an earlier investigation, the same author provided a report in which personal involvement was much more pronounced. In it the subject 'dreamed' of travelling on the underground in London:

> I came off at a certain station and for some reason tried to cross the line. I stepped on the electrified line and received a shock. I screamed, and several hands reached down to pull me up. Just then another train came rushing into the station and just as it was on the point of touching me I shook myself and realized I was not asleep but only imagining the situation. The image was much more vivid than an ordinary dream.[12]

At the turn of the century, Miller described a number of complex hypnagogic dramas consisting of various scenes unfolding in front of her while she was still aware of, and could respond to, her environment.[13] The following is typical of this kind of experience although not as rich and long as those reportd by Miller (see chapter 8 for her case):

> Quite frequently, and particularly when resting in the afternoon, I experience dreams. They do not appear to be dreams in the true sense of the word in that I am conscious of all that is going on around me. Yesterday afternoon, for instance, I 'dreamed' that I was bidding for a large house at an auction. When I walked out of the house, I saw a truly superb seascape, which even now I can visualize in detail. It was certainly not reminiscent of anything I have seen in a picture nor along any of our coasts. Whilst I was looking at this scene, a man came up and stood beside me. He repeated a quotation: 'Only that which is retained in the heart can . . . ' – the rest I have forgotten. The foregoing is the most recent but only one of many such 'dreams' I have had in this twilight state.[14]

In the last century, Saint-Denys claimed to have been able to observe hypnagogic experiences turning into dreams, in which he participated, 'without any interruption in the chain of ideas – without, as it were, any intellectual hiatus between the two states', i.e. the states of wakefulness and sleep. Below are three extracts from Saint-Denys's diary which clearly support his claim:

I have just wrenched myself from my first sleep in a moment of vivid recollection and, remembering the observations I wished to make, I thought it a good idea to write down what I have just experienced. At first it was like a kind of drowsiness during which I thought in a confused way about the people who dined with us today, and about Mrs de S.'s pretty face. Her face didn't appear to me clearly at first; afterwards I began to see her better, and then, without being able to tell how it happened, it was no longer she I saw but her cousin, Mrs L., who was sitting with a piece of tapestry-work in front of her. The design she was working at represented a beautifully coloured garland of flowers and fruit, which I could see perfectly well, as I could all the details of the room and Mrs de S.'s costume. It occurred to me that I had just fallen asleep and was dreaming, so I shook off my sleep by an effort of will, and picking up my pencil I immediately noted all this down as indicating how a dream begins. I am sure there was no distinct gap between the ideas I had in my head as I dozed off and these last images, which were so complete and distinct that they were definitely part of a dream.

Today I had the great satisfaction of capturing my whole dream in its entirety, from the last thought I had while still awake to the idea which occupied me at the moment of waking, without losing anything of the different things I thought I saw, heard or did successively in between. This is what happened. While still awake, but on the verge of sleep, I thought vaguely of the visit we were to make the following morning to the Château d'Ors., and I remembered the great avenue of chestnut trees along the approach to the château. First I saw it as if in a mist. Then I could clearly make out some trees, their bright green leaves perfectly outlined. However, now it wasn't the chestnut avenue at Ors. but, I think, an avenue in the Tuileries or in the Luxembourg. There were many people walking there. I recognised Mr. R. with Alexis de B. and began to chat to them. During this time some gardeners or tree-fellers were occupied uprooting a large dead tree. They shouted to us to get out of the way because the tree might fall towards us. Immediately, before we had been able to move out of the way, the tree fell on my companions, and the shock of the experience woke me up.

I close my eyes to go to sleep, thinking of some objects I noticed this evening in a shop in the rue de Rivoli. I remember the arcades of the street in question, and I catch a glimpse of something like luminous arcades forming repeatedly in the distance. Soon a serpent covered with

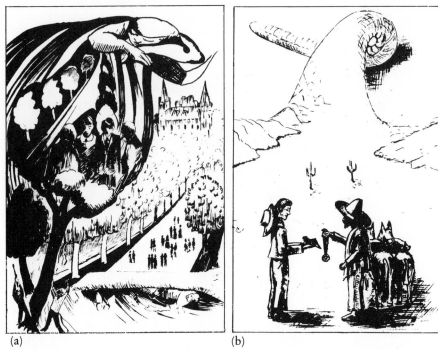

(a)   (b)

Figure 4.1 (a) and (b) *Saint-Denys claimed to have been able to observe hypnagogic experiences turning into dreams without a break in consciousness, merely by calling up past experiences which were then used as links to gain entry into a dream state.* (illustrations of second and third extracts)

phosphorescent scales appears before my mind's eye, surrounded by innumerable ill-defined images. I am still in the period when things are confused. The images fade and re-form very quickly. The long fiery serpent has turned into a long dusty road burning under the summer sun. I immediately see myself travelling along it, and my memories of Spain are revived. I talk to a muleteer carrying a *manta* (blanket) on his shoulder; I hear the bells of the mules; I listen as he tells me a story. The countryside matches the central figure; at this moment the transition from waking to sleep is complete. I am completely taken up in the illusion of a clearly defined dream. I was offering the muleteer a knife, which he seemed to like, in exchange for a fine antique medallion he showed me when I was suddenly brought out of my sleep by an external cause. I had been asleep for some ten minutes, as far as the person who woke me could tell.[15]

At other times, Saint-Denys notes, the transition from the waking to the dreaming state is effected through 'the memory of sounds', such as when, while falling asleep, we think of a conversation between ourselves and some other person who then gradually takes on a vivid appearance and thus constitutes the first element of a dream.

Other examples of hypnagogic dreaming come from laboratories where subjects learn, through biofeedback, to enter a 'theta' state which is characterized by psychophysical relaxation and 7 cps (theta) EEG, both of which are, as we know, typical components of hypnagogia. For example, having had some training in 'theta' feedback one subject decided, like so many others in a similar situation, to 'practice theta' without feedback. Towards the end of her second session she 'vividly experienced this scene':[16]

> I was in a curious place. It was a corridor, well-lighted, . . . Off the corridor on the left . . . were rooms, also lighted as far as I could see, in which I felt there must be people and scenes. I saw into only the first of these rooms, and I saw myself and someone else, together but doing I know not what. I really peered into the room for a few seconds, then withdrew and stepped back into the corridor. I had something in my hand . . . it may have been a rag doll, and there were coins on the floor . . . big shiny ones, not like money as we know it, but more like big ancient coins of gold and silver. Suddenly, as the conscious-I became aware of this scene . . . , the I-in-the-scene looked up at the conscious-I and halted what she was doing, as if she were being spied upon; she stopped and looked at 'me', seeming to say, Well, so what do *you* want; yes? can I help you? . . . And for a brief instant there were three of me: one in the room, one looking into the room, and one looking at the first two. In this moment the scene froze, then faded.

With a feeling of a sense of 'unfinished business', reminiscent of the many cases of ordinary awaking from a sleepdream followed by a refalling into sleep or a halfsleep state in which the threads of the previous dream are picked up again, this subject returned to the laboratory a few days later where she had the following experience:

> I saw myself as a tiny mannikin standing before a huge blank wall; that won't do, I told myself, you mustn't stand *off* and *look* at yourself . . . ; get down there into the figure, be the figure: And then I travelled down and merged with the figure so that 'I' was staring at the blank wall. . . . Then I saw a door, tall and wooden, standing slightly ajar in the midst of deep, velvety blackness. Brilliant light streamed from the other side of the door, radiating into the velvety blackness and clearly illuminating the form of the door, its hinges, frame, knob. The image persisted; I found it very attractive, still, solemn, flowing, beautiful . . . then I had the idea of going through it, that there I might find the corridor. So I went through and there indeed was the corridor and the other me frozen into the exact same attitude of 'Yes, what is it?' in which I had left myself some days ago. . . . Again I tried to be active: Don't just look at her, I told myself, be her; so I went over and tried to

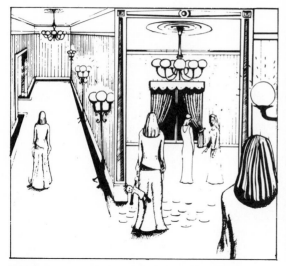

(a)

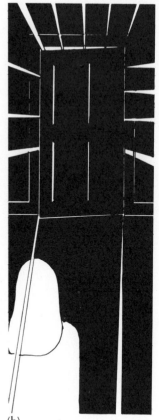

(b)

Figure 4.2 (a), (b), (c),
(d) *A 'theta' dream.*

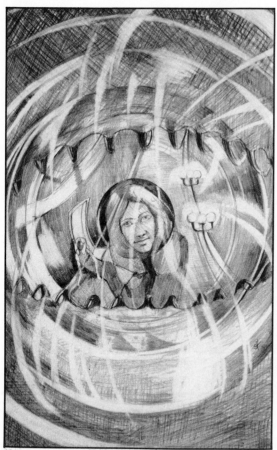

(d)

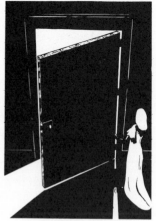

(c)

merge with this figure of me as I had done earlier with the mannikin. Okay, now, I said, let's look again into the first room, c'mon, look; and let's look more at the corridor . . . but I couldn't do so; I couldn't make out anything in the room and, instead, the me-of-the-corridor just sank down slumped against the wall – exactly like a limp rag doll: she was inanimate, without consciousness. . . . So I didn't push anymore . . . I just let it be. . . . And then I became aware of a huge eye; a beautiful eye, filling my entire visual field. It lingered quite a while; it just looked, its lid blinked naturally; but what was most beautiful, most enthralling, was the pupil: It was golden – an alive, moving, vibrating, changeful gold. I looked at the eye, and it at me, quietly, solemnly, benevolently, compassionately, beautifully – for a long time.

One of his subjects, McKellar writes, claimed that he could step into his hypnagogic visions 'as an actor may walk onto the stage' and 'act the part of a magician and transform the action, even change the characters'.[17] On one occasion, moreover, a subject dreamed of changing into an animal:

the imager found himself a member of a group of sheep standing outside a slaughter house. He told me, 'I was one of them. We moved up the gangway. I could feel what all the sheep felt'. In the image, he saw the slaughterman's face and the expression on it. The image was very frightening indeed.[11]

Foulkes and Vogel, too, have shown that 'the typical hypnagogic dream seems no less well-organized than its REM-period counterpart',[18] and that, seen in a psychoanalytic perspective, is often shown to be, like a 'REM-period' dream, 'primary process' in that it contains displacement and condensation which makes its images bizarre and symbolic so that they become susceptible to depth-level psychoanalytic interpretation.[19] The frequently reported brevity of hypnagogic dreams, these workers further point out, is probably the function of an interesting and revealing characteristic which is also often, but not always, present in sleepdreams, namely 'the omission of visual continuity, so that the subject reports that his visual imagery was something more like a succession of snapshots than like a movie . . . , the continuity residing in the dreamer's "understanding" rather than in his visual imagery'.[20] But the same study has also shown that although on the whole hypnagogic dreams appear to be shorter than sleepdreams, the former can be, and sometimes are, comparable in length to the latter, displaying continuity and duration of events similar to that observed in waking life.

Dreams and shades of dreams

Indeed, it is now fairly well established that dreaming takes place not only during emergent stage 1 but also in the absence of REMs,[21] during continuous alpha EEG, and during descending stages 1 and 2,[22] that is, in addition to the fact that dreaming does occur at sleep onset, evidence argues that it also takes place in the absence of sleep as well as during those epochs of 'quiet' sleep which are generally thought to be devoid of dreaming.[23] In view of this, it would be grossly misleading to speak of dreaming as if it were a singular and uniform activity admitting of no variations or species within the boundaries of its definition. In fact, it was just over seventy years ago when van Eeden enumerated no less than nine different kinds of dream, three of which are of particular interest to my present discussion, viz. the initial dream, the lucid dream, and the wrong waking up.[24]

Although van Eeden protests that the initial dream is not a hypnagogic experience, his description of it belies his protestations. He says that

> it occurs only in the very beginning of sleep, when the body is in a normal healthy condition, but very tired. Then the transition from waking to sleep takes place with hardly a moment of what is generally called unconsciousness, but what I would prefer to call discontinuity of memory.

This sounds very much like Saint-Denys's reports of hypnagogic experiences turning into dreams without a break in the chain of ideas. Van Eeden continues:

> In hypnagogic hallucinations we have visions but we have full bodily perception. In the initial dream type I see and feel as in any other dream. I have a nearly complete recollection of day-life, I know that I am asleep and where I am sleeping, but all perceptions of the physical body, inner and outer, visceral or peripheral, are entirely absent. Usually I have the sensation of floating or flying, and I observe with perfect clearness that the feeling of fatigue, the discomfort of bodily overstrain, has vanished. I feel fresh and vigorous, I can move and float in all directions; yet I know that my body is at the same time dead tired and fast asleep.

What van Eeden is describing here is an unusual form of hypnagogic dream, the induction and utilization of which is advocated by yogis and occultists as a means of achieving continuity between waking and dream life.[25] The hypnagogic core phenomenon of the LEBs is especially noticeable in the experiences of floating and flying, and in the feeling of freshness and invigoration.

The lucid dream, a term coined by van Eeden himself, had already been noted by Aristotle who wrote that 'often when one is asleep, there is something in consciousness which declares that what then presents itself is but a dream'.[26] On occasion, having become aware of dreaming, a person may retain this 'lucid dream' state of mind well into the, eventually, ensuing waking state, thus achieving a continuity of consciousness that bridges the gap between sleepdreaming and wakefulness. Descartes, for one, appears to have made accidental but profound use of such a state. It occurred to him during one night in 1619 when, in a series of three dreams interrupted by wakings, he conceived his 'greatest discovery', namely the unity of all the human sciences. As his biographer records, at the end of the third dream, but still asleep, 'wondering whether what he had seen was dream or vision, he not only decided while sleeping that it was a dream, but also interpreted it before sleep left him.' Soon, however, 'doubting whether he dreamt or meditated, he woke up without emotion and continued the interpretation of his dream on the same lines with his eyes open'.[27]

More recent research has not only confirmed but also experimentally elaborated and analysed lucid dream experiences.[28] The lucid dream is not unlike the initial dream in terms of mental state. They differ from each other mainly in the fact of their temporal occurrence: the initial dream occurs early in the sleep cycle whereas the lucid dream takes place at the tail end of it, 'in the hours between five and eight in the morning' as van Eeden noted. In a lucid dream the subject becomes aware that he is dreaming, whereupon he either awakes or his waking mentation *appears* to be reinstated while he continues in the dream state, i.e. he appears to himself to be awake in a dream.

My qualifying of the state of the subject by saying that it *appears* to him that he is awake in his dream is prompted by two considerations. First, in the cases where the awareness that one is dreaming results in wakefulness it has been noted that the important contributing factor to the termination of the state has been an 'overcritical' attitude of mind. This might be interpreted as implying that the reported sense of awareness in a dream is not sufficient to guarantee the full presence of waking mentation, in which case it might be argued that awareness that one is dreaming is only apparent. This leads to the second observation that often, although the subject is fully certain of being 'awake' in a dreamworld, he soon 'awakes' to tell someone of his lucid dream only to discover that eventually he *does* wake up and realizes that he had been having dreams within dreams. Lucid dreams are thought by some workers to take place during short periods of hallucinatory wakefulness.[29]

As can be seen in the above, lucid dreams tend to grade imperceptibly into false awakenings or wrong waking up, the latter being a dream experience in which the subject imagines himself waking up and getting on with his normal morning routine. McKellar reports the case of a subject who dreamed of getting up and making breakfast for her husband who was leaving on a journey that morning, only eventually to wake up in reality and find her husband kissing her goodbye having already made and eaten his own breakfast.[30] (See chapter 2 for other cases.) The same author reports another interesting case in which the subject having 'woken up' and found himself in a bathtub as deep as his height noticed on the sides of the bath hypnagogic images such as he experienced regularly. He then 'woke up' for the second time having full memory of his previous state and the added ability of flying, which he practised for a while before 'waking' for the third time to find himself in the kitchen in front of an unusually elaborate meal. Finally, he made his way from the kitchen to the bathroom whereupon he awoke properly.[31]

A personal incident recorded by Leroy brings hypnagogia and false awakening so close together that their distinction is hopelessly blurred. Leroy reports that about 5.30 one morning, having woken to answer a call of nature, he returned to bed, lay on his back and closed his eyes to find that when, after a while, he wanted to open them he could not do so although he still felt fully awake and aware of the fact that it was daylight and that only a few minutes earlier he had been up. The attempt to open his eyes merely resulted in his seeing beautiful geometric figures, and although the dreadful thought of having gone blind occurred to him this did not detract from his enjoyment of the visions. His attempt to force his eyelids open with his hand simply led to an intensification of the luminosity of his mental visual field. When he finally managed to open his eyes he found that both his arms were, in fact, under the blankets where they presumably had been all along. He concludes, 'I was in a condition which was not properly the hypnagogic state yet seemed to be both the hypnagogic state and the dream state.'[32]

A phenomenon related to hypnagogia and to the three types of dream discussed above, and which further strengthens the relationships and similarities of these experiences, is what is known in the parapsychological literature as an out-of-the-body experience (OBE). This is the experience of finding, or projecting, 'oneself' outside one's body. That is, the person becomes 'aware' that his consciousness and his physical body are not spatially coincident and that 'he' can move around outside his physical body. Although this subject is discussed in more detail in chapter 6, it is brought up at this point of our exploration both because of its tendency to occur in hypnagogia and its phenomenological similarities with the initial dream and the lucid dream of van Eeden. Tart, for example, found that his OBE laboratory subjects tended to spend a great deal of time in a 'borderland state'. He reports that the OBEs of one of his two subjects seemed to have occurred in conjunction with stage 1 sleep.[33] Yet this subject sharply distinguished his OBEs from his dreams. In addition, there were no clearly developed delta waves in any of the subject's EEG patterns. Tart concludes that such experiences appear to be a mixture of dreaming and 'something else'. This 'something else' is subjectively expressed as the awareness (false or otherwise) that one is awake in one's dream or dreamlike state.

Returning to feedback-induced hypnagogia for a moment, we find Oliver differentiating between three 'layers' of consciousness in this state.[34] He notes that in the 'deepest' level he is not aware of the room or of the sound of the feedback and that his awareness is filled with a dreamlike experience over which he has no control, save for that required to arouse and report, even though this too is sometimes lost, leaving him entirely dependent on the laboratory observer who then arouses him sufficiently to enable him to report. In the next 'higher' level he is able to review the dreamlet although

Figure 4.3 *OBEs in hyp-nagogia are thought by some workers to be a mixture of dreaming and 'something else'.*

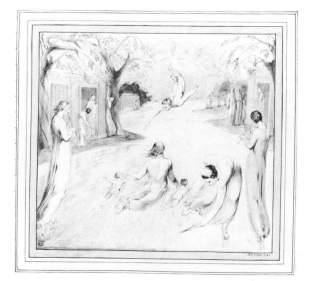

still unable to speak and still unaware of anything in the room. In the third 'higher' level he is aware of sounds in the room and can verbally report. In this latter state he also experiences bodily disconnections and distortions as well as distortions of perception of time and of his relationship to objects in the room. We can see here that in Oliver's experience the 'deepest' level is not at all dissimilar, in terms of reality testing, to the sleepdream state, that in the second 'higher' level being able to take stock of what has occurred in fairly 'realistic' terms he is probably in a lucid dream state, and that in the third 'higher' level he is in a split-consciousness state which borders on waking reality, deep daydreaming, and abnormal or paranormal perception.

Another interesting variation of hypnagogic dreaming is one in which the subject wakes momentarily from a sleepdream and then returns to it, this time retaining a vestige of waking consciousness. This phenomenon shares both the character of the hypnopompic state, in that it is a continuation of a dream after the subject has woken, and that of the hypnagogic, in that the experience is a 'going into' a dream state from a waking or halfwaking one. It is also a form of lucid dreaming in that the person is aware that a dream is taking place. Critchley has referred to this fairly common experience as 'a sort of "inter-dormitum"'.[35]

Interestingly enough, hypnagogic visions and the dreams of the in-between states were explored a long time ago by the little understood genius of Swedenborg, whose publications on the subject came under the misguided critical attack of the philosopher Kant.[36] In one of his books, having spoken of 'the vision which comes when one is in full wakefulness, with the eyes closed', Swedenborg continues:

Nay, there is still another kind of vision which comes in a state midway between sleep and wakefulness. The man then supposes that he is fully awake, as it were, in as much as all his senses are active. Another vision is that between the time of sleep and the time of wakefulness, when the man is waking up, and has not yet shaken off sleep from his eyes.[37]

Towards the end of the previous chapter we saw how Archer, among others, was able to watch himself dreaming in the hypnopompic state. But undoubtedly one of the greatest explorers of this side of hypnagogia *as a dream state* still remains the Russian Ouspensky.[38] Prompted by the haunting feeling of 'interesting and enthralling' childhood dream experiences, Ouspensky set out to study the nature of dreams, and the methods of his investigations as well as the results and conclusions he arrived at merit the attention of any serious worker in this area. Of particular relevance to the study of hypnagogia is his finding that by far the best, indeed the only, way of observing and experimentally investigating dreams is by learning to preserve consciousness in them, that is, 'to know while dreaming that one is asleep and *to think consciously* as we think when awake', and that the most efficacious method-state to this end is hypnagogia – indeed, the very fact of being conscious in a dream, he found, turned the dream state itself into hypnagogia, or, as he preferred to call it, 'half-dream state'. He apparently chose the use of the latter term because in this state he 'both slept and did not sleep at the same time'.

As he came to realize, early on in his research, that if he allowed his attention to dwell on these 'half-dream states' at sleep onset he 'could not sleep afterwards', he decided that it was much easier to observe them in the morning, 'when already awake but still in bed'. Wishing to create these states, he continues, 'after waking I again closed my eyes and began to doze, at the same time keeping my mind on some definite image, or some thought.' Soon, however, these hypnopompic states began to occur spontaneously, 'without being preceded by any visual impressions', but giving rise to a 'feeling of extraordinary joy'. The fact is, he significantly notes, that

> in 'half-dream states' I was having all the dreams I usually had. But I was fully conscious, I could see and understand how these dreams were created, what they were built from what was their cause, and in general what was cause and what was effect. Further, I saw that in 'half-dream states' I had a certain control over dreams. I could create them and could see what I wanted to see, although this was not always successful. . . . The dreams, observed in this way, became gradually classified and divided into definite categories.

He proceeds to give examples of these categories, one of which is of special interest to our discussion as it appears to be the hypnopompic dream equivalent of Silberer's autosymbolic phenomenon. This is the 'recurring dream', which often haunts people with feelings of premonition, prophecy,

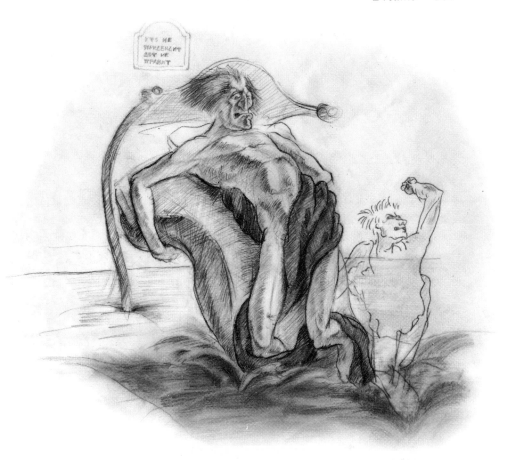

Figure 4.4   *A recurring 'mud' dream which Ouspensky, while in hypnagogia, was able to identify as being caused by the sensation of his legs becoming entangled in the bedclothes.*

and hidden or allegorical meanings. According to Ouspensky, such feelings are entirely unfounded. For instance, in one of his recurring sleepdreams a quagmire or bog would appear before him on the ground or even on the floor of the room, without any association with the plot of the dream. Although he did his utmost to avoid this mud, not to step into it, even not to touch it, invariably he got into it and it sucked him up to the knees. With great effort he sometimes succeeded in getting out of it, but then he usually awoke. It was very tempting to interpret his dream allegorically, as a threat or a warning, Ouspensky notes, but when he began to have it in the hypnopompic 'half-dream state' he found that it had a very simple explanation: the whole content of the dream was created by the sensation of his legs being entangled in the blanket or sheets, so that he could neither move nor turn them, and if he succeeded in turning over and escaping from the mud in his dream he invariably awoke because of the violent movement he had made in bed. While in this state, he was also able to trace the 'peculiar' character of the mud to the imaginary 'fear of bogs' he had in childhood. He offers various other examples of recurring dreams, some more complex than the above, the simple nature of which he was able to understand when they occurred to him also in the hypnopompic state. Some caution, however, is called for here since not all dreams experienced in hypnagogia, not even all recurring dreams, are explicable along these lines, as can be seen from the evidence adduced in other chapters of this book. Also, although undoubtedly one can learn to retain waking consciousness in one's hypnagogic dreams, and even control and transform one's dream imagery as Ouspensky and other workers have shown, it is not by any means an easy nor an altogether certain task to avoid falling into a state of *dreaming that one is conscious in one's dreams*. I shall have more to say on this later in this chapter and in chapter 11.

An intriguing theory put forward by Ouspensky to explain the genesis and structure of Maury's well-known hypnagogic dream wherein the latter

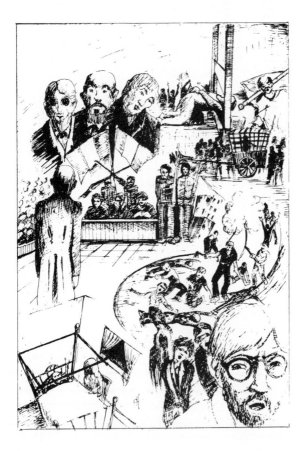

Figure 4.5 *Maury's dream. Is this, as Ouspensky suggests, an example of dreaming a dream in one order of events and re-membering it in another?*

imagined himself being condemned by the Revolutionary Tribunal and beheaded at the guillotine (see chapter 2) involves both the transforming-incorporating character of hypnagogia and the proposition that dreams can develop in reverse order although they are remembered in what we believe to be the right (rationalized) order. While Maury himself explains the almost instantaneous experience of his dream as due to the speed with which imagination works, Ouspensky suggests that the fall of the rod on his neck roused Maury into a halfsleep state in which, terrified by the strange and guillotine-like event, he imagined himself being beheaded; this image in its turn gave rise to the vision of the scaffold, which led to the Paris streets, the crowds, the Tribunal, scenes of massacre, i.e. the appearance of one image gave rise to another, and so on, by association and as an answer to Maury's bewilderment and shock. Thus, when Maury awoke properly the last item of his hypnagogic dream was 'scenes of Massacre', from which he thought forward to the scene of the execution, reconstructing the dream in an *orderly* manner, never even imagining 'the possibility of dreaming a dream in one order of events and remembering it in another'.

Even though no experiments have as yet been carried out to test this hypothesis – and it would be very difficult to see what would constitute verification in this case – the suggestion that some mental phenomena, viz. certain hypnagogic dreams, may transpire in a spatiotemporal world very different from, if not entirely contrary to, the three-dimensional, linear, unidirectional world of 'wakefulness', not only can it be easily accommodated within the bounds of the general viewpoint adopted in this book but may also shed light on various 'psychic' and 'creativity' phenomena to be examined later (see chapters 6 and 8). It is also of interest to consider in passing that, despite Ouspensky's general anti-occult arguments, several schools espousing occult disciplines recommend the practice of 'remembering backwards' as a means of breaking away from the straitjacket of 'wakeful' thinking and of acquiring 'psychic' flexibility.[39] All this, however, is neither to exclude the possibility that Maury's dream developed in a foward but 'telescoped' manner in which visual continuity was omitted nor to deny that most hypnagogic experiences, including hypnagogic dreams, unfold in this latter way, as proposed by Foulkes and Vogel.[20]

Some philosophical implications and general remarks

The discussion so far in this chapter has shown that hypnagogic experiences can sometimes be full-blown dreams and that such dreams may take place while the subject retains awareness of his environment, the latter claim being demonstrated either objectively (e.g. the person may respond correctly to environmental stimuli) or subjectively (e.g. the person 'knows' that his body is asleep). It has also been shown that there is more than one kind of dream and that there are at least certain cases in which the distinction between hypnagogizing, dreaming, and being awake is critically blurred.

Although it is not my intention at this point to enter into a detailed philosophical discussion concerning the status of sleep, dreams and wakefulness, the above observations carry certain implications which I would like to discuss in brief, mainly in reference to Malcolm's views on the subject.[40]

The central thrust of Malcolm's arguments concerning dreaming hinges on two suppositions: first, a person can only dream while asleep, and second, while asleep a person cannot intelligibly be said to have experiences. From these two suppositions flow statements such as 'if a man had a dream it follows he was asleep', which clearly contradicts the evidence presented above showing that a person in hypnagogia can have a dream while retaining awareness of his environment, that is, while he is not asleep. Malcolm further states that 'if anyone holds that dreams are identical with, or composed of, thoughts, impressions, feelings, images and so on . . . occurring in sleep, then his view is false', and that it is impossible to establish that someone is aware of anything at all while asleep. What Malcolm is saying here is that dreams are not experiences. Of particular relevance to my discussion is his assertion that dreams are not composed of images. But what are they composed of then? According to Malcolm, they are composed of nothing: 'The statement "I dreamt such and such" implies that such and such did not occur.'

Both Sullivan[41] and Malcolm deny the possibility of 'experiencing' a dream. Sullivan asserts that 'one never under any circumstances, deals directly with dreams. It is simply impossible. What one deals with . . . are recollections pertaining to dreams.' Similarly, Malcolm argues that 'statements of the form "I dreamt so and so" are always inferential in nature'. Again, these statements fly in the face of evidence that dreams *are* experiences and that, as shown with hypnagogic dreams, they can be dealt with directly and not inferentially. That they are immediate experiences and not inferences is also very powerfully shown in nightmares where the person may wake up displaying all the physiological and psychological signs of fear and remain hypnopompically in the dream state for an appreciable space of time.

Malcolm further denies the occurrence of lucid dreams, arguing that

> The sentence 'I am asleep' no matter how respectable in appearance . . .
> [is] an inherently absurd form of words . . . the very notion of judging
> that one is asleep is unintelligible. . . . If 'I am dreaming' could express a
> judgment it would imply the judgment 'I am asleep', and therefore the
> absurdity of the latter proves the absurdity of the former. . . . the idea
> of someone's making *any* judgment while asleep is unintelligible, and
> this result holds of course for the supposed judgment that one is
> dreaming.[42]

Again, these conclusions, however validly they are arrived at, are drawn from premises which are clearly not true.[43] We have seen that people can and do have dream experiences in which they are aware of being asleep and dreaming. In chapter 6 are also presented reports of subjects who claim that they can see their physical body lying in bed asleep. One might, of course, argue that such reports are mere 'dreams', that a person dreamt that he was aware that he was asleep and therefore his judgments might be erroneous. But this possibility, too, is unjustifiably denied by Malcolm because, as he says, 'one who is asleep cannot make judgments and therefore not erroneous judgments.'

The question of judging or deciding that one is asleep and dreaming revolves round the presentation of criteria for the objective confirmation of the occurrence of such a judgment. In this respect, evidence is now emerging that the subjective awareness of dream lucidity can be confirmed by means of objective correlations. It has been shown, for instance, that sleeping subjects are able to communicate to an experimenter their having a (lucid) dream by clenching their fists or moving their closed eyes to a preplanned pattern, and that they can respond volitionally to external stimuli, and initiate, carry out and report complex experiments involving memory and muscular and perceptual activities.[44] That the subjects are indeed asleep at the time is attested by the 'electrophysiological signs of unambiguous stage REM sleep' displayed throughout the experiences.[45] Similarly, there is some evidence to support the view that suitably trained subjects may acquire the ability to retain so-called reality testing while deeply asleep, as, again, attested by recordings showing the subject to be in NREM stage 4 of sleep with EEG activity at 4 cps.[46] But before looking at the questions raised by such reports, I should like to consider the validity of the often raised objection against the employment of confirming techniques *in* the dream itself.

No doubt, as noted above, to speak of being aware that one is asleep and dreaming may amount to no more than saying that one is dreaming such a state of affairs. However, to say this without any qualifications is to carelessly throw out the baby with the bath water, to ignore both the employment of often validly chosen 'internal' criteria and the fact that, when dreaming, a person functions in a world governed by its own particular laws which can be investigated while the dream is in progress. The criteria chosen (or, sometimes simply discovered) vary from one individual to the next, and some seem better than others. For instance, some people may suddenly, and for no apparent reason, become aware that they are dreaming, whereupon they might proceed to experiment with their imagery in order to test the 'fact' that they are dreaming. An example of this kind of testing is given by Ouspensky who, in one of his hypnagogic dreams, found himself with a black kitten in a large empty room. On becoming aware that he was dreaming, he decided to test the situation by transforming the black kitten into a large white dog, which he did, the reasoning being that since in a waking state this would be impossible, if it came off it would mean that he was asleep and dreaming. Another technique is to train oneself to seize upon some incongruity or anachronism in the dream and use it as a means of realizing that one is dreaming. Fox gives an example of a dream in which he suddenly became aware that the slabs on the pavement outside his house were arranged in the opposite direction to the way they were in waking reality.[47] Other people, including myself, seize upon phenomena which are impossible in the physical world. From my own repertoire, flying, and breathing underwater, are stock examples. (In agreement with Fox, I find that being aware that I am dreaming endows me with a feeling of exaltation and power and renders the environment enormously vivid and 'mystically beautiful'.)

Another approach is to construct a mental picture into which one steps at sleep onset, thus initiating the dream and retaining consciousness that one is dreaming[48] – though 'reality testing' is often lost or consciously suspended. Examples illustrating this method are to be found by the score in occult practices where, in fact, they constitute one of the easiest and safest techniques for consciously entering the ('astral') dreamworld. This approach may also be employed, incidentally, for therapeutic purposes, with apparently greater benefits than one would gain from sleepdreams and ordinary or guided daydreams.[49] We have also seen Ouspensky's method of re-entering hypnagogia at the hypnopompic end. On the same level, other, more 'objective', criteria may be sought for along the lines of shared dream experiences, that is, of experiences in which two or more individuals are aware of participating in the same dream and who can thus confirm each other's reports. Some pioneering work involving hypnosis has also been done in which subjects were instructed to hypnotize each other thus creating hypnotic dreams which they shared.[50] Objections to the above methods on the ground that they constitute mere dreams within dreams are wide of the mark: they confuse the *logical context* of the statement 'I am conscious that I am dreaming' with its *experiential status*. In the former, the statement is readily translatable into 'I am dreaming that I am conscious that I am dreaming', but not so in the latter. The experience of being conscious in one's dream has a very different status from that of dreaming that one is conscious in one's dream. I shall return to this below.

The arguments in the preceeding paragraph are meant to direct one's attention to the realities of the dreamworld itself. My concern at this point is to indicate that dream life need not always be directly related to waking life, and that although a person's state of consciousness must, of necessity, alter in order for him to function in a dream, it need not alter to the extent of his not being able to tell that he is dreaming. This has the corollary that when dreaming a person is implicitly cognizant of the fact that he is acting in an environment very different from that of wakefulness (as witnessed by his readiness to accept strange and impossible phenomena as natural). To be aware that one is dreaming is to make explicit to onself what one has already implicitly accepted. An important point also to bear in mind is that a dream state requires a person to withdraw from the physical reality, to lose interest in it. Thus, it can be argued that awareness that one is dreaming need not refer to the physical world for its confirmation. This is not, however, to say that no such reference should be made. As already shown, a person in hypnagogia may be dreaming and yet be aware of his physical environment. Philosophical objections to such evidence want to argue that if a person is aware of his environment then he is not fully asleep and therefore cannot be dreaming.

Now, the important problem presented to us here is that dreaming has hitherto been associated with sleep, and so it is thought that, by definition, one has to fall asleep in order to be able to dream. This is an assumption rising from a confusion of the character and function of *sleeping* and *dreaming* and their relationship to each other. As I discuss this topic in some detail in chapter 11 I shall confine myself here to what is directly relevant. Dreams are often defined as hallucinations experienced during sleep, and are distinguished from wakeful hallucinations. But this immediately raises two important questions: first, how 'awake' are people when experiencing so-called wakeful hallucinations, and second, how 'asleep' are they when dreaming? There is sufficient evidence to show that, in respect to the first question, hallucinatory experiences transpire in a climate of dreaminess or other-worldliness in which the attention of the subject is, at the very least, temporarily absorbed in a reality other than that of wakefulness. The second question may be answered in two ways: to begin with, we have the evidence from numerous hypnagogic reports that some dreams, however they are defined, do occur in a state of double-consciousness, i.e. in a state in which the subject retains awareness of his immediate physical environment and may respond to it appropriately, and on other occasions, although he loses immediate contact with his physical environment, is nonetheless cognizant of the fact that his experiences transpire in a non-physical world. This mental state is sometimes referrd to as *hallucinosis*, to distinguish it from the state in which the subject is thought to be completely taken in by the imagery and believes it to transpire in the physical world. Then, we may look at the question from the position of the definition of sleep itself. Sleep is generally defined in terms of the syndromic presence of certain physiological, behavioural and subjective (psychological) parameters. But neither the syndrome as a whole nor the parameters individually appear to be necessary for the occurrence of dreaming. Indeed, in certain cases the parameters themselves are at variance with one another. For instance, 'under conditions of extreme sleep deprivation, the EEG can indicate "deep sleep" when the subject is awake, at least by the usual standards – talking, responding to instructions, etc.'[51]

The relationship of sleeping to dreaming seems to be basically that of providing conducive conditions for the latter's occurrence. The only psychological point on which the two traditionally meet is that of loss of reality testing. But this, as pointed out above, is not always the case, that is, in hypnagogia a person can have dreams in which he may or may not participate but which he is clearly aware of as not being physical events. To demand, on definitional grounds, that a person must be asleep, i.e. lose reality testing, in order to be able to dream, is entirely arbitrary. The truth of the matter is that there are many kinds of dream not all of which answer the same exact definition, and whose relationship to the parameters of sleep varies widely – so much so that sometimes sleep may be said to be absent. What is of great significance here is that practically all forms of dreaming are to be encountered in hypnagogia. Moreover, the latter brings forcefully to the fore the need to consider carefully our use of the concepts *reality testing* and *wakefulness*.

It is usually taken for granted that all experiences must have reference to the physical world for validation of their status, i.e. all criteria having regard to experience must ultimately be grounded in, or derive from, the laws of the physical world. But, again, this ignores the fact that for certain experiences 'reality testing' is not only unnecessary but altogether inappropriate. Many experiences in everyday waking life are of this character. For example, when we watch a movie we do not as a rule dissect it in terms of camera angle, lighting, direction, acting, etc., or in terms of realistic temporal continuity. On the contrary, having accepted certain conventions we think it quite natural that one hundred years may be condensed in the space of a few minutes, and not infrequently we become moved to anger, tears, exhilaration, and so on by the film's contents, knowing full well that the whole thing is fictitious – not to mention our intellectual elasticity in implicitly accepting the conventions of a cartoon movie. And yet, we do not question ourselves as to whether we are 'awake' at the time, nor do we constantly hold back telling ourselves that what we are watching is not 'real'. Dreams are not dissimilar, in this respect, to such experiences. Moreover, in a hypnagogic dream we may experience a sense of awareness which encompasses both the feeling of wakefulness and the knowledge that we are dreaming, and this without feeling the need to make particular reference to the physical world in order to confirm or validate the experience. In the physical world we confirm a state of affairs basically by means of combining two methods, namely by comparing the results of our own observations, which we carry out by varying a number of relevant conditions, with those obtained by other people. We do this usually without appeal to a world outside the physical. The experiences of hypnagogia suggest that a similar approach may be appropriate for the study of dreaming, in that we can study the processes of the latter without direct reference to the reality of the physical world – which, of course, does not mean that we should abandon our search for physiological and behavioural correlations, or refuse to see possible physiological causes in certain types of dream.

Nonetheless, what appears to be the strongest objection to studying dreams from within, namely that such a study is doomed from the start because dreams can imitate waking reality in all respects, has the paralysing implication that we can never know, at any given moment, whether we are awake or dreaming, that is, however we attempt to verify our being awake *now* we can never be certain that we are not dreaming that we are awake and carrying out these tests: at every step of our experiments we shall be haunted by this possibility. And it is no good saying that we can tell we are not dreaming because dreams always come to an end, since we may simply be having dreams within dreams so that every time we think we are awake we may be dreaming that we are. This makes nonsense of the concepts of 'wakefulness' and 'dreaming'. But, as noted above, in hypnagogia we are sometimes in the position of experiencing the feeling of wakefulness while knowing that we are dreaming, which is very different from either being awake (and wondering whether we are dreaming) or dreaming (and believing that we are conscious that we are dreaming).

5 · Meditation

In respect to meditation and its relationship to hypnagogia it would promote clarification and facilitate comparison if I began by noting the main features of the traditional eight stages of Patanjali's 'Yoga Sutras'.[1] The stages are: *yama, niyama, asana, pranayama, pratyahara, dharana, dhyana, samadhi.* The first four stages deal with the reduction of psychophysical distraction – the first two are concerned with the quietening of emotions and desires, and the next two with the reduction and elimination of exteroceptive and proprioceptive 'noise'. The fifth cultivates and deepens psychophysical withdrawal: attention is detached from sensorial input and psychological concern with the environment. The sixth stage involves concentration of attention on an object or image for a certain period of time. Whereas in this stage attention may be allowed to fluctuate within the confines delineated by the features of the object or image, in the seventh stage (*dhyana*: often translated as 'meditation') attention is further limited within the object or image and concentration is of a longer period. Finally, in *samadhi* there is a continuous maintenance of attention which 'is said to be "absorbed" in the object and there is a dissolution of subject-object differentiation which is associated with an experience of transcending space-time'.[2] Patanjali called the last three stages *Samyama* and said that in practising them a yogi acquires *siddhis* or paranormal powers.

On the physiological side, this tuning out of the environment and turning of the attention inwards (psychological withdrawal) is correlated with significant decreases in oxygen consumption, heart rate and blood lactate, and increases in skin resistance and EEG alpha rhythm activity.[3] Moreover, it has been observed that both advanced yoga meditators and Japanese Zen masters display a typically hypnagogic progression of EEG during their exercises: first a continuous alpha rhythm is observed followed by a decrease in alpha activity towards the alpha-theta range which eventually gives way to pure theta.[4] This progression is known to be correlated with decrease of ventilation and a switch from abdominal to thoracic breathing (see Appendix II). It is, of course, well known that breath control constitutes an essential part of some forms of yoga. Gastaut wondered whether meditation might not be 'a pre-hypnagogic state which does not progress to sleep'.[5] In fact the view that meditation is hypnagogic in nature is strongly supported by evidence that even trained meditators appear to fall asleep during their practices.[6] Bagchi and Wenger speculated that 'meditation may represent a twilight state in which stimulus-response reflex probably functions . . . below the cortical level'.[7]

The hypnagogic nature of meditation

Referring back to my very brief sketching of Raja Yoga stages, it will be observed that both the physiological switch to parasympathetic activity as well as the psychological withdrawal are necessary features of hypnagogia. Indeed, the first five stages of Patanjali's yoga are none other than the hypnagogic factors of psychophysical relaxation and withdrawal; the difference is only that they are induced consciously and deliberately instead of occurring spontaneously. It will also be remembered that absorbed attention leading to fascination, wherein contemplation or reflective thinking is inapplicable, is a distinctive mark of the deep stages of hypnagogia. In meditation, however, attention is 'focused' on an object or image instead of being merely diffuse as in hypnagogia: it is, nonetheless, not focused analytically, that is, it is not directed to analysing or dissecting the object or image but merely to 'observing' or watching it. Perhaps the term 'focused' should not be employed at all in this state of affairs since the attending of the meditator is primarily used as a means for maintaining withdrawal and intensifying concentration. It is of interest, in this respect, to note that 'it is axiomatic in most branches of mysticism and occultism, that the ego – or the conscious mind, or the cortex of the brain – is the "dragon in the way"', and that the mind, as 'the slayer of the Real', must, in its turn, be slain by the disciple.[8] It is also noteworthy that during meditation there occur body alterations, numbing of parts of the body, buzzing, tinglings all over the body, dizziness, light-headedness, pulsations of energy flowing from head to toe, a wonderful sense of ease and release, and that, as certain sounds become internally audible, '*the mind becomes fascinated by them*, being drawn to them irresistibly'[9] (my italics).

Writing on Swedenborg, van Dusen says:

> Since childhood Swedenborg had a personal practice that happens to be one of the ancient Hindu Yoga and Buddhist ways of enlightenment. . . . He would relax, close his eyes, and focus in on a problem with total concentration. At the same time his breathing would nearly stop. Awareness of the outer world and even bodily sensation would diminish and perhaps disappear. His whole existence would focus on the one issue he wanted to understand. . . . The problem he was concentrating on would blossom out in new, rich and surprising ways.[10]

Swedenborg himself refers to his method of concentration as 'a kind of passive potency'[11] which, van Dusen explains, 'is an attentive receptiveness as in meditation'. Of the hypnagogic nature of meditation, van Dusen writes:

> In meditation, first the mind wanders off. . . . The effort to call the mind
> back sets up an internal split: the person trying to concentrate and a
> host of other odds and ends appearing. The observant person may be
> beguiled into one of these mental perambulations only to find later that
> he wandered off into a dream and sleep. Zen monks doing this same
> sort of thing sit up with eyes fixed on a spot to prevent sleep. . . . Next
> the observer learns to watch inner processes. Much that disturbed the
> meditator earlier was the first surfacing of these inner processes. The
> observer watches feelings, ideas, faint images, words, sentences, and
> later whole scenes come and go. He is watching mental processes occur
> spontaneously. It is common that the observer, seeking inner events,
> overreacts upon seeing or hearing something. This overalertness tends
> to knock out the spontaneous processes emerging from the psyche,
> which are delicate and faint at first. A balance needs to be learned
> between the responding observer and spontaneous phenomena that turn
> up. *At this level the original meditation has deepened into the
> hypnagogic state.*[12] (my italics)

The observation in the above quotation that over-alertness tends to put an
end to the process points clearly to the receptive attitude required for its
maintenance and to the learning to balance oneself in this state – arguments
put forward earlier in my analysis of the necessary conditions required for the
induction, prolongation and exploration of hypnagogia. More importantly,
Van Dusen sees a natural series in these processes: meditation, hypnagogia,
sleep, and that it often does so if the meditator does not take the appropriate
steps to prevent it. Such prevention, on the other hand, leads to a state of
trance in which

> inner experiences are no longer delicate and faint, but are clear, intense
> and real. Personal awareness still exists, but bodily awareness is less or
> lost altogether. . . . Suddenly there is a feeling of intensified conscious-
> ness but a paralysis of the body.[13]

It would seem obvious that, given the data we have on hypnagogic dreams,
and bearing in mind earlier arguments on internal attention states in
hypnagogia (in particular, absorption and fascination), trance – at least the
kind or stage referred to here – is nothing more than an intensified and
deepened hypnagogia, and the experiences therein hypnagogic dreams.
Van Dusen sees a natural series in these processes: meditation, hypnagogia,
trance. Indeed, the series as a whole may be viewed as a deliberate
hypnagogic induction which, prevented from its natural tendency to lead into
sleep, leads instead via trance to the final stage of meditation, *samadhi* or
enlightenment.

In his experimental studies on meditation, Deikman, adapting a procedure
from Patanjali's Yoga, instructed his subjects to adopt an attitude of 'passive

abandonment' as they concentrated on a blue vase. His instructions ran:

> By concentration I do not mean analysing the different parts of the vase, or thinking a series of thoughts about the vase, or associating ideas to the vase; but rather, trying to see the vase as it exists in itself, without any connections to other things. Exclude all other thoughts or feelings or sounds or body sensations. Do not let them distract you, but keep them out so that you can concentrate all your attention, all your awareness on the vase itself. Let the perception of the vase fill your entire mind.[14]

Again, these instructions can be recognized as directions for psychophysical withdrawal and diffuse and absorbed attention which, as we saw earlier, are marks of hypnagogia. The instructions to attention and concentration can be seen as directions for the deliberate induction of a state of fascination that presents itself spontaneously in hypnagogia, and can be further prolonged and deepened in the latter by attending to and concentrating on the imagery. The relationship between hypnagogia and meditation becomes even closer when the object of concentration is an internal image. In the latter case, instead of the subject becoming fascinated by emerging hypnagogic imagery, as is the case with hypnagogia, the procedure is reversed and an image is visualized and used to fascinate the subject. As Deikman points out,

> the active phase of contemplative meditation is a preliminary to the stage of full contemplation, in which the subject is caught up and absorbed in a process he initiated but which now seems autonomous, requiring no effort. Instead, passivity – self-surrender – is called for, an open receptivity.[15]

This would lead, as we saw with hypnagogia, to an increase in the vividness of the image, to its acquiring self-like qualities, and to its becoming 'electrochemically' related to the subject – all characteristic changes reported by Deikman's subjects in his experiments on meditation. Thus, typical reports speak of merging with the object of attention, of being unable to organize perceptions (everything, both in the foreground and background, seems to 'clamour for attention at an equal intensity, resisting visual organization'), of the environment exhibiting 'a kind of luminescence'.

Deautomatization

Deikman interprets these changes as part, or the result, of

> a 'deautomatization', an undoing of the usual ways of perceiving and thinking due to the special way that attention was used. The meditation exercise could be seen as withdrawing attention from thinking and reinvesting it in percepts – a reverse of the normal learning sequence.[16]

He borrows the concept from Gill and Brenman who explain that 'deautomatization is, as it were, a shake-up which can be followed by an advance or a retreat in the level of organization'.[17] To the extent that hypnagogia is also a form of deautomatization, its study may furnish us with insights into the mental processes occurring in mentally abnormal people, e.g. schizophrenics, as well as in creative individuals, in that the 'shake-up' – an effect of the LEBs – is symptomatic of both (see chapters 7 and 8).

During meditation a percept or image is attended to the exclusion of everything else, and 'attention for abstract categorization and thought is explicitly prohibited . . . the active intellectual style is replaced by a receptive perceptual mode.'[15] The resulting deautomatization is thought to be 'a shift toward a perceptual and cognitive organization characterized as "primitive", that is, an organization preceding the analytic abstract intellectual mode typical of present-day adult thought'. Deikman notes both that the perceptual and cognitive changes that occurred in his subjects were consistently in the direction of a more 'primitive' organization, and that the phenomena reported fulfilled completely Werner's[18] criteria of the functioning of imagery when the latter has not yet become an instrument in reflective thought whereby of necessity it loses its sensuousness, fullness of detail, colour and vivacity. Werner's studies of the imagery and thought in children and people of primitive cultures revealed that these are '(a) relatively more vivid and sensuous, (b) syncretic, (c) physiognomic and animated, (d) dedifferentiated with respect to the distinctions between self and object and between objects, and (e) characterized by a dedifferentiation and fusion of sense modalities'.[15] It is significant to note that these features are also present in hypnagogia, and may thus relate, through the latter, the mystical with the primitive. They also link with my earlier discussions on regressivity, and in later sections they will be correlated with oldbrain activities, thus arguing for the placing of hypnagogia, the primitive, and the mystical at a very early stage of evolution. Although this might not seem all that original at first sight, its explicit argumentation would bring out empirical and philosophical issues in respect to the actual function of these states – and of hypnagogia in particular – and enable us to make inferences as to the possible structure of the environment and of human needs, capacities, and mental attitudes and modes of experience in the remote past.

The attitude of renunciation adopted by many religious meditators is sufficient, Deikman argues, to produce deautomatization. In addition, he points out that the long-term practice of meditation may create temporary stimulus barriers producing a functional state of sensory isolation. In respect to hypnagogia, it can be likewise argued that hypnagogic induction is an implicit renunciation both of the external world and of the intellectual, rational or 'cortical' kind of thinking, and that psychological withdrawal as an important feature of hypnagogia produces a similar functional state of sensory isolation. (The relation of sensory isolation to hypnagogia is discussed in more detail in chapter 9.) In fact, most manuals on meditation suggest it should be practised in quiet and darkened surroundings to assist psychological withdrawal. Indeed, religious hermits, as the word itself indicates, are people who withdraw physically and psychologically from the external world, and in the East some even wall themselves up in caves thus cutting out completely visual, and, to a critical extent, other sensory stimulation – a practice clearly conducive to hypnagogia.

Relevant to the study of hypnagogia are what Deikman proposes as the five principal features of the mystical experience: (a) intense realness, (b) unusual sensations, (c) unity, (d) ineffability, and (e) trans-sensate phenomena.[19] In what follows I shall examine these features and relate them to the experiences of hypnagogia.

Sense of reality

The first feature is an intense feeling of reality which attests for the individual the truthfulness of the experience. Deikman argues that in meditation

> (a) the *feeling* of realness represents a function distinct from that of reality *judgment*, although they usually operate in synchrony; (b) the feeling of realness is not inherent in sensations, per se; and (c) realness can be considered a quantity function capable of displacement and therefore of intensification, reduction and transfer affecting all varieties of ideational and sensorial contents.

Thus, during perceptual and cognitive deautomatization, 'the quality of reality formerly attached to objects becomes attached to the particular sensations and ideas that enter awareness'. In this process 'stimuli of the inner world become invested with the feeling of reality ordinarily bestowed on objects. Through what might be called "reality transfer", *thoughts and images become real.*' These statements are of particular importance to the study of hypnagogic imagery and mentation as they might explain how, in full or partial deautomatization in hypnagogia, a variety of experiences takes place ranging from raised sensitivity to external stimuli to the reduction and fading out of this sensitivity through reorientation leading to full investment of attention in internal activities and giving rise to the phenomena of partial and full dissociations appearing in this state.

In Part One we saw how the sense of reality experienced in respect to hypnagogic imagery may range from (a) the awareness that imagery is vivid but not real, to (b) the awareness or belief that it is just as real as physical reality, to (c) the conviction that it is true and objective to the exclusion of physical reality. The sense of reality in (a) and (b), as we have already seen in relation to contemporaneous reporting of the experience, places the subject in a state of double-consciousness, and (c) may lead to dissociation. Realness itself might be a function of a decrease of cortical and increase of subcortical activities. If rational thinking and interpretation of the environment are cortical activities, then, as we shall soon see in some detail, mystical experiences are clearly not cortical (at least not in the same sense), and the same will be true of hypnagogic experiences. Cortical activity, as we know it, is differentiating, analysing, and interpreting. By contrast, in (b) and (c) above, and in the late stages of meditation, none of these activities are possible – images and thoughts are either just as real as the normally perceived physical environment or they are the only real 'objects' around. Rationality imposes a barrier between the subject and the world; but the sense of reality *per se* is 'irrational', distinct from reality judgment, as Deikman put it, i.e. it is not dependent on reality judgment – indeed, it might be argued that any form of judging tends to reduce the intensity of the feeling of reality with which hypnagogic (and mystical) experiences are endowed. The fact that mystical experiences are often described as 'infantilism' or 'return to Adamic innocence', i.e. to a stage prior to the maturation and predominant use of the cortex, and the description of hypnagogia as 'regressive', point to the same direction, that is, to the predominance of oldbrain activity. The mental and neurophysiological processes by which realness is increased, decreased, or reoriented, and whose study might facilitate our understanding of numerous normal, abnormal and paranormal behaviour and cognitive attitudes (e.g. normal perception and cognition, epileptic and schizophrenic mentation, psi experiences) are, it will be argued in later chapters, to be found in practically all their variations in hypnagogia.

Unusual percepts

In reference to the second principal feature of the mystical experience, that of unusual percepts, Deikman says that many of these phenomena can be understood as representing *an unusual mode of perception* rather than an unusual external stimulus. He quotes part of the report of one of his subjects who experienced a strong sense of motion and a shifting of light and darkness during the experiment:

> Now when this happens it's happening not only in my vision but it's happening or it feels like a physical kind of thing. It's connected with feelings of attraction, expansion, absorption and suddenly my vision pinpointed on a particular place and . . . I was in the grip of a very powerful sensation and this became the centre.

Another of his subjects reported, 'when the vase changes shape . . . I feel this in my body and particularly in my eyes . . . there is an actual kind of physical sensation as though something is moving there which recreates the shape of the vase.' In both of these reports the kind of electrochemical relationship between subject and object discussed earlier as occurring in hypnagogia during the processes of internalization and empathy is clearly present. With regard to the first report Deikman suggests that the perception of motion and shifting light and darkness may have been the perception of the *movement* of attention among various psychic contents (whatever such 'movement' might actually be). 'Attraction', 'expansion', 'absorption', would thus reflect the dynamics of the effort to focus attention – successful focusing is experienced as being 'in the grip of' a powerful force.

There are two points worth noting in respect to the above statement. First, Deikman's interpretation of the experience of 'attraction', etc., as reflecting the dynamics of the effort of attention, is very similar to Silberer's 'functional (effort) phenomena' encountered in hypnagogia. These are defined by Silberer as the

> autosymbolic experiences which represent the conditions of the subject experiencing them or the effectiveness of his consciousness . . . they have to do with the mode of functioning of consciousness (quick, slow, easy, difficult, relaxed, gay, successful, fruitless, strained, and so on).[20]

The second point is that the subject's description of being in the grip of a very powerful sensation points to a state of absorption and fascination very similar to that taking place in hypnagogia: Deikman's interpretation of being 'in the grip of' a powerful force as the experience of successful focusing of attention points to the same state of fascination.

In regard to the second report, quoted above, Deikman says that

> [this] subject might have experienced the perception of a resynthesis taking place following deautomatization of the normal percept; that is, the percept of the vase was being reconstructed outside of normal awareness and the *process* of reconstruction was perceived as a physical sensation.

He refers to this hypothetical perceptual mode as 'sensory translation' and defines it as 'the perception of psychic *action* (conflict, repression, problem solving, attentiveness, and so forth) via the relatively unstructured sensations of light, colour, movement, force, sound, smell or taste'. He relates this concept to Silberer's autosymbolic phenomena but points out that it differs in its referents and genesis:

> In the hypnagogic state and in dreaming, a *symbolic* translation of psychic activity and ideas occurs. Although light, force, and movement may play a part in hypnagogic and dream constructions, the predominant percepts are complex visual, verbal, conceptual, and activity images. 'Sensory translation' refers to the experience of nonverbal, simple, concrete perceptual equivalents of psychic attention.

It is debatable, however, whether Deikman's description of hypnagogic contents as 'complex' is justified – in fact, he is cautious enough to qualify this description by the use of the adjective 'predominant'. As we know from the study of the phenomenology of hypnagogia many people experience sensations of falling, drifting, swelling, sinking, flickering or flashing light, swirling clouds of colours, explosions of sounds, etc. Whether these too are to be seen as autosymbolic phenomena, as van Dusen tentatively suggests, does not preclude them from also being translations of psychic activities, or indeed of being the actual 'inner' perceptions of such activities. If a point of difference is to be made between the experiences of Deikman's subjects and those of hypnagogists, it is that in the former the meditators were concerned with the perception of an external object whereas in the latter, once psychological withdrawal has been achieved, the subject is involved in the 'internal perception' of imagery. This difference, as we shall see, changes character when the object of meditation is an internal image instead of an external object. If the subject in meditation were to begin with an inwardly turned attention directed at an internal image, 'sensory translation' might then appear in the familiar hypnagogic forms of ideoretinal light, swirling colours, drifting, falling, etc. It would be an oversimplification, and at the same time an oversight, to argue that all functional autosymbolic phenomena must be of a complex nature. We must bear in mind that Silberer's observations were carried out under conditions of (a) drowsiness and (b) effort to think. But if the second condition is not present, as is the case both in meditation and in the normal hypnagogic process, then the presence of attention which is both non-analytic and does not seek an object outside the subject may be experienced as a series of 'simple' kinesthetic, visual, auditory, and other sensations such as drifting, shifting, expanding, flashes of light and explosions of sound.

An important point to be borne in mind here is that the electrochemical relationship between the subject and object may enable the subject to so internalize the properties of the object as to experience them 'in himself': alternatively, in this state of consciousness the subject's thoughts, intentions, etc., towards the object-image may be experienced as kinesthetic and quasisensorial perceptions of alterations of attention. A shift of awareness to another object-image would, in this respect, also be *felt* in a similar manner, that is, as a pulling away from the first image (or the second image becoming enlarged and/or moving towards the subject). An extreme example in the opposite direction would be the termination of this absorbed state of attention by a sudden and loud sound: the subject would then *feel* this sound internally, literally *in his gut* (which is, incidentally, an indication of how non-analytic and deep attentional states may be related to the 'visceral brain': see chapter 10).

In addition, since there must be some form of correlation between psychological and physiological states or processes, it may not be at all improbable that some of these quasiperceptual experiences of sensory translation might be, as Leary argued in respect to hallucinogenic-drug experiences, a 'direct awareness of the processes which physicists and biochemists and neurologists measure',[21] that is, cellular and electron activities which may collectively (in groups) correspond to psychological processes. However extreme in scope and speculative this idea might seem prima facie, it might not sound all that unlikely when seen in its proper perspective. This could be achieved if we allowed ourselves to view hypnagogic images as a conglomeration of 'solidified' electromagnetic waves which, in the last analysis, they must be. Whether we are indeed dealing with the emerging into consciousness of a personal subconscious or a Universal Unconscious, we are faced with experiences which are compounded of fluidic impressions, intuitions, feelings, certainties, awareness of significance, and more 'objectified' (turning into object-based experiences) images. 'The contents of conscious experience', as Koestler observed, 'have no spatio-temporal dimensions; in this respect, they resemble the non-things of quantum physics which also defy definition in terms of space, time and substance.'[22] The comparison may be more literal than metaphorical. Hypnagogic visual images have been observed by many researchers both to form themselves out of specks and clouds of what is argued to be ideoretinal light and to dissolve again into it. It has been pointed out that such observations take place at those stages of hypnagogia nearest to ordinary wakefulness. This implies that the deeper a subject is involved with hypnagogic experiences the less likely he is to observe their possible ultimate speck-like nature. It remains, of course, debatable whether the 'specks' are indeed of ideoretinal origin.

Figure 5.1 (a), (b), (c) *Photographs of 'exposed electricity'. Note the similarity with hypnagogic sparks, specks, clouds, 'frog's eggs'. Are hypnagogic experiences of this kind perceptions of electrical activities in one's body?*

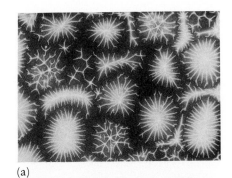

(a)

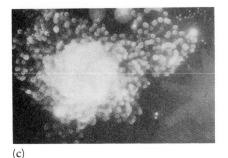

(c)

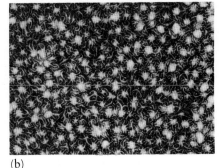

(b)

Experiments in electrical stimulation show that imagery can be elicited by stimulating parts of the visual pathways beyond the retina, as well as by stimulating other areas of the brain. Although it can still be argued that such stimulation may, in its turn, lead to ideoretinal stimulation and thus present the subject with schemata appearing in the retina, two problems need to be answered, namely (a) how is it that many subjects 'miss' the specks and clouds and report only seeing defined objects, and (b) if ideoretinal light is involved how is it (i) that images can be moulded out of this substance and projected in front of the subject not only when his eyes are shut, but, more importantly, when open, and (ii) that the images arise simultaneously in both eyes and are thus not only moulded and projected simultaneously in both the eyes but also are perceived binocularly? A further argument in respect to the last point would be that, even if the eyes were shown to converge when the subject is seeing an image, an explanation has still to be found in order to account for both the fact that the whole of a hypnagogic picture is seen in sharp focus and yet has depth, and its illumination is non-directional. But, if we bear in mind the indication that specks and clouds are seen at the stages of entering and coming out of hypnagogia, and if we remind ourselves of the states of consciousness a subject is in (a) as he enters and exits hypnagogia and (b) as his attention is more deeply drawn when in a deeper hypnagogic stage (as he becomes fascinated), we might then be able to appreciate how consciousness itself may perceive 'thought substance' now as specks and clouds and now as more object-like imagery. The more one becomes involved (absorbed) in hypnagogic imagery the greater it exhibits emergent properties, the more it unfolds into further activity. Conversely, as one observes it analytically it disintegrates into specks and disappears.[23]

It can thus be argued that both in meditation and in hypnagogia the subject may find himself, due to the prevailing attentional state, in the position of being able to experience (a) the shifting and qualitative changes of attention as kinesthetic and quasiperceptual sensations, and (b) the actual electro-chemical and electromagnetic activities in his body sometimes as specks and clouds of colour and on other occasions as object-like images. In respect to the latter, one of Leaning's correspondents – Professor Romaine Newbold – stated that on two or three occasions he caught glimpses of what he took to be the convolutions of his own brain. On one occasion, he says,

> [I saw] something like a starfish, but the arms were but slender threads springing from projections of the central body. . . . Both the centre and the arms glowed with brilliant light, like that of a full moon. . . . I recognized it instantly as one of the 'giant starshaped cells' of the nervous system. . . . A thrill of excitement went through me – and instantly all disappeared.

The same correspondent also reported that he frequently experienced flashes of light and explosions of sound before falling asleep.[24]

But these arguments are, of course, in no way to deny other aspects of

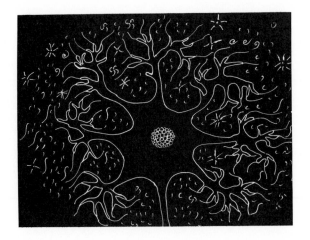

Figure 5.2 *A giant star-shaped cell as believed to have been seen in a hypnagogic vision.*

hypnagogic imagery, such as its symbolic nature and its connection with other types of imagery. Both in hypnagogia and in meditation the human entity is presented with multilevel organizations of internal activity, the interrelationships of some of which, e.g. electrochemical activity and symbolic imagery, appear incongruous to the waking mind. Consider, in this respect, the concept of a *symbol* as a picture, an act, a sound, etc., that stands for some other thing or things (pictures, ideas, emotions, etc.). This is open to more than one interpretation. By this I do not simply mean that a symbol can be made to stand for, or is interpreted as standing for, different things, but that it may *correspond* to different things at different levels of organization in much the same way that steam and ice are different aspects of water, that is, they correspond to, or represent, water (H_2O) in different states. In a similar respect strong correlations between psychological and physiological events or processes may enable them to stand as 'symbols' to each other. Moreover, a person may be able, as argued above, to switch his perspective from one series of aspect-symbols or organizations to another, or, as in meditation and hypnagogia, he may perceive-cognize two or more organizations simultaneously.

As Deikman points out, the 'illumination' mystics talk about may be more than just a metaphor, it 'may be derived from an actual sensory experience occurring when in the cognitive act of unification a liberation of energy takes place, or when a resolution of unconscious conflict occurs, permitting the experience of "peace", "presence", and the like.' The notion of energy being liberated during hypnagogia is also a view held by yogis and occultists,[25] and may be explained in respect to this state as the result of relaxation, of the 'letting go' of tension produced by the intense application of the active mode.[26] Deikman states that

> sensory translation may occur when (a) heightened attention is directed to the sensory pathways, (b) controlled analytic thought is absent, and

(c) the subject's attitude is one of receptivity to stimuli (openness instead of suspiciousness) . . . the general psychological context may be described as *perceptual concentration*. In this special state of consciousness the subject becomes aware of certain intra-psychic processes ordinarily excluded from or beyond the scope of awareness.

In the case of hypnagogia, condition (a) is always in reference to internal imagery into which attention becomes absorbed, while the latter two conditions are typically part of the hypnagogic syndrome. But it must be reiterated that sensory translation as defined by Deikman may not be present throughout hypnagogia which includes other, more complex, experiences such as autosymbolic phenomena, perseverations, memories, novel imaginal constructions, etc.

Unity, ineffability, and trans-sensate phenomena

Deikman discusses his third principal feature of the mystical experience, that of unity, in the light of three hypotheses, viz. as regression, as the perception of one's own psychic structure, and as the perception of the real structure of the world. The first has been discussed above. The second, which has also been discussed in relation to the second principal feature of the mystical experience, argues that if 'the actual *substance* of the perception is the electrochemical activity that constitutes perception and thinking', then 'the contents of consciousness are homogeneous' and therefore the idea and the experience of unity would 'constitute a valid perception in so far as it pertained to the nature of the thought process'. In other words, one would be experiencing one's thought processes as electrochemical activity without the intervening sensations-and-associations-of-memories from which one infers the nature of the stimulus – and this would constitute an experience of unity. In contrast to this 'solipsistic' hypothesis, the third theory argues for a 'perceptual expansion' resulting from a reversal, or temporary suspension, of the learned automatization operating in the individual since his infancy and responsible for the selection of some stimuli and stimulus qualities to the exclusion of others.[27] Deautomatization would thus permit aspects of reality, which were hitherto blocked from awareness, to become accessible.

As argued above and earlier in this book, the first and second hypotheses may stand as good explanatory notions of various stages of hypnagogia and are not mutually exclusive. The third hypothesis also provides useful explanatory concepts and acts as a qualifier to the theory of regression: in addition, it relates to Deikman's fourth feature of the mystical experience, that of ineffability.

Deikman distinguishes between three kinds of ineffable mystical experience. The first kind 'is probably based on primitive memories and related to phantasies of a preverbal (infantile) or nonverbal sensory experience . . . very suggestive of the prototypical "undifferentiated state", the union of infant and breast.' This is a 'regression in thought processes' brought about by renunciation and contemplative meditation, a main effect of which is functional sensory isolation that contributes to an increase in recall and vividness of such memories.[28] According to Schachtel, the ineffability of these memories may be due to the fact that the normal adult mind is conditioned by 'categories (schemata) of memory which are not suitable vehicles to receive and reproduce experiences of the quality and intensity typical of early childhood'.[29] The relevance of these phenomena to hypnagogia lies in three sets of hypnagogic features: (a) the abandoning of analytic thought and the return, or reorientation, of the subject to an earlier mode of cognition, (b) the intensification of this earlier mode due to fascination, (c) the experience of comfort, security and conviction. In this state of non-analysis, fascination and conviction, the hypnagogist's experiences may be ineffable in two senses: first, if they are of infantile origin, they are probably unstructured, and second, as argued in chapter 3, they may not be remembered due to fascination and the inability to rehearse-memorize the experience.

The second kind of ineffable mystical experience is very different from the one above in that its ineffability may be due to the 'revelation' being too complex to verbalize. As James put it, 'states of mystical intuition may be only very sudden and great extensions of the ordinary "field of consciousness"' going beyond verbalization.[30] This type of experience is also often reported as taking place both in drug-induced states and in hypnagogia. The experience is 'a revelation of the significance and interrelationships of many dimensions of life'; the subject 'becomes aware of many levels of meaning simultaneously and "understands" the totality of existence.' Although it is not to be argued that all hypnagogic experiences are of this kind, it is doubtless the case that some hypnagogic experiences are of this nature as we shall presently see.

In agreement with Ehrenzweig,[31] Deikman proposes that in this state of consciousness 'a new "vertical" organization of concepts' takes place, that is, an organization of the non-linear 'logical' kind which permits interrelationships of extensive, and normally entirely unrelated, and diverse schemata. This view is similar to the one I expressed above in respect to my interpretation of symbolism. The notion of 'vertical' organization of concepts may account for the apparent 'irrationality' of statements made by mystics, psychotics, LSD-users, hypnagogists and creative individuals. In respect to hypnagogia, many reports emphasize the 'irrelevancy' of one image to the next, the synesthetic relationships among data of different sense modalities, the apparently unjustified feelings of conviction in regard to connections among seemingly unrelated ideas, the 'solutions' of problems which may or may not hold true in the light of later analysis (see chapters 6, 7, and 8 for discussions on the crossing and syncretization of frames of reference emerging from the new matrix created by the subject's LEBs).

The third kind of ineffable mystical experience Deikman relates to his fifth principal feature of the mystical experience, viz. the trans-sensate phenomena, in which 'the experience *goes beyond* the customary sensory pathways, ideas, and memories': although 'filled with intense, profound, vivid perception' the experience is '*unidentifiable*, hence indescribable'. Deikman maintains that such experiences are the result of the operation of a new or undeveloped or unutilized perceptual capacity responsive to dimensions of the stimulus array previously ignored or blocked from awareness, and that 'the meaningfulness, and the intensity reported of such experiences, suggests that the perception has a different scope from that of normal consciousness', that it is not associated with reflective consciousness, loss of 'self' being characteristic of the trans-sensate experience. Ehrenzweig argues that 'owing to their incompatible shapes [these images] cancel each other out on the way up to consciousness and so produce in our surface experience a blank "abstract" image still replete with unconscious fantasy'. This 'full emptiness' is encountered in hypnagogia as a strong sense of realness, certainty, and conviction.

Van Dusen suggests that the deepest level of hypnagogia

> is a kind of satori or enlightenment. Suddenly the questioner and the answerer are one. This one breaks into infinite images of all its representations. The individual awakens as though from a trance, puzzled by what was suddenly seen and experienced.[32]

He gives an example in which he experienced 'a gigantic mandala' in the shape of 'an intricately and deeply carved Oriental wood design of a fourfold form' whose centre was 'an empty hole through which the fearsome force of the universe whistled'. Poe said of his hypnagogic images that

> [they] have in them a pleasurable ecstasy, as far beyond the most pleasurable of the world of wakefulness, or of dreams, as the heaven of the North-man theology is beyond its hell. I regard the visions, even as

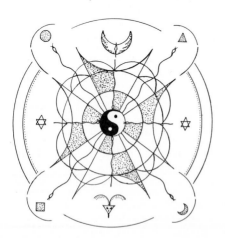

Figure 5.3 At a deep hypnagogic level the ecstatic subject may be presented with a condensed pictorialization of the psychophysical universe in the form of a mandala.

they arise, with an awe which, in some measure, moderates or tranquillizes the ecstasy – I so regard them, through a conviction (which seems a portion of the ecstasy itself) that this ecstasy, in itself, is of a character supernal to the human nature – is a glimpse of the spirit's outer world; and I arrive at this conclusion – if this term is at all applicable to instantaneous intuition by a perception that the delight experienced has, as its element, but *the absoluteness of novelty*. I say the absoluteness – for in these fancies – let me now term them psychal impressions – there is really nothing even approximate in character to impressions ordinarily received. It is as if the five senses were supplanted by five myriad others alien to mortality.[33]

On the hypnopompic side, Sherwood writes:

I have sometimes come back to consciousness with great reluctance, still exhilarated with an inspired poem I am reading, the last strains of which are still ringing in my ears. The lines are too lovely and important to be lost and I make frantic efforts to retain them through the mists of returning consciousness. Perhaps I succeed, yet, when they are examined in the cold light of day, I am blankly astonished to find that all virtue has gone out of them. The lovely fragment is meaningless although my other self was so lately moved by its rarity to something approaching ecstasy.[34]

Wambach, reporting on the work of some fellow psychologists, says that

when their subjects were hooked to biofeedback machines, and were registering between zero and four cycles per second, they were unable to recall when they awoke what they had said. They had been 'asleep'. But when they were questioned when in this deep state, they often reported mystical insights. It seemed that in this deep state material could be reached that was not normally available to the conscious mind.[35]

Other remarks include 'exquisite peaceful joy', 'a feeling of extraordinary joy', and the inability to identify certain visual hypnagogic 'perceptions'.[36]

The mystical standpoint

A wider understanding of the occurrence of these 'mystical insights' in hypnagogia could be gained if we took a closer look at what might be called the *mystical attitude* and the *mystical epistemology*. If we look at Zen Buddhism, for instance, we learn that it 'aims at changing the experience of a person to that particular view of himself and the world which is called "enlightenment"'.[16] This end is achieved by an attitude of non-striving, non-analysing-categorizing, non-separateness (non-mindedness, as Suzuki[37] would put it) which a Zen monk would cultivate by regular and prolonged meditation practices and in everyday life. The concept of a separate self exemplified in the application of the striving action mode is gradually and deliberately abandoned. Whether this is viewed as a return to the unity of a Universal Unconscious or a leap into a superconsciousness, its achievement would require the explicit or implicit assumption, present in one form or another in all kinds of personal abandonment, that *nothing can go wrong* because *there is nothing to go wrong* in the first place. This attitude of letting go is, as we have seen, a receptive mode attitude, and this shift in functional orientation is an essential precondition for the occurrence of hypnagogia and a necessary condition for its prolongation or introduction to sleep. There is here the important absence of fearful concern for the Future: the mystic's aim is to demolish the concepts of both space and time and live (in whatever sense 'living' is to be understood in this state) in the Present. This analysis might partly explain the sense of spatial and temporal *immediacy* with which hypnagogic experiences are generally endowed: as in the mystical experience, hypnagogia calls for the abandoning of spatial and temporal concern, and, as images appear, the released personal concern (a concern we carry about with us as somatic and psychological 'schemata', i.e. as a collective schema of the 'self') becomes reinvested in the imagery which then acquires a self-like quality.

It is interesting to note that two of James's[38] four defining marks of mysticism, viz. transiency and passivity, are also shared by hypnagogia. In addition, his description of a fivefold gradation of mystical experience includes the 'sudden feeling which sometimes sweeps over us of having "been there before"', or the *déjà vu* experience, which is significantly correlated with hypnagogic phenomena[39] and even argued by Ellis to be a regularly occurring phenomenon within hypnagogia itself as a form of paramnesia.[40] Also interesting and very relevant to my discussion is Stace's approach to mysticism in which he makes the pertinent distinction between the mystical experience *per se* which is genuine and authoritative, and the interpretation given by mystics which 'may be either true or false'.[41] This is an important marker also shared, as we saw earlier, by the deeper stages of hypnagogia. In chapters 7 and 8 we shall further see how hypnagogia may throw light, by means of its accompanying awareness of significance and the feeling of certainty, on both schizophrenic and creative mentation, a distinction between the two heavily depending on the ability or inability of the subject to interpret the experience – and test it in the light of 'waking' consciousness – as 'true or false'.

The fully developed mystical experience, Stace tells us, 'when projected onto the logical plane of the intellect involves three things, viz., 1. that there are no distinctions in the one, 2. that there is no distinction between object and object . . . 3. that there is no distinction between subject and object.'[42] Whilst hypnagogia generally falls short of the fully developed mystical experience it is clearly the case, as we saw in chapter 3, that diffuse and absorbed attention tends to lead to a weakening and dissolution of distinctions between subject and object, and among objects themselves as 'similarity' turns into 'sameness'. In the same respect, viz. that of diffuse and absorbed attention wherein rational analysis is unobtainable, we can see relationships between hypnagogia and mystical states as the latter are described by various mystics. For instance, in one of his sermons Eckhart writes that 'if you are to know God divinely, your own knowledge must become as pure ignorance, in which you forget yourself and every other creature'.[43] In *The Cloud of Unknowing*[44] we are told that 'contemplation in its perfection' is only achieved 'when all other things and activities have been forgotten (even your own)' and self-awareness is relinquished ('Contemplation' is here clearly used not in the same sense employed earlier by Sartre to convey a differentiating, analytic, attitude, but in the opposite sense of pure abstraction.)

Don Juan, in Castaneda's *Tales of Power*,[45] distinguishes between two main modes of perceptual activity and experience: the Tonal and the Nagual. The former corresponds to the rational consciousness whereas the latter can neither be described nor made to fit any known intelligible cognitive mode: it can only be hinted at. In the Nagual 'there are no thoughts involved; there are only certainties.' On one occasion Don Juan says to Castaneda, 'You want to explain the nagual with the tonal. That is stupid. . . . You know very well that we make sense in talking only because we stay within certain boundaries, and those boundaries are not applicable to the nagual.' Here, as in hypnagogia, the presence of certainty renders reflective thinking unobtainable: a state of affairs asserts itself and the hypnagogist, the mystic, or, in the case of Don Juan, the sorcerer, knows, in a 'fascinated' manner, that state of affairs to the exclusion of alternatives. Moreover, Don Juan's insistence on not using the tonal type of experiencing to describe the activities of the nagual suggests a similar distinction to that of the active and receptive modes and may thus further enable us to obtain an insight into the paralogical mentation of hypnagogia in so far as it suggests that the logical rules of the tonal (active mode, waking consciousness?) may not be applicable *within* the nagual experience, that is, it suggests not so much a dissolution of consciousness as an organismic reorientation to a different kind of reality.

Mystics in general talk of the existence of more than one reality. Koestler, too, refers to three orders of reality: the perceptual, the conceptual, and the mystical – the second pervading the first, and the third all-pervading.[46] Sri Aurobindo distinguishes between matter, life, mind, and supermind or mystical mind.[47] Castaneda talks of the tonal and the nagual. In the Vedas we come across two levels of truth: 'the lower level is the empirical level of everyday experience, while the higher level is reserved for the Absolute.'[48] The Advaita philosopher Vidyaranya says in regard to Maya (appearance), 'Maya is understood in three ways: by the man in the street as real, by the logician as undeterminable, by the follower of the scripture as non-existent.'[49]

Without making the same high claims for hypnagogia, one might, however, argue for a different reality wherein different rules are applicable. In hypnagogia, as in a mystical state, if we try to make 'objective' sense of the experiences (or utterances) we may end up by either considering them unintelligible or allowing that they may hold good in some 'other' kind of reality. But it is doubtful whether we can truly hold that we are able to clearly and definitively draw the limits of intelligibility. In classical logic, for example, the law of the excluded middle is a valid part of the system, but in some logics, e.g. Brouwer's intuitionistic logic, this law is no longer valid. What is unintelligible according to one system may be clearly intelligible in another.[50] In the words of Suzuki, 'to understand it [the Zen experience] one must have the experience, and at the same time there must be a specially constructed logic . . . to give to the experience a rational or an irrational interpretation. The fact comes first, followed by an intellectualization.'[51] In the fully developed mystical experience intellectualization can only take place in what Underhill has called the 'afterglow', a state in which the mystic finds himself immediately after the actual experience and which is like a reverberation of the experience.[52] In hypnagogia this resembles Poe's startling himself into wakefulness and then analysing the experiences having recollected what took place during the experience itself.[53]

The problem of comprehending both the hypnagogic and the mystical experience is, however, twofold. It is not merely the case that one must first have the experience and then reason about it, but also that the experience itself often appears to equip one with the ability to 'think' in a way that seems to transcend common rationality, i.e. a 'right' kind of reasoning seems to be integral to the experience itself. What kind of reasoning this might be was hinted at by Aristotle who said of the initiates in the Eleusinian Mysteries that they not so much acquired knowledge (propositional knowledge) from the Mysteries as 'suffered', 'felt', and 'experienced' 'certain impressions and psychic moods' that led to their becoming perfected and 'fulfilled' (τετελεσμένοι).[54] Thus, a main difficulty in discussing the status of hypnagogia and adjacent states (including the mystical) is not only that the experiences appear to unfold in a universe of discourse which has rules different to those of everyday waking consciousness, but, most importantly, that *the meaning and use* of these rules seem to be different, that these experiences carry *in themselves* both their own reasoning and method of verification. In this respect, to say, for instance, as some philosophers do in reference to mysticism, that 'so long as there is no intelligible proposition before us, there is nothing to discuss'[55] may simply be an irrelevant argument, a mere tilting at windmills, since 'intelligible proposition' implies an epistemological methodology which is, if my analysis is correct, inapplicable in these states.

Crichton-Browne's lectures on 'Dreamy mental states' may shed some extra light on the present discussion especially as they bring together phenomena and states of consciousness encountered in mysticism, mental illness, and creativity. For instance, Crichton-Browne cites a personal account of the Renaissance historian J.A. Symonds who reports:

> Suddenly in church or in company, when I was reading, and always, I think, when my muscles were at rest, I felt the approach of the mood. Irresistibly it took possession of my mind and will, lasted what seemed an eternity and disappeared in a series of rapid sensations which resembled the awakening from anaesthetic influence. One reason why I disliked this kind of trance was that I could not describe it to myself. I cannot even now find words to render it intelligible. It consisted in a gradual but swiftly progressing obliteration of space, time, sensation, and the multitudinous factors of experience, which seems to qualify what we are pleased to call ourself. In proportion as these conditions of ordinary consciousness were subtracted, the sense of an underlying or essential consciousness acquired intensity. . . . The apprehension of a coming dissolution, the grim conviction that this state was the last of the conscious self, . . . stirred, or seemed to stir, me up again. The return to ordinary conditions of sentient existence began by my first recovering the power of touch.[56]

It is noteworthy that Symonds's 'mood' was preceded by muscular relaxation and an inward turning of attention. Also, his comparison of the ensuing state to that of 'anaesthetic influence' points to the presence of a paralytic numbness and loss of body awareness: the return to the ordinary waking state was, likewise, marked by the return of tactile sensations and the re-establishment of body schema boundaries.[57] But, unlike a mystic, or a normal hypnagogist, Symonds fought the experience: he was apprehensive of a coming dissolution and an ending of the conscious self, he disliked 'this kind of trance' because he could not describe it to himself. Later in the same report he exclaimed, 'I wish and I cannot will; I cannot concentrate myself on an end of action.' Symonds is here clearly unwilling to accept a naturally occurring shift in functional orientation (which takes place spontaneously in normally occurring hypnagogia, and is deliberately induced in meditation), thus setting the two modes against each other, viz. the active mode against the receptive.

In a similar vein, Deikman points out that the onset of many cases of acute schizophrenia is preceded or marked by mystical experiences.[16] This, he argues, is probably due to the abandoning of a desperate struggle and 'a sudden, sharp and extreme shift to the receptive mode'. But, again, unlike the mystic whose long training has prepared him for the experience, and the hypnagogist who normally enters hypnagogia gradually (and whose state of alertness and cortical activity is usually relatively subdued), the psychotic is neither prepared nor equipped for it. 'In the case of acute mystical psychosis', Deikman argues, 'a crucial rejection of life impasse triggers a collapse of the action mode and a sudden rush of receptive mode cognition and perception ensues for which the person is unprepared and unsupported.' This 'shift to the receptive mode may arouse great anxiety and a compensatory attempt to control the receptive mode experience, an attempt that is an action mode response.' Similarly, in respect to hypnagogic trance, van Dusen argues that 'in contrast to the capable seeker who deliberately enters a trance, the psychotic usually does not seek and cannot control the eruption of this material into awareness. . . . The difference is an impaired ego, not under- standing or wanting these processes.'[58] The abandoning of oneself to 'ego death', as Deikman points out, is what a mystic is trained to do and a schizophrenic finds most difficult. Likewise, full entrance into hypnagogia, and a prolongation and exploration of this state, require the absence of fear of ego loss, a difference between normal hypnagogia and the mystical state, in this respect, lying in the implicit lack of fear of ego loss in the former, and the explicit seeking of ego dissolution in the latter.

6 · Psi

Several and disparate sources of evidence appear to suggest that hypnagogia is significantly conducive to paranormal events,[1] that spontaneous psi events occur in experimental hypnagogia,[2] that developing psychics experience an increase in hypnagogic phenomena,[3] that hypnagogic visions might be an early form of clairvoyance,[4] and that some hypnagogic images might be precognitive.[5] A number of workers have also obtained significant psi results in hypnagogic-ganzfeld studies.[6]

The word 'psi' is commonly employed as an umbrella term to encompass all kinds of so-called paranormal phenomena. It is used in this chapter, and throughout the book, in reference only to telepathy, clairvoyance, clair-audience, psychometry, out-of-the-body experiences (OBEs), and some forms of trance, as a term of convenience. In what follows I propose to examine the relationship between the above psi states and hypnagogia and show that these are related in their respective psychophysical induction and phenomenology, and that hypnagogia is indeed conducive in the production of psi states, and, vice versa, the deliberate/experimental induction of psi states tends to render the latter hypnagogic. I shall, further, discuss the presence of hypnagogic experiences in psi, religious, and mystical events and view psi reports in the perspective of the subjects' set and setting. Finally, I shall return to this latter theme in the process of a brief examination of some theoretical formulations regarding both psi and hypnagogic mentation.

In general, support for the existence of close relationships between psi and hypnagogia comes from the practices and literature of occultism, the literature on controlled psi experiments, and spontaneous cases. Confirmation of psi-conducive relationships also comes from my own studies which encompass interviews with psychics, observations made at spiritualist development circles, and reports from two groups of people I instructed in relaxation and meditation over two periods of thirty two-hour weekly sessions (see Appendix III). All the phenomena of hypnagogia were observed in the second and third studies and partly confirmed by the first. It is worth noting that in both the second and third studies snoring was not an infrequent auditory phenomenon! thus demonstrating the hypnagogic nature of these practices. In a different approach, Leaning's examination of crystal visions also revealed that these were phenomenologically indistinguishable from the hypnagogic type.[7]

Psychophysical induction of psi

Individuals involved in the production of psi, irrespective of their theories and beliefs as to the nature of psi phenomena, advocate psychophysical relaxation as the first step in the induction of the psi-conducive state. Sinclair, for instance, writes:

> relax completely your mental hold of, or awareness of, all bodily sensation. . . . Relax all mental interest in everything in the environment. . . . Drop your body, a dead weight, from your conscious mind. Make your conscious mind a blank. . . . To make the conscious mind a blank it is necessary to 'let go' of the body; just as to 'let go' of the body requires 'letting go' of consciousness of the body.[8]

Butler, writing on the conditions for developing clairvoyance, says that physical relaxation and emotional calm are of utmost importance.[9] Roberts advises that the medium 'should be freed of all worry and responsibility whilst the sitting is in progress. He (or she) should be allowed to fall into a trance, go to sleep, or simply rest.'[10] Similarly, Edwards writes that would-be psychics must learn to 'place their minds into a condition of receptive abandonment'.[11] Bennett notes that the best time and place to begin psychic training is 'in bed at night' when one becomes naturally relaxed.[12] Huson also instructs that 'the ideal time . . . is before falling asleep at night, but not when you are overtired'.[13] Numerous other investigators, practitioners, and subjects have variously pointed out the need for calmness, inactivity and absence of expectation, disinhibition, lack of self-consciousness and conscious interference, 'high carelessness' and placidity.[14]

White identified the following five steps in the ESP process: '(1) Relaxation, (2) Engaging the Conscious Mind, (2A) The Demand, (3) The Waiting, the Tension, and the Release, and (4) The Way the Response Enters Consciousness'.[15] Steps (1), (2), and (2A) contain in essence the symptoms of what was later defined by Honorton[16] and Braud and Braud[17] as the psi-conducive syndrome.

Honorton's markers are '(a) a sufficient level of cortical arousal to maintain conscious awareness; (b) muscular relaxation; (c) reduction of exteroceptive input from peripheral receptors; and (d) deployment of attention toward internal mentation processes'.[18] The Brauds propose that the psi-conducive syndrome involves the following seven major characteristics: (a) physical relaxation, (b) decreased arousal, (c) reduced sensory distraction and increased concentration, (d) a more inward focusing of attention, (e) decreased action mode/left hemisphere functioning along with increased receptive mode/right hemisphere functioning, (f) an altered world view, (g) momentary importance of psi.

It can be seen that Honorton's model is here covered by the Brauds' (a), (c) and (d) features. The Brauds' fifth feature arguing for a close positive relationship between right-hemisphere functioning and receptive mode in the production of psi is debatable.[19] The Brauds' second feature, that of decreased arousal, although not specific enough, appears to be pointing to a generally agreed upon direction, a difference with some other workers lying in the specification that a moderate level of arousal or activation seems optimal for psi performance.[20] It is thus argued that the optimal low arousal level conducive to psi activities is one of deep relaxation accompanied by alphoid EEG.[21] The Brauds' 'reduced sensory distraction and increased concentration', and 'a more inward focusing of attention', seem to overlap with White's step (2), that of engaging the conscious mind. However, a close look at these marks is called for as none of them appears to be explicit enough or clearly understood and agreed upon by all subjects and workers. Moreover, an analysis of the mode of inducing and maintaining these marks may be seen to relate closely to hypnagogia.

In White's paper it is pointed out that the second step is induced or achieved by two apparently diverse methods, viz. either by concentrating on a mental image until all perceptual, physiological and mental distraction is reduced or entirely prevented, or by making the mind a blank.[22] White notes that both methods 'accomplish the same purpose: to engage or distract the full attention of the conscious mind'. Summarizing the main features of step (2), she says that these 'seem to be lack of strain, passivity, a blank mental screen, persistence, and – paradoxically – concentration in one form or another'. Concentration, however, is not of the active, analytic, kind but of the passive or receptive type. As Sinclair points out, in ESP activities 'a part of concentration is complete relaxation.'

In contrast to Rhine's argument that 'sleepiness' and 'dissociative factors' lower ESP ability,[23] many workers in the psi area have pointed out that fatigue and drowsiness are favourable conditions for telepathy,[24] and that 'some of the best telepathic cases seem to involve dissociation'.[25] For instance, Gibson noted that during psi experiments his subject seemed to be in a semi-dissociated state,[26] and Tyrrell reported that his subject was quite definitely aware of 'almost losing consciousness of her surroundings'.[27] As Murphy points out,

> we may find, for some purposes, that the conditions of fatigue and drowsiness, or even of ill health, give us exactly that mechanical basis for dissociation which we desire, . . . and that the condition of *falling asleep* or of *waking up* gives sufficient dissociation, while permitting the individual to grasp more clearly, at the conscious level, the paranormal impression for which he has been reaching. . . . In the records of spontaneous cases we find dozens of examples of very light sleep, or drowsiness, or transition states between waking and sleeping.[28]

In non-spontaneous cases, that is, in those cases where the subject deliberately sets out to induce a psi state in himself, he typically concentrates relaxedly on a mental image or thought such as a rose or blankness until a state of 'fascination' is achieved (cf. chapters 3 and 5). Significantly, this state is clearly hypnagogic both in phenomenology and in the fact that it tends to lead into sleep. For instance, Sinclair instructs, 'After you have practised the exercise of concentrating on a flower – *and avoiding sleep* – you will be able to concentrate on holding the peculiar blank state of mind which must be achieved if you are to make successful experiments in telepathy'[29] (my italics). Similarly, Warcollier notes that this concentration 'cannot be long maintained without provoking *a state of approaching sleep*, betrayed by the appearance of [hypnagogic] images', and that 'it is not a question of merely thinking of a certain flower, but of seeing it appear inwardly as *a hypnagogic image*'[30] (my italics).

At this point some psychics would 'demand' that the appropriate picture or message appear to their consciousness. Most psychics, however, would not make the 'demand' a separate step in their procedure but formulate their intention for the psi performance at the inception of the experiment and retain it diffusedly throughout the session. Nonetheless, at this point, White argues, a 'tension is produced because the percipient is trying to straddle two opposites: consciously, he is concentrating exclusively on an image which he knows is *not* what he seeks, while simultaneously he is entertaining an awareness of a void, wherein lies the sought-for answer!'

There are two important points to be noted at this juncture. The first point relates to the attitude of the subject towards the target. Sinclair again instructs, 'Keep the eyes closed and the body relaxed, and give the order silently, and with as little exertion as possible.'[31] Beyond this, White notes, one simply 'hopes and waits'. This is strongly reminiscent of Leaning's remark that control of hypnagogic imagery is achieved not so much by 'willing' as by 'wishing', McKellar's hypnagogist who 'requested' the appearance of particular hypnagogic images, van Dusen's observation that one can enhance hypnagogia by entering into 'conversation' with it, Delage's waiting in hypnagogia 'in a state of expectation to catch the images that might occur', Ardis and McKellar's description of the state of the hypnagogic subject as one of 'alerted attention' as opposed to 'close scrutiny', and Green *et al.*'s description of the same as 'detached effortless volition'[32] (cf. my analysis of hypnagogic control in chapter 3).

The second point arises from White's remark that step (3) includes 'tension', and that this tension is the result of holding into one's mind both an 'irrelevant' image and an awareness of a void in which the sought-for answer eventually is to appear. In respect to her first remark, not all psychics speak of 'tension'. On the contrary, of all of White's quotations in respect to step (3) only one psychic, Carlson, and one investigator, Tyrrell, make reference to 'tension'. All the others speak of 'waiting patiently' and 'expectantly' for a picture to appear. What is perhaps meant by 'tension' under these circumstances might be better understood if we take note of

Carlson's own remark that this might be 'equivalent to "friction"'. Now, 'friction' is not necessarily 'tension'. It might, in fact, constitute the psychic's somesthetic sensation of internalization and absorption: an 'empathic' state reached after the initial relaxation, meditation, and psychological withdrawal. The same line of argument will also be directed against White's second remark: the percipient's mind is not tensed between an irrelevant image and a void. What is probably happening here is that concentration on a mental image is employed to achieve psychological withdrawal, absorption, fascination – a singular narrowing of attention hemmed in by internal and external stimulus barriers.[33] Having achieved this degree of internalization one then simply waits receptively, avoiding falling asleep. If some form of tension is to be accepted as being present here this might be the result of waiting, when the latter, due to the non-appearance of the desired target, becomes long and sometimes tedious.[34] For those who aim at 'blanking' directly without the intermediary of a mental image, there can clearly be no presence of tension as proposed by White.

In the above we can see that the psychological state reached so far by the psi percipient is essentially that of hypnagogia which has been both deliberately induced and prevented from reaching sleep – instead, it becomes internally intensified resulting in a state of light trance wherein the percipient almost loses consciousness of the surroundings. In this state, White's step (4), the entering into consciousness of the telepathic response, takes place, and I shall be discussing the character of this response in a wider examination of psi phenomenology in the next section.

Perceptual, quasiperceptual, and cognitive-affective phenomena during psi

In this section and the next we shall see that, first, all the perceptual, quasiperceptual and cognitive-affective phenomena encountered in psychic studies are also to be found in hypnagogia, second, the circumstances under which they occur are the same (this constitutes a continuation of arguments presented in the previous section), third, the order in which they occur is the same, and fourth, phenomenologically their differences are mainly inter-pretative, i.e. they are dependent on set and/or setting. I shall begin by examining the phenomena of clairvoyance, telepathy, and trance, setting aside the examination of those accompanying ecsomatosis (OBE) which I propose to undertake in the following section.

The first argument above constitutes a blow-by-blow comparison of hypnagogic and psi phenomena. To begin with, since both hypnagogia and psi states share the same inducting conditions, viz. psychophysical relaxation, it is not at all surprising to find that they display the same somatosensory phenomena. As with hypnagogia, there are reports of drifting, floating, body schema alterations such as shrinking, expanding or disappearing of parts of the body, and body dissociations. Roberts writes that during sittings for psychic development the would-be psychics may feel 'a cold shudder', have 'a sensation of heat' or 'a feeling of extreme drowsiness', 'feel as if they were floating' and 'become aware of colours, light, spirit powers'. She further describes what is clearly identical to Leroy's and Sartre's observation of the hypnagogic self-induced paralysis and the well-established hypnagogic body schema alterations: 'There may be occasions when the medium will feel as if the body is completely inert, or as if the throat cannot speak. Another sensation is that of feeling minutely small, or enormously large.'[35] My own notes from observations made at psychic development circles include reports such as 'I felt my body growing bigger', 'I felt heaviness, and then parts of my body dissolving; and then my arm started shaking', 'my face was as if covered by cobweb', 'half my face disappeared', and 'I felt the features of my face changing as though a mask or another face were being impressed on them'. Garrett notes that

> all the sensory faculties are called into play in telepathy. . . . I have known that in the telepathic experiment the senses of taste and smell were serving me as keen agents in knowing that a telepathic state was functioning. . . . The percipient may feel a faint electric tingling or warmth. There is tactile response and 'gooseflesh may appear on the skin'.[36]

Interestingly, and in relation to Arnold-Foster's and Ornitz *et al.*'s observation that in the hypnagogic state the subject's senses become more acute,[37] Roberts says that 'small bodily discomforts quickly become accentuated when the psychic power sensitises the medium' and 'every medium who experiences trance control will notice how the senses seem to become more acute, so that a quiet cough sounds like a thunderclap and the rustling of clothing like a hurricane.'[38] Likewise, Northage notes that a 'sudden noise can give a most dreadful physical shock'.[39]

To the self-posed question 'How can I be sure that it is a state of trance control and not just a submerged part of my mind which has become active?', Roberts responds:

> To answer this question, the medium must examine the results of the controlled communications. Are you able to say things which were not previously in your mind? Do you become aware of things about people which you did not know before? Do you 'see' vivid pictures while under control which you do not recognise in the normal state? . . . Do you feel different? Does the body become hotter or colder? In short, does the controlled state differ from the normal one?[40]

However, a positive answer to the above questions puts the developing medium's experiences well within the phenomenological span of hypnagogia. Again, the phenomena of clairvoyance, as described by Roberts, are indistinguishable from those of hypnagogia:

A clairvoyant vision is generally discerned when the ordinary consciousness is at rest. Sometimes it will consist of a complete figure or a face of a person; or it may be a nebulous form which appears to be hidden in a cloudy substance. Often it is in the form of beautiful scenery or brilliantly coloured symbols. The onset of the opening of clairvoyant vision is frequently heralded by clouds of delicate colours which seem to be swirling within the head of the sitter. These experiences of the inward consciousness are often thought to be purely imaginative. There is one test by which the medium can prove whether they are psychic or imaginary: In imaginary pictures the thinker visualises the picture before it is seen; if the image is of psychic origin it is 'seen' first and then thought about – indeed, the medium is often surprised by the fact that he (or she) has seen something which is so unexpected.[41]

Similarly, Garrett writes that attempts to build figures imaginatively and make them act as in clairvoyant vision always fail; 'they never hold together, and continually change and fall away from their type. But the clairvoyant image "happens". You come upon it.'[42] Sinclair notes that in telepathy

fragments of form appear first. For example, a curved line, or a straight one, or two lines of a triangle. But sometimes the complete object appears; swiftly, lightly, dimly drawn, as on a moving picture film. These mental visions appear and disappear with lightning rapidity. Then one must 'recall' this first vision. . . . It is necessary to recall this vision and make note of it, so as not to forget it.[43]

As with hypnagogia, there are also reports of megalopsias and micropsias.[44]

In my interview with Northage (see Appendix III), she spoke of the clairvoyant vision as having 'a peculiar light, quite a distinctive light that comes out of the whole picture, as if the whole picture is motivated by light', and that psychic colours are much brighter than physical ones: 'It's not so much colour as light: imagine colour full of light.' She further remarked that visions are always 'perfect in detail', they move very fast and seem to be both in front and yet 'all round me', and that one can 'see' behind images as if they were transparent – compare this with Collard's hypnagogic vision (chapter 2) wherein she found herself inside a 'crystal' corridor which she was simultaneously viewing both from the inside and the outside, and with Leroy's hypnagogic image in which he could 'see' the rib of a parasol that 'should be hidden by the cloth and by the body of the funnel, both of which are opaque'.[45]

During a 'demonstration', Northage further remarks, she ceases to be analytical and loses self-consciousness almost entirely, she becomes so deeply absorbed in the psychic reality that she does not even recognize familiar people in the audience. When speaking in trance, although she hears her voice 'it's almost like talking in another language', nothing really registers – as with visions, words come and go and are forgotten the moment they are spoken, 'it's like having gas at the dentist's': you do not lose consciousness altogether but you are not particularly concerned with what goes on.

Instructing on how to develop ESP, Huson, having pointed out the conduciveness of hypnagogia to such enterprise, notes that after the initial stages of psychophysical relaxation one finds oneself staring into what feels like three-dimensional space:

> In this depth the 'imaginals' (as I named them) appear dimly at first, but more solidly and clearly with practice. These may be things you know in daily life like books or bottles or flowers, or they may be large abstract shapes, often architectural in appearance. Keep your mental gaze on them and you'll notice that they are continually growing and` evolving into something else, like a speeded-up film of a plant growing. When I saw my first surrealist painting as a child, I knew exactly what the artist was portraying.[46]

By this time, Huson explains, one has travelled two-thirds of the way to achieving true clairvoyance: the next step is to learn to 'hook' the ESP target. Later on in the same work he explicitly states that 'hypnagogic dreams can and do become channels for ESP scanning'.

In the above examples it can be seen clearly that visual psi experiences are practically indistinguishable from those occurring in hypnagogia both in their content and in their nature. Also, the mental state of the subject appears to be the same.

The following quotation from Butler will shed extra light on some of the points presented so far and reveal more phenomenological similarities between psi states and hypnagogia. On this occasion Butler is describing the technique of scrying in a black mirror. After the instructions for the preliminary psychophysical relaxation, the subject gazes quietly into the mirror there to see the surface of the mirror first clouding over with what looks like mist which then breaks out into whirling clouds and brilliant sparks of light. He continues:

> If you can keep your mind in the quiet state, then the appearance in the mirror may begin to increase and to take other forms. Fragmentary glimpses of brilliantly coloured landscapes, faces grave and gay, and luminous coloured clouds may all show themselves. . . . These pictures are the first cousins to those curious little pictures which are seen by some people during the entry into sleep and again when awakening from sleep. The psychologists call them hypnagogic images, and assume that they are made and projected by the subconscious. This is true enough, but in our present case, they may be more than just images; they may be message-carrying images, bringing information which has been received by the inner senses. They are, as it were, waking dreams, and have their own definite meaning.
>
> When you have reached this stage, you have begun to develop

clairvoyance. You will discover for yourself the curious trick of holding the mind in a poised and yet relaxed condition; something which seems impossible at first. Many times you will become suddenly excited at what you see, and the whole vision will close down immediately. You will find that your visions begin to divide into two distinct groups. . . . One set of images will be of normal everyday things, and the other will present symbolic forms to you. You will also find that the symbolic vision seems to be associated with a positive questioning attitude of your mind. The literal vision appears to be reflected into your mind without any effort on your part; it is a passive vision. . . .

Now as you proceed with your development, you will find that certain images have a symbolic value, and are the code which your inner self is using. You will have to learn from your visions what such symbolic forms *mean to you*. We have stressed these three words, for they are very important. What a symbol means to the inner self of one person is not necessarily the meaning it has for another.[47]

There are a number of very interesting and relevant points to be brought out of this lengthy quotation. To begin with, the point is made once more that psi states, just like hypnagogia, are dependent on psychophysical relaxation, that the slightest degree of excitement would bring them to a halt.

Second, if it were not for the psychic set and setting within which the imagery referred to appears, there would be no justification phenomenologically for calling it psychic and not hypnagogic. Butler refers to the images under discussion as 'first cousins' to the hypnagogic imagery, but the only distinction he draws between them is that the former may be 'message-carrying images'. Elsewhere, he proposes that hypnagogic images on the whole belong in the occult type called 'images rising' whose emergence pertains to the magical method of the 'Evocation of Images'.[48] However, the 'message-carrying' feature appears to be neither an intrinsic nor a distinguishing characteristic of the phenomenology of the state. As already noted, hypnagogic experiences can and do become channels for ESP scanning. On the other hand, imagery emerging in a psi state has not been conclusively shown to be always 'message-carrying'. Thus, once again, the distinction is primarily one of 'set'.

Third, we encounter here the well-known autosymbolic hypnagogic phenomenon. Butler appears to be distinguishing between literal visions and symbolic visions. The latter he importantly connects with 'a positive questioning attitude' or an 'effort' on the part of the subject. If we pursue the argument that a psi state is essentially a hypnagogic state (minus set and setting), then the introduction of 'effort' (Silberer's 'effort to think') might lead to the appearance of the autosymbolic hypnagogic phenomenon wherein one's questioning attitude is represented in the emerging symbolic imagery. Fourth, emerging symbolic imagery is said to have a specific meaning for the individual. This is precisely the point made by Silberer and Slight in respect to hypnagogia and discussed in chapter 3.

That often the only features distinguishing psi from hypnagogic phenomena are those of set and/or setting can be seen from a juxtaposition of reports from both areas. For instance, Butler gives the following typical 'reading' of a type of psychic activity called 'psychometry':

> I see before me a wide expanse of water – I think it is the sea. Yes, I feel it is the Atlantic Ocean. I am standing on the deck of a ship – it seems to be a wooden ship – it is a warship of some kind, for I see guns – muzzle-loading guns of Nelson's time or thereabouts. . . . [49]

Compare this with one of Archer's hypnagogic visions: 'I see a picture of a calm, oily sea; no land is visible, but there is an idea in my mind that it is the Irish Sea near Dublin.' Archer also reported seeing the hypnagogic image of a Red Indian and, on other occasions, hearing the irrelevant sentences 'Agnes enjoyed her punch' and 'Charlie writes suggesting we should meet here at Gipsy Hill'.[50] Leroy reported hearing hypnopompically the sentence 'George is dead'.[51] Had such experiences taken place in a 'psychic' setting or had they occurred in subjects with appropriate beliefs, they might have easily been interpreted as messages from some supernatural source.

The following example from Garrett is of double importance as it not only argues for a possible psi activity in a clearly hypnopompic state but also reveals some very strong psychological similarities with one of Slight's hypnopompic experiences to be discussed below:

> I was awakened from sleep one night by a strong feeling that somebody had something urgent to tell me. So vivid was the dream that someone had been urging me to listen to him that I got up, and went to the door of my apartment, certain that I had been awakened by knocking. However, there was no one there. I went back to bed, and heard a very quiet voice say, 'You won't remember me, but I met you years ago with Lawrence.' The same voice continued, 'I am Lawrence. I wish that they would realize that I am decently dead, and finished with the ways of man.' The voice ceased at that point. . . . In the morning I had a letter from a friend in Dorsetshire, who wrote asking the question: 'Do you believe that Lawrence of Arabia was killed in a motorcycle accident, or was that a story given to the press to hide some important piece of work that he is doing at the moment?' I should mention here that the night before I had had no thought in my own mind of Lawrence of Arabia, but had thought, rather, of D.H. Lawrence; but I then remembered that I once met Lawrence of Arabia through a very well-known and high-ranking English officer who had admired D.H. Lawrence, and who had introduced me to both of the Lawrences on the same day.[52]

It is important to note that although Garrett had not thought of Lawrence of Arabia the night before, she had, however, thought of D.H. Lawrence. The two Lawrences were related in her mind not only by name but also by the fact that she had been introduced to both of them on the same day – indeed, in Garrett's example it would appear that the two Lawrences became identical and interchangeable thus pointing to the already observed tendency in hypnagogia to transform similarity into sameness.

Slight reported the following hypnopompic-hypnagogic experience which, had the appropriate psychic set and setting been present, would most certainly have been attributed to a psi state and/or some supernatural agency:

> The next example occurred in the morning while half awake. During the previous day I had been much impressed by the change in appearance of a lady whom I had not seen for some time. Later in the day I conversed with some friends on the topic of how a man aged gradually whereas a woman aged rapidly and was exposed to influences from which a man was exempted, as child bearing, the menopause, the burden of the family and the like.
>
> I had begun to pursue this line of thought in the half awake state when suddenly I found myself spelling out the letters B-R-O-W-N, and dimly aware of a bell tolling with each letter. After the N the name Marguerite came rapidly to mind and only then did I piece the letters together and realize they formed a name known to me. Then I became fully awake and heard a bell tolling, which occurred every morning at this time. . . .
>
> I relapsed into a half waking state and began to turn the matter over in mind. First I remembered being informed – though I had long forgotten – that although Miss Brown was now unprepossessing and even ugly in appearance she had been handsome and beautiful before the onset of her illness, and miraculously changed after the onset. It seems that Miss Brown had formed a splendid example to illustrate the previous train of thought but I still felt unsatisfied and then the image of another lady appeared – a relation who had personal connections with Miss Brown which fact dawned on me as if for the first time.
>
> Realization came that here lay the real interest and the previous line of thought also applied to the latter lady. Miss Brown had formed a double bond since she provided an ideal illustration of such change in a woman and at the same time was connected with a personal interest.
>
> The name Marguerite was a mystery since I had never heard Miss Brown's christian name and it had no connection with the other lady. No association would come to this name and I was left with the feeling that possibly further elements lay behind it which might give a deeper interpretation. Later in the day I discovered that Miss Brown's christian name was Marguerite and on reflection found that there had been only a few fleeting occasions on which I might have learned this fact.[53]

Besides the similarity in the manner in which the Lawrences in Garrett's case and the two women in Slight's case were related, in Slight's example there is implicit a method of introspective probing or questioning which is in essence the same as that employed by psychics in their psi activities. Indeed, Slight touches on two aspects of this method. The first aspect illustrates the technique of posing questions or probing the process. In both hypnagogia and psi states it is required that in order to gain a response from the process one must pose a mental question or adopt a questioning attitude without, however, interrupting one's receptive mode. This is demonstrated in the present example by Slight's observation, 'I still felt unsatisfied and then the image of another lady appeared.' That is, he adopted an attitude of questioning to which the hypnagogic process responded by bringing forth another image. This, as we have seen, is at times autosymbolic. Indeed, the same appears to be fully appreciated by Slight when he says, 'It seemed that Miss Brown had formed a splendid example to illustrate the previous train of thought.' This latter feature (autosymbolism) may, in fact, be due to the current specific mental attitude of the subject. For instance, it may be autosymbolic only when the questioning is related to oneself or to some abstract ('egocentric') material, whereas, when the questioning is directed to a more precise 'external' object – be it an image or a 'thing' – the outcome may be a further unfolding of imagery related to the original image but also containing novel elements some of which may be facts concerning the object and which may be argued not to have been known to the subject prior to this experience.

This, as stated above, is a line of questioning advocated and pursued by most psychics. Roberts writes, 'The medium should not be satisfied to receive one name such as "Mary" but should ask which "Mary", "What is her other name?" When the double name is given, then the medium should ask for the name of the town in which she lived, and so forth.'[54] In my interview with Northage I asked her to describe her reaction when she gives some information to a 'sitter' which he does not accept as veridical. She said:

> I go back and say to myself 'How did I get that?' That's the first thing I do. I retrace my steps, I go back and find how I got it, first of all, because I could have inadvertently changed it. Or, I ask [my spirit communicators] for more information: if I know I'd given it out accurately then I say 'They [i.e. the 'sitter'] don't understand that, explain it', and it may be that something added to it makes it clear.

And we must bear in mind that when a psychic engages in ESP activities and describes his/her imaginal experiences, 'he should try to do this without emotion and try to hold the attunement gently, allowing the thought impression to continue.'[55] This is identical to observations in respect to hypnagogia, viz. that one may engage in a concurrent description of one's hypnagogic experiences so long as one remains receptive towards both the imagery and one's physical environment.

The other aspect of the method of both hypnagogizing and engaging in psi activities touched upon by Slight is found in his remark that after his initial hypnagogic experience he became fully awake and then 'relapsed into a half waking state and began to turn the matter over in mind'. Likewise, Sinclair's wife describes how after the extra sensory perception of the image of a drawing and the sketching on paper of what she received, she returns to the ESP state of mind in order to continue with the experiment. In respect to hypnagogia, the ability to oscillate in and out of this state is a strong indication of how easily it can be abstracted from its setting, thus becomming indistinguishable from psi and similar states.

A further observation relating to the above is the *sense of realization*, as if for the first time, that such and such is the case in regards to the nature of an image or idea. This experience of *jamais vu* cuts across both hypnagogia and psi states. In the example under discussion reference to it is made at least twice – in the second paragraph: 'only then did I piece the letters together and realize they formed a name known to me', and the third paragraph: 'which fact dawned on me as if for the first time'. A possible third reference may be in the opening of the fourth paragraph. In the psi literature this is pointed out as the characteristic feature of novelty, of the knowledge of new facts regarding a psi object about which the percipient did not or could not have known. These facts appear to the percipient as if for the first time – see, for instance, Robert's response to her self-posed question quoted above.

This element of novel realization is of more than passing interest. It is, of course, a matter for debate whether the presence of the character of novelty is to be interpreted as a mark of the extrasensory acquisition of new facts. In the present example Slight does not remember ever having heard Miss Brown's first name and he seems to doubt whether such an event occurred on the few fleeting occasions on which he might have learned it. However, he does not clearly impute a paranormal character to his experience, thus leaving open the possibility of a forgotten experience. Indeed, the fact that the presence of the experience of *jamais vu* should not be taken as a mark of acquisition of knowledge extrasensorially is illustrated by Slight's observation that the existing personal connection between his relative and Miss Brown dawned on him as if for the first time. The manner in which *recognition* may be taken as *cognition* of new facts in hypnagogia is further illustrated by his observation that having spelled out the letters B-R-O-W-N 'the name Marguerite came rapidly to mind and only then did I piece the letters together and realize they formed a name known to me' – obviously, had he not recognized the name, the piecing together of the letters would have been taken as yielding knowledge of a new fact. But again, the seeming acquisition of new knowledge in this state may turn out to be the reviving of a long-forgotten memory as evidenced by Slight's observation that he remembered being informed, *though he had long forgotten*, about Miss Brown's former beautiful appearance.[56]

Related to the above is the feeling of significance or conviction, of the 'hunch' or '*knowing* as apart from *thinking*',[57] which often, but not always, accompanies the imaginal experience of a psychic. Thus, Butler points out that, although 'there is always a background of impressional sensing which accompanies the pictures seen or the sounds heard, and this background is important in enabling you to interpret that which you perceive', nonetheless, at the early stages of a psychic's development 'sometimes the pictures arise without any surrounding impressions.'[58]

Garrett remarked that 'the beginning clairvoyant' passes through a stage of perceiving 'doodlings' or random images. These are elements which can be formed gradually into 'word-designs':

> As an example of these word-designs, he might say '"I have a feeling" that the images suggest "Happiness"'. 'I see the lines forming the letters "H..a..p..p..y.."' – but the letters slowly spelled out (at times, even pronounced as an integrated word 'Happy'), or the feeling of 'Happiness' will have no concrete significance for him, although the word may have a clear meaning to the agent with whom he is working.[59]

It has, of course, already been suggested in respect to hypnagogia that the appearance of lines and simple geometric designs may belong to a relatively light stage of this state, and that sometimes images may carry a 'feeling', an awareness of their significance, whereas on other occasions they may appear irrelevant to the subject. From our discussion of hypnagogia so far it becomes clear that the mark of irrelevancy may be due to the presence of two conditions either of which may appear separately or in conjunction: the first condition relates to the stage of hypnagogia, viz. light stage, and the second to the degree of facility, 'training', or 'practice' one has had with hypnagogia. As van Dusen pointed out, even simple hypnagogic images may convey a meaning and thus be significant if the subject allows himself to become involved in his hypnagogic imagery and enter into a 'conversation' with it. But clearly, in order to achieve this, his attention must be absorbed in the unfolding of the imagery, that is, he must become 'fascinated' by this internal activity and, to a considerable extent, withdraw psychologically from his environment. Similarly, in regard to clairvoyance, Garrett talks of switching to a different reality, which Le Shan refers to as the 'psychic reality';[60] and Northage remarks that when the latter is active her physical environment recedes and the psychic becomes predominant; she becomes absorbed in it. And in both the hypnagogic and psychic activities the imagery may have 'no concrete significance' for the subject, i.e. it may appear irrelevant, until one learns to 'question' it.

Furthermore, in the example of 'word-designs' given by Garrett we may note, first, how a 'beginning clairvoyant', just like a hypnagogist, may have a feeling of significance concerning his imagery, second, that letters may appear and spell out a word or a name (cf. Slight's example), and third, that both the feeling of significance and the word may relate to each other but still remain irrelevant to the subject. In respect to the third remark, the difference between a hypnagogist and a clairvoyant would lie in the manner of their facing their 'irrelevant' imagery: the former would generally dismiss it as simply irrelevant, or at most as having something to do with his subconscious, whereas the clairvoyant, as Garrett points out, would seek for possible relevance in the experiences and personality of the observer or agent with whom he is engaged in a clairvoyant experiment.

Stanford argues that

> the strong sense of conviction often associated with cognitive-'perceptual' ESP cases likely derives not from the intrinsic nature of such events but from the circumstances that the ideas, feelings, images, etc., psi-mediated into awareness in such instances are so unusual or inappropriate in the life-context in which they appear that the person experiencing them is inclined to impute to them an unusual or psychic origin.[61]

It seems to me, however, that in his above argument Stanford is placing the cart before the horse. This is, in fact, an occasion where the sense of conviction or accompanying awareness of significance encountered in hypnagogia may throw light on the occurrence of the same or similar feeling in 'cognitive-"perceptual" ESP cases'. It is a matter of observation that the feeling of conviction occurs both in ESP and in hypnagogia when (a) the subject's analytical mind is completely subdued, neutralized or otherwise engaged, (b) a fully receptive state is achieved, and (c) attention is absorbed. In hypnagogia these conditions are found fully present in the deep stages in which also awareness of surroundings is either completely lost or greatly diminished. These very same conditions are also present when, in ESP, a percipient experiences a 'strong sense of conviction' – indeed, as we saw earlier in this section, various psychics explicitly reported that a hypnagogic state must be reached and sustained if a successful extrasensory experience is to take place, the latter often being accompanied by a sense of conviction. This analysis indicates that the sense of conviction, whenever it occurs in hypnagogia or in psi states, is intrinsic to the state and that it is not derived from the current circumstances. On the contrary, the imputation of a psychic origin to such events may be due, as already alluded to in this section, to the percipient's set of beliefs. It is of course to be expected that the percipient in a psi experiment should impute such origins to his imaginal experiences since they derive from the setting itself with his own set of beliefs in psychic phenomena added (cf. the Brauds' 'altered world view' and 'momentary importance of psi').

Ecsomatic phenomena and the conduciveness of hypnagogia to their occurrence

The psi-conduciveness of hypnagogia is further evidenced by the tendency of ecsomatic experiences (OBEs, ecsomatoses, exteriorizations, astral projections) to occur spontaneously at sleep onset and at waking from sleep, and by the fact that subjects with long experience in ecsomatosis not only report having had most of their experiences at such times but also advocate the induction of hypnagogia as a necessary step to the achievement of such events.

Green reports that 'both "just after going to bed" and "before getting up in the morning" are mentioned by different subjects as favourable times, the former predominating'.[62] Typical cases read: 'while lying on my back in bed with my eyes closed, preparing to go to sleep I find myself moving upwards', or 'these out-of-the-body experiences occurred at night when I was in bed in a semi-conscious condition, that is, almost asleep, or on the verge of waking.' Green further reports that out of 176 cases, 66 per cent were reported as having taken place while the subject was lying down and 20 per cent as while sitting, that is, 'in the position of least muscle tone'. Although only about 37 per cent of the subjects said that they noticed they were relaxed during their ecsomatosis, and about 21 per cent said they were the 'same throughout' and 31 per cent expressed no opinion, in the case of the latter two groups it may be argued that they felt no difference because they were already relaxed prior to their experience. In fact, several subjects emphasize that 'the degree of relaxation which they experienced in the ecsomatic state was abnormal for them, saying, for example, that they were "relaxed completely; more than usually", or "extremely relaxed, quite the reverse of my conscious state"'. The case is more so with those who induce their ecsomatosis. One subject, for instance, writes:

> I had to lie down on the floor, in a fairly warm atmosphere, not cold and concentrate on putting my whole body to sleep, breathe deeply, two or three times, and let my body completely go. . . . I sort of drifted away. . . . I opened my eyes, and I was looking down at myself laying on the floor.

Many subjects, however, report that deep relaxation merely resulted in their falling asleep, until, that is, they achieved some proficiency at keeping themselves poised between wakefulness and sleep.

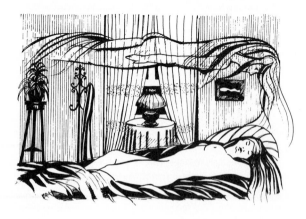

Figure 6.1 *Early attempts at achieving an OBE usually lead to sleep, but by gaining a proficiency at balancing oneself in hypnagogia a person may suddenly find himself/ herself floating in the air and looking down at his/ her body lying on the floor or bed.*

Instructions on how to induce exteriorization encountered in the occult and psychic literature explicitly recommend hypnagogia as a state highly conducive to the induction of such experiences. Monroe, for instance, says of exteriorization in hypnagogia that 'this is perhaps the easiest and most

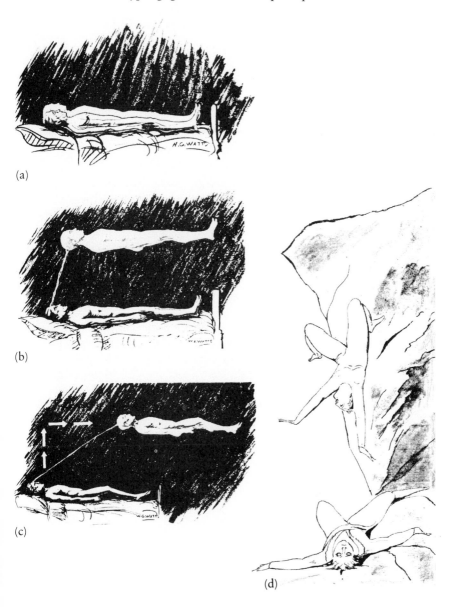

Figure 6.2   *Muldoon's representation of how the 'phantom' exteriorizes following a hypnagogic induction: (a) 'phantom' rising, (b) above the body, (c) projecting into a flying dream. The latter often comes to an end as a falling dream (d).*

natural method and usually ensures relaxation of both body and mind simultaneously'.[63] Muldoon writes, 'I would awaken between one and four o'clock in the morning, usually, and the astral body would begin to "rise", as I entered sleep again; but, on other occasions . . . the projection would begin in the hypnagogic state when emerging from sleep.'[64] He instructs that if a subject wants to achieve an OBE the easiest way to effect it is

> in the hypnagogic state, when going to sleep – if he will but concentrate his attention upon himself and try to see what is really happening, as he enters sleep. In other words, if he will but train himself to keep the balance between consciousness and unconsciousness – while slightly favouring the former – without tension in mind – and will maintain this well into the hypnagogic state, he will feel the discoincidence, as the phantom [psychic 'double'] enters the zone of quietude, usually as a falling sensation.[65]

Similar instructions are given by numerous other investigators,[66] some of whom have also offered detailed lists of hypnagogic phenomena occurring during ecsomatosis. These include: the seeing of lights, images, figures, landscapes, the hearing of various sounds all the way from inarticulate noises to beautiful strains of music, the hearing of one's name being called, the feeling of being touched. It is also noteworthy that Fox's 'vibrating circles', the 'vibrating curtain of circular cells' or 'frog's eggs' seen in his hypnagogic visions (see chapter 2), are encountered in his OBEs too 'beneath the golden glow suffusing the room'.[67]

Many of Green's subjects commented on the brightness and vividness of the imagery experienced in the ecsomatic state. As in hypnagogia, they also remarked on the illumination being apparently sourceless and diffuse as if the objects seen are 'lit from the inside'. The senses are said to be 'heightened', 'enhanced', 'more acute', and the visions are 'crystal clear' with minute visual details being perceptible; in some cases the subjects reported as seeing not with their eyes but with 'something else' or 'with whole consciousness'.[68]

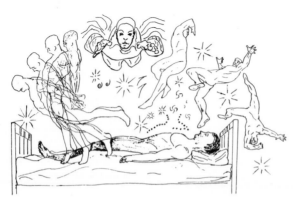

Figure 6.3 *An OBE accompanied by visual hypnagogic phenomena and the sensations of floating, drifting, whirling, sinking.*

Typically, ecsomatic subjects report kinesthetic experiences of falling through the bed, floating upwards, sinking, drifting, or whirling. Often these experiences are accompanied by paralysis or catalepsy. Significantly, this condition of paralysis, which occurs naturally in hypnagogia,[69] is specifically sought for by occultists who utilize it to achieve ecsomatosis and who otherwise would have to induce it in themselves by means of deliberately producing a hypnagogic state. The problem at hand is, as Fox puts it, 'to put the *body* to sleep while the mind is kept *awake*'. He instructs: 'Favourable times to experiment are after a substantial repast or when we wake in the morning feeling very loath to arise; for the body is then naturally disposed to enter the trance state.'[70] For purposes of comparison, the reader is referred back to chapter 2 to descriptions of hypnagogic experiences provided by Collard which strongly link the deliberately induced ecsomatoses of psychics and occultists with those that occur naturally in hypnagogia.

In relating hypnagogia to ecsomatosis four important observations present themselves in connection with the affective-cognitive state of the subject.

The first observation concerns the psychological calmness and detachment frequently reported as experienced by ecsomatic subjects. As with hypnagogia, it is often pointed out that both the induction and the ecsomatic experience *per se* are characterized by 'a perfect balance in the mind', and that 'the occurrence of emotional disturbance or conflict almost invariably leads to the termination of the ecsomatic state'.[71] Green reports that, both in experimental and spontaneous cases, subjects describe themselves as being calm, relaxed, detached or indifferent, as feeling what would appear to be an impersonal kind of curiosity, and although some of them may profess a great and agreeable interest in what goes on they do not seem to become emotionally involved in the outcome of events beyond feeling 'objective interest and fascination'.[72]

The second observation is closely related to the first and refers to the fact that 'ecsomatic subjects do not appear to be inclined to engage in analytical thought; their attitude appears, generally, to be that of an alert but usually passive observer', an 'interested spectator sort of thing!', as one subject put it. The experience is often likened to 'watching a cinema film' where the subject feels just like 'an interested observer of something which seemed to arouse no surprise' in him.[73] The 'film-watching' attitude may be related more widely to the general tendency of the subject to accept as perfectly reasonable phenomena that are clearly not so and which he would certainly be more critical of in the waking state. As we know, the same attitude of detachment has also been noted in hypnagogia by many investigators.[74]

The third observation refers to remarks by subjects that while in the ecsomatic state they experience the feeling that 'they could obtain an answer to any question they chose to formulate'. This is a 'feeling of "all-knowing and understanding"', a feeling that one knows things without thinking, and that everything is easy and possible.[75] It is worth noting, and remembering for later reference (chapters 9 and 10), that this feeling of omniscience and omnipotence is not only also encountered in hypnagogia[76] but is to be found in other, related states as well, and, most significantly, in the reports of near-death experiences and the experiences of individuals who survived 'clinical death'.[77]

The fourth observation refers to the hypnopompic trance accompanied by what Fox has called False Awakening,[78] and which has been reported, as we saw in chapter 4, by a number of workers in the hypnagogic area. Fox connects this both with a concurrent state of paralysis which is accompanied or followed by ecsomatosis and with the awareness that one is dreaming which leads to what he calls Dream of Knowledge (also known as lucid dreaming: see chapter 4).

Hypnagogic experiences as psi, religious, and mystical events

In this section belong what Green and McGreery have called 'informational' or 'warning' cases in which 'the information conveyed may be the solution to a problem with which the subject has been consciously occupied for some time, or it may be a spontaneous "warning" of a danger which the subject has not previously thought about'. For instance, one subject reports that she was awakened suddenly one night to see her dead grandfather standing by her bedside. While wondering why such a phenomenon should take place, she went downstairs to look at her husband's dinner in the oven. 'As I went downstairs and opened the door at the bottom', she reports, 'I gasped. The house reeked of gas.'[79]

In their classic investigation, Gurney *et al.* reported numerous cases of people who at sleep onset saw and/or heard the visions and voices of friends and loved ones, or were woken in the middle of the night by such sounds and visions, to be conveyed information vital to them. Often, the visions were of people known to be still alive but who subsequently were found either to have died at the time of the recorded 'visitation' or were in a very stressful or dangerous situation and had called out to the subject. Some cases involved pacts between two people to the effect that whoever died first would 'appear' at his moment of death to the surviving partner. Occasionally, even the circumstances of a loved one's death were purportedly 'seen' by the living party. On a more cheerful note, these authors presented a case of telepathy in which the father of a young woman saw hypnagogically (as he lay next to her dozing) what his daughter was visualizing while reading a novel.[80]

In fact, this latter kind of phenomenon appears to occur much more widely than investigators in the area are prepared to concede. In my research into 'development circles' I came across it on numerous occasions. On the whole, such phenomena were spontaneous but I soon found that I was able at times to inject into them a measure of experimental intentionality. For instance, on one occasion I dozed while a member of a particular 'circle' I was participating in was doing psychometry – an exercise-experiment in which a person holds in his hand an object such as a ring, a cross, or a wrist-watch that usually belongs to another member of the 'circle' (as a rule he does not initially know who it belongs to) and, concentrating relaxedly over this object, reports his impressions (which can be visual, auditory, somesthetic, etc.). As this would-be psychic – let's call him Peter – described his mainly visual impressions, I began to 'see' very vividly various scenes. This went on for a while when I suddenly became aware that what Peter was describing were the very scenes I was seeing with my eyes shut. I observed this for a while longer and then proceeded to experiment by altering my visions. And, lo and behold, Peter followed suit – he began to describe my altered visualizations. I then 'fed' him with words and thoughts which he promptly 'picked up' and reported. Later, when I began to hold evening classes in 'Altered States of Awareness', I made the experiment a more straightforward one by visualizing a complex scene and asking the members of the class to pick up its contents telepathically. Although the results were on the whole not statistically significant, some reports were too accurate to dismiss as mere chance (see Appendix III). In connection with hypnagogic ecsomatic phenomena, Collard also states that 'these experiences can be shared' and that when she and her brother were children they 'used to "go expeditions" together'.[81] Other reports, too, speak of 'shared' hypnagogic experiences, as in the case of a person who, at sleep onset, saw vividly 'the face and form' of a friend and had a brief conversation with her, only to hear from her a few days later that at precisely the same time she had had 'an identical experience' in a 'vivid dream'.[82]

In my interview with Northage she recounted to me hypnopompic experiences which she explicitly considers to be paranormal in nature. Garrett, too, gives various personal examples of telepathy and clairvoyance that took place on retiring to bed at night or waking up in the night or in the morning.[83] Green and McCreery mention a number of apparitional cases that

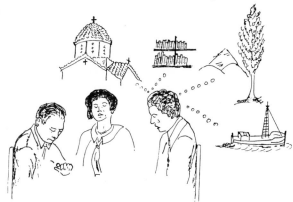

Figure 6.4 *My experiment with Peter. As Peter talked I 'fed' him with mental pictures which he promptly picked up and described: 'The owner of this ring is a very religious person. . . . He, or she, likes books a great deal. . . . He is also very fond of the country-side, and of nature in general. . . . He likes the sea and is very keen on boating. . . . '*

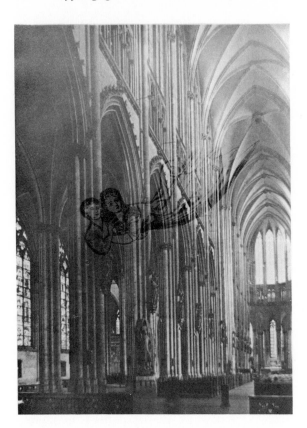

Figure 6.5 *Going expeditions together.*

took place in hypnagogia, and note that in many of these experiences 'the subject, who is awake at the time, temporarily loses his awareness of his normal environment, and seems to be perceiving a different one'. They call these experiences 'waking dreams' by analogy with sleepdreams and class both as 'metachoric', that is, as 'experiences in which the subject's field of perception is completely replaced by a hallucinatory one'.

Along with the many spontaneous psi cases reported as having taken place during hypnagogia, in this section will be included those cases to which their experients impute supernatural or religious import.[84] For instance, Forman considered his hypnagogic visions of mountains and hills rolling against him as sent by heaven to warn him of future difficulties, Iamblichus referred to them as 'god-sent', and Poe spoke of their spiritual nature.[85] Various workers have drawn attention to the strong possibility that mythology and folklore may have their genesis in such phenomena,[86] and Maury proposed that many visions of the saints were hypnagogic experiences.[87]

In contrast to Maury's remark, which is clearly meant to argue against imputing a supernatural character to many of the (hypnagogic) visions of the saints, Tappeiner, a theologian, considers the experiences of hypnagogia as 'a psychological paradigm for the interpretation of the charismatic phenomenon of prophesy'.[88] Without relinquishing the belief in the ultimate spirituality of the prophetic phenomena, Tappeiner employs the concept of the unconscious which he equates with 'the domain of "spirit" in which the Holy Spirit functions', and the phenomenological and cognitive-experiential state of hypnagogia, to explain how prophesying (a 'spontaneous utterance . . . for purposes of upbuilding, encouragement, and consolation') takes place. According to Tappeiner, a person in a religious group enters a 'revelatory state of mind' by focusing attention upon spiritual reality and quieting the ordinary busy consciousness. Along with these latter two markers there is also in operation a type of unconscious processing of the material presented in the meeting. Then, in the revelatory state, the material is suddenly crystallized in hypnagogic imagery which emerges in the form of 'seed-thought', 'beginning phrase', or 'vision', the latter being 'an inner picture or "cartoon" which simply emerges suddenly, whole, and with no previous conscious consideration of it'. The contents of such experience are often shared by a number of people in the group, that is, two or more people may have, for instance, the same vision. It is not to be understood, however, that all hypnagogic experiences are 'prophetic' or spiritual in any sense, but only that the act of prophesying, which is thought to have its genesis in Spirit, registers and expresses itself through the psychological mechanism operating in hypnagogia.[89]

That hypnagogia constitutes a state in which religious and mystical experiences can be had appears also to be a view held by many sufi mystics who, according to Abbé Rouguette who made a study of Moslem secret societies in Africa, believe that the truth reveals itself in all its glory through hypnagogic visions of corals, plants, trees, animals, autoscopies, and the form of the disciple's 'Sheikh'.[90] Similar views, including techniques for utilizing hypnagogia for the attainment of mystical experiences, are expressed by Tibetan yogis[91] (see also chapter 5).

Psychological observations and theoretical formulations

REGRESSIVITY As in the case of hypnagogia, investigators in the psi area often compare psychic mentation to childlike, primitive, mystical or magical modes of thinking. In both cases the subject may return (or 'regress') to earlier modes of cognizing and feeling accompanied by a sense of being protected or 'cocooned' characteristic of early childhood. Garrett, for instance, made use of hypnagogia to develop a 'passivity-consciousness' that enabled her to return to childhood and to the child's 'initial knowing', and would employ this 'process of going to the child-me' whenever she felt the need to understand or explain psychic phenomena.[92] What is of great relevance here is that certain important points of relationship or similarity between hypnagogia and 'regressive' types of thinking are the same as those pointed out as existing between the latter and psi mentation. Let us look at them point by point.

To begin with, not only are we told that Garrett's telepathic functioning is that of the 'child-me' but also that the original induction of this state or type of mentation was achieved by developing a 'passivity-consciousness' as she lay in bed at twilight. Second, psi researchers, like many workers in hypnagogia, identify in telepathic imagery the presence of dynamics such as condensation (syncretism), dissociation (fragmentation), inversion, and the phenomenon of neologism[93] (which are also to be found in the thinking and languages of primitive people, children, schizophrenics, and the experiences of 'drug' takers). Third, Warcollier remarks that, like a child, the telepathic percipient does not attach to the same elements the same importance as the agent does, and that, as in tachistoscopic perception, fragmented and dissociated details are revealed which are 'entirely irrational'. Now, if the importance the agent attaches to the elements of a picture are taken as 'rational', the whole contention appears to argue for an 'entirely irrational' fragmentation and assemblage of details. This is in agreement with the observations of hypnagogists who repeatedly remark on the fragmentariness and irrelevance of their imagery. Moreover, it is in agreement with my hypothesis that the irrelevancy of hypnagogic imagery may be due to the fact that hypnagogic mentation surfaces from frames of reference not coincident with 'waking rationality'. Fourth, the same writer compares telepathic mentation to a child's attitude of taking in an experience as a whole and feeling himself part of it. This has clear parallels in the hypnagogic absorption and fascination wherein the subject lacks the ability or inclination to analyse and differentiate. The fifth point is an extension of the fourth: in hypnagogia imagery is often not merely perceived but felt in a kinesthetic manner, as if some unseen internal lines of connection between the subject and the image were in operation. Likewise, Garrett notes, 'The beginning of telepathic reception makes itself felt in my body; my mind as such never seems to play any part.'[94]

A further but very important observation may be added. In my review and analysis of hypnagogia, subjects on the whole emphasize the 'externality' of their imagery, that is, of its seemingly taking place outside them. At the same time it is reported that the induction and prolongation of hypnagogic imagery is dependent on an attitude towards it characterized by acceptance, curiosity, 'passive' attention, interest, friendliness, empathy, that very often the imagery is experienced kinesthetically, and that strong emotions (e.g. disgust, fear) bring the experience to an abrupt ending. This same apparent contradictoriness between empathy and objectivity (externality) are also encountered in psi activities. Garrett, for instance, writing on clairvoyance, says:

> The perceiver's sense of unity with what he perceives, and at the same
> time the complete objectivity and lack of response of all that he shares in

so intimately – together, these two factors, which are somehow contradictory, constitute a puzzling problem for thought after the experience.[95]

THE SUBCONSCIOUS LEVEL AND PARALOGICAL TYPES OF ASSOCIATION It is generally thought by workers in the psi area that successful psi activities are carried out at an unconscious level, and that many *partly* successful telepathic experiments are due to interference from the conscious and subconscious (preconscious) levels, the latter apparently lying between the conscious and the unconscious and comprising temporarily forgotten experiences and dissociated memories which, given the appropriate conditions and stimuli, may rise to consciousness. The unconscious is by definition an unknown and unknowable mental level, whereas subconscious mentation can be, and indeed is, experienced in dreams and dreamy states.

The main relevance of this theory to my discussion of hypnagogia lies in the observations that, first, where the conscious and subconscious merge into each other known rules of association, logic, and memories may be operative, and second, where conscious, wilful, mentation is the least present (approaching the unconscious) rules of association, logic and memories appear to operate in a very different frame of reference. (See chapters 7 and 8 for more detailed expositions of such implications.)

The first observation may be related to the light stages of hypnagogia wherein imagery changes may result from conscious or semiconscious associations following known rules of association, such as contiguity, resemblance, contrast, etc. For instance, one of Galton's correspondents reported the hypnagogic visual image of the beak of a bird changing into the barrel of a gun as a result of associations of shape and, perhaps, game shooting.[96] Similar changes have often been observed in telepathic experiments. For example, Warcollier reports an experiment in which the percipient saw the image of the trunk of a tree, then a branch of a tree, then a gun barrel, the form of a finger, and finally a bundle of faggots, the actual image 'transmitted' being a painfully tightly bandaged finger.[97]

The second observation we may relate to the deeper stages of hypnagogia wherein irrelevancy of associational links is most striking. Here, if any associations are to be postulated at all, these are mediate associations. Again, in respect to psi, Warcollier offers a number of cases of telepathic experiments in which he believes mediate associations were in operation. Related to this hypothesis of unconscious or mediate associations is Alexander's argument that although hypnagogic images may be analysed into their respective constituents they are complete in themselves and inexplicable, 'they contain "two and two", but they *are* "four" – and the addition remains to be accounted for. The addition is the *mental* fact of their making; *a fact which has never been a conscious fact.*'[98]

Alexander also makes another important remark, namely that as hypnagogic images 'have no associational *points d'appui* they are almost impossible to remember'. This remark is significant in two respects. First, it suggests a possible explanation of the occurrence of phenomena such as paramnesia, *déjà vu*, and *jamais vu* in hypnagogic and psi states. It may also point to an explanation of the often expressed inability of a psychic reporting a paranormal perception to tell whether the experience refers to the past, present or future. In a similar respect, we have the report in which 'a photograph of the percipient was once used as a target, and the percipient described the photograph in detail without recognizing himself'[99] – compare this with Slight's hypnopompic example. Also Muldoon, reporting on a hypnopompic experience preceding an ecsomatosis, describes the phenomenon in which, he says, 'I was aware that I existed, but *where* I could not seem to understand. My memory would not tell me.'[100]

Second, the absence of 'points of support' is clearly in reference to associational links operant in the waking state, which does not necessarily rule out the possibility that different rules of logic and/or a frame of reference entirely foreign to the waking self is in operation here. Indeed, in discussing hypnagogic images Alexander argues that these are 'mental constructs' which 'are not constructed in consciousness', from which he infers that 'they are the work of mind that is not conscious'. He continues:

> Further, my experience leads me to believe that these images are the work of a highly differentiated mental compartment. I find little connection between my ordinary thought and imagination and the work of my hypnagogic agent – whatever it may be. To formulate the points of difference: (1) There is almost no associational connection. (2) There is certainly no volitional connection, the images are spontaneous and self-willed. (3) There is no emotional connection. In short, the images are the work of an agent that does not share in my interests, aims or feelings.[98]

(Although Alexander did not make a study of his hypnagogic experiences by stage, it appears that most of them have taken place at an advanced hypnagogic stage wherein, as we know, the subject is deeply withdrawn from his physical and psychological environment (from his 'interests') and is emotionally relaxed (no emotional links) and passive (no volitional connection)).

Whether, along with Alexander, we postulate the existence of an 'agent', or propose a drastic change of the frame of reference, we are here dealing with a realm of experience in which the known rules of association appear to be non-operant. Or, if they are operant, they are so in a mediate way. Moreover, in the process of transferring such experiences to a waking, analytical frame of mind, the subject may often lose (forget) the experience altogether or bring forth into consciousness distorted fragments accompanied by memory peculiarities (*déjà vu*, *jamais vu*, etc.). In respect to paranormal perception, Le Shan similarly proposes that 'the apparent triviality, tangentiality, and superficiality of much of the sensitives' production is due to the data being translated from one system to another'.[101] Likewise, Heywood refers to Niels Bohr's observation that 'the part of the self which is, so to speak, in focus during an ESP-type experience is not the part which later tries to analyse it'.[102]

It thus appears that at a certain level of 'consciousness' both hypnagogic and psi activities occur within a frame of reference or mode of experiencing which has different laws of logic, unities, relational systems, etc., than the waking mode. Van Dusen, in respect to hypnagogia, and Le Shan, in reference to clairvoyant reality,[103] both support the view that the subject of such experiences usually maintains a distinction between the two modes by means of setting, viz. the hypnagogist usually has his experiences within the setting of going to sleep, and the clairvoyant or medium may employ forms of setting such as the trance, automatic writing, scrying, etc. – this observation also throws incidental light on psychotic experiences where the person usually loses the ability to distinguish between phenomena that come from different modes of experiencing (see chapter 7).

SET AND SETTING REVISITED Two possible points of difference in antecedent conditions between experimental psi (as distinct from spontaneous) and hypnagogia need to be examined at this juncture. These are thought to lie in the facts that in the former there is *usually* a period of 'blankness', or of intentional visualization followed by 'blankness', before psi activity, and that there is always on the mind of the subject the diffuse awareness that he is involved in a psi activity. A third point may lie in the sense of mental alertness felt by many psychics when in a psi state.

In respect to the first feature, the difference may be only apparent and due to the fact that in psi performance the percipient in the 'old method' is aware – indeed, he makes a point of being so – of the steps taken and the state(s) he shifts into. Thus, he is aware of his induced state of blankness, a state which is primarily the result of psychological withdrawal. It must be noted, however, that: (a) if the subject concentrates non-analytically on a specific image he inadvertently induces in himself a hypnagogic state which, if the appropriate steps are not taken, results in sleep, and (b) if the subject 'blanks' his mind he, in effect, initiates in himself a process of drastic quantitative reduction (and, arguably, elimination) of 'normal' thought formation which, as Vihvelin pointed out, constitutes the initial stage of hypnagogia, and which is inevitably followed by qualitative thought changes. Thus it transpires that various psi activities occurring under conditions prevailing in (a) comprise, in essence, phenomena taking place in a sustained hypnagogia, and those occurring under conditions prevailing in (b) argue that psi phenomena tend to occur naturally in a state of hypnagogia.

In regard to the second feature, viz. that of awareness that one is involved in a psi activity, this clearly constitutes the subject's mental set. By itself it would undoubtedly 'bias' the interpretation of any phenomena that might appear during the experiment or psychic exercise. This is not to depreciate the fact that results in psi experiments often reach high levels of significance, but to point out that if psi and hypnagogic experiences are phenomenologically the same then the most important distinguishing factor might be the percipient's or subject's mental set. In which case the calling of a phenomenon a hypnagogic experience or a psi event may be seen purely as a label we employ to indicate the type of functional significance we ascribe to it at the time of its occurrence.

The third feature, that of feeling alert during paranormal activities, is clearly referring to the mental state of the subject in respect to his imaginal environment and not to his physical surroundings – it resembles more a state of being awake in a dream or dreaming while awake rather than of ordinary wakefulness. It may thus be closely related to the sense of certainty or conviction referred to by both psi and hypnagogic objects. Significantly, this state of alertness is reported as occurring *after* the process of induction of psychophysical relaxation, quantitative reduction of thought processes, and elimination of analytical thinking. This process, however, would in most cases, as we saw, lead to sleep unless it is checked.

It might be objected to at this point that even if psi induction is in essence hypnagogic it ceases to be so when, at this stage of withdrawal, the process is prevented from leading into sleep. Against this argument, there are two important sets of observations. The first comes from our knowledge that a person in hypnagogia, having become aware of the unfolding hypnagogic imagery, may become further interested in it, a fact which, as Alexander pointed out, 'tends to prolong the hypnagogic period and so to multiply the number of the images'.[104] Thus the prolongation of hypnagogia and its prevention from leading into sleep may happen naturally in a non-psi climate. Moreover, the longer the hypnagogic period the greater is often the resultant *internal alertness*. We may remind ourselves of Monroe's remark that the practice of holding the borderland state 'indefinitely without falling asleep' results in 'consciousness deepening'.[105]

The second set of observations argues that the production of hypnagogic imagery is not necessarily linked with the process of falling asleep.[106] This apparent contradiction in terms argues in essence that 'falling asleep', just like 'engaging in psi', constitutes the set and setting of the subject and that all the known hypnagogic phenomena may take place in the absence of such set and setting. This may widen the function of hypnagogic imagery, or rather of those phenomena studied under the set and setting of hypnagogia, in that they can be seen to occur in other states under circumstances that need not be 'hypnagogic'.

Subject-state interface and other considerations

The above arguments are in no way to contend that psi activities are always and in all subjects hypnagogic in the sense of *necessarily* tending to lead into sleep. As in the case of hypnagogia whereby attending, or learning to attend, to one's imagery prolongs the phenomena and increases internal alertness, one can learn to enter a psi state simply by evoking the appropriate mental attitude – 'tuning-in' or shifting to another reality, as it is often put. In this manner, physical relaxation becomes a mere concomitant of the subject's absorption into internal space: as in double-consciousness in hypnagogia, the person in this psi state is awake, i.e. retains reality testing, but primarily attentive to, or absorbed in, another reality. But just as in hypnagogia a person normally needs a certain amount of practice in order to learn to balance himself between wakefulness and sleep and achieve a state of dreaming while awake, so the aspiring psychic too goes through a period of hypnagogizing, and often falling asleep in the process, before learning to retain wakefulness throughout the experience.[107]

It is thus of great importance to take into account the amount of training a person has had (or his natural aptitude or ability, which amounts to the same thing). This is a question of subject-state interface. Ignoring this often gives rise to confusion as to whether during a psi activity a psychic is relaxed, absorbed, fully awake, or whatnot. The values of the psi-conducive syndrome as a whole are highly dependent on this interface. So much so that a person who is, for example, by temperament very relaxed may need little or no 'shift' in this direction when entering a psi state. Similarly, if one is able by nature or training to 'tune-in' at an instant, the shift in these values may be hardly noticeable both to the observers/experimenters and to oneself. The situation invites parallels from other fields, such as the comparison between the effort required on the part of an average individual to balance himself on a tightrope as opposed to the almost effortless balancing of a trained acrobat, or the enormous effort expended by the average individual again to solve a particular problem whose solution is immediate and embarrassingly too obvious to the mind of an Einstein or a child prodigy.

Then we have those cases of psi functioning during states of great excitement, danger, fever or overpowering desire, none of which can be said to be conducive to falling asleep. These are cases of extreme activation of the active mode which leads to a 'jamming of the circuits' and a sudden switch to the receptive mode (see chapters 3 and 5). In the previous chapter the suggestion was made that certain mystical experiences are of this nature, and that the same is probably true of some forms of psychosis. (The latter argument will be further developed in the next chapter.) What is of relevance here is not so much the presence or absence of sleep-inducing conditions as such as the clear presence of a modal shift to a state which resembles in many respects that of wakeful dreaming.

7 · Schizophrenia

Comparisons between hypnagogic and schizophrenic mentation have been drawn by various authors, all of whom would agree that the study of hypnagogia should enhance our understanding of both pathological states in abnormal individuals and of 'abnormal' states in the normal population. As McKellar and Simpson put it in pointing to the phenomenological similarities between schizophrenic and hypnagogic experiences, 'to understand abnormal mental occurrences more fully, it may be necessary to examine abnormalities themselves in terms of *seemingly* abnormal experiences which a psychotic merely shares with many nonpsychotic normal individuals.'[1] Hypnagogia is arguably the only naturally occurring state of consciousness in which sane people can get at least an insight into the nature of insanity.

In what follows I shall confine myself mainly to the task of identifying phenomenological features common both to hypnagogia and schizophrenia, and examine briefly arguments suggesting that hypnagogic experiences are pathogenic in nature. I shall not argue for a complete phenomenological identification of schizophrenia with hypnagogia. This is partly because the term schizophrenia is a collective one comprising a group of disturbances not all of which can be said to have the same aetiology and phenomenology.[2] I shall, however, continue to use the term as a convenient umbrella to cover a number of symptoms that may loosely represent the core of an entity. For the sake of clarity I shall begin by briefly outlining the four major types comprising the clinical picture of idiopathic schizophrenia and their generally correlated six principal disturbances, and seek to identify the latter in the phenomenology of hypnagogia.

Schizophrenic disturbances and their features

The six principal disturbances in schizophrenia, according to Mayer-Gross *et al.*, are: (1) disturbance of thinking, (2) disturbance of emotions, (3) disturbance of volition, (4) catatonic symptoms, (5) primary delusions, (6) hallucinations. These disturbances are readily correlated with the four types comprising the clinical picture of schizophrenia, viz. simple, hebephrenic, catatonic, and paranoid:

> Loss of affective response is the leading symptom of simple schizophrenia. Thought disorder, emotional abnormalities and volitional weaknesses constitute, in varied distribution, the hebephrenic form. Catatonic symptoms predominate in the catatonic type, often accompanied by volitional and emotional disturbances. Primary delusions followed by secondary delusional interpretations may be present in all types except in the simple schizophrenic.[3]

Ever since Kraepelin's bringing together of a number of symptoms to describe the collective disease entity dementia praecox, workers in this area have been trying to identify a fundamental disturbance that would characterize the illness. Stransky proposed 'intrapsychic ataxia' as the basic symptom and described it as a lack of co-ordination between thinking (noö-psyche) and emotions (thymo-psyche), now generally referred to as incongruity of affect.[4] Bleuler saw the 'splitting' as primarily a thinking disturbance appearing as the result of the loosening in the association of ideas through which repressed complexes and unconscious wishes emerge to gain the upper hand and disrupt the personality.[5] Jung considered schizophrenia to be psychologically identical with dreams and hysteria.[6] Berze pointed out as the primary disturbance 'insufficiency and lowering of psychic activity'.[7] Mayer-Gross *et al.* comment that

> The lowered mental activity may prevent the making of a clear distinction between what is real and what is imaginary, so that the schizophrenic indulges in delusional ways of thinking and behaving. Other authors have used as a comparison the half-waking state of the normal person going to sleep. A person in this state may have similar difficulties . . . in distinguishing between reality and imagination.[8]

Cameron proposed as an essential symptom an overinclusiveness in thinking, defined as 'an inability to preserve conceptual boundaries, resulting in incorporation of irrelevant ideas leading to vagueness and confusion of thought'.[9] Payne held that this might be the outcome of a breakdown in a 'filter' mechanism which screens out stimuli that are not relevant to a task at hand.[10] McReynolds considered overinclusiveness to be the result of a high level of unassimilated percepts which 'tends to reduce the degree of rigorousness or strictness which the patient habitually requires for assimilating percepts' [viz. perceptions and images].[11]

Although I shall examine some of these theories in more detail later, it is in place to draw attention here to the above observations and hypotheses arguing for 'dissociation', 'loosening of associational links', 'overinclusiveness', 'breakdown of a filter mechanism' and the laxity of categorizing, as they also typically apply to hypnagogia. Let us now look at the schizophrenic disturbances and their relationship to hypnagogic mentation and behaviour.

The main anomalies of the thought process in schizophrenia may be grouped as follows: loosening in the association of ideas, dissociated thinking, overinclusiveness in conceptualization, thought blocking and thought withdrawal, pressure of thought, thoughts spoken aloud or *echo de pensée*, and thoughts 'put into' the patient's mind. Mayer-Gross *et al.*, having pointed out that schizophrenic thought disorder is an abnormality of the thought process and not an abnormality of the ideas which may be expressed by the patient, further note that it 'has other aspects than a simple disconnection of thought or the putting together of overtly disconnected ideas', viz.:

> In early cases it often appears as a 'woolly' vagueness, or as an inconsequential following of side-issues which lead away from the main topic of conversation. . . . The patient's thought is directed by alliterations, analogies, clang associations, associations with the accidents of his environment, symbolic meanings, and the condensations into one of several, perhaps mutually contradictory ideas. The effect is sometimes like that of wit, and indeed may be on occasion genuinely witty; and the patient may therefore appear facetious or jocular when speaking about serious subjects. Words are used out of context, as it were, a concrete meaning being employed when the abstract would be more appropriate, and vice versa.[12]

Below are two examples of schizophrenic thinking from Mayer-Gross *et al.*, the first being a verbal report and the second an excerpt from a letter showing 'schizophrenic thought disorder, with incoherence, tangentiality, neologisms and ill-defined confluent paranoid delusional ideas':

> I feel that everything is sort of related to everybody and that some people are far more susceptible to this theory of relativity than others because of either having previous ancestors connected in some way or other places or things, or because of believing, or by leaving a trail behind when you walk through a room you know. Some people might leave a different trail and all sorts of things go like that.

> It is a tragedy perhaps, I find practically all the foreign human beings had this knowledge, and perhaps at least certain of our own Nationality such as myself and not, even my friends, comrades, where aware of the State Authorities must have been, which I feel you will accept as to be Sts – in all aspects revalent to delibirary to try and induce, such as been my lot, constant body, head, Activation numerical strong, and distant Voice face and body barrage.[13]

The authors add that the first patient 'claimed that this statement was a clear one, and showed signs of anger when asked to elucidate it'.

Another example, from Jaspers, illustrating the phenomenon of *flight of ideas*, is the response of a patient to her doctor's inquiry as to whether she had seen any changes in herself in the past year:

Yes, I was dumb and numb then but not deaf, I know Mrs Ida Teff, she is dead, probably an appendicitis; I don't know whether she lost her sight, sightless Hesse, His Highness of Hesse, sister Louise, His Highness of Baden, burried and dead on September, the twenty-eighth, 1907, when I get back, red-gold-red. . . . [14]

Describing 'Deborah's' state of mind while in a mental hospital, Hannah Green refers to her use of a language (Yri) 'whose metaphors used "broken" to mean "consenting" and "third rail" to mean "complying" . . . *Uguru* . . . was "dog-howling" and meant loneliness'. She speaks of 'the Yri logic and frame of words' which, although incomprehensible to the doctors and nursing staff, were perfectly meaningful to her, e.g.:

'*Recreat*', Deborah said, '*Recreat xangoran temr e xangoranan. Naza e fango xangoranan. Inai dum. Ageai dum.*' (Remember me. Remember me in anger, fear me in bitter anger. Heat-craze my teeth in bitterest anger. The signal glance drops. The Game' – Ageai meant the tearing of flesh with teeth as torture – 'is over.')

Another example from the same source reads:

'*There was a gear* . . . ' she cried aloud, and it came in Yri loud and mingled with strange words which were not hers. '*There was a gear all teeth, two at least world-caught. And now nothing, nothing engages with the world!*'[15]

Some shorter examples from other sources read: 'Do you know nase I'm sitting here . . . nice log . . . do I say those things . . . right a good nay . . . do you know what appetch I don't know . . . whaw appetch. That is a phona'; 'That means feling absence and rodential job'; 'Because it is a sort of hydrantic evering'.[16]

Schizophrenic-hypnagogic features

Practically all of the schizophrenic thought disturbances are encountered in hypnagogia. For instance, McKellar reports the case of a subject who at the end of an hour-long hypnagogic experiment was asked to explain the meaning of the proverb 'Too many cooks spoil the broth'. 'In her drowsy state', McKellar says, 'she was unable to do this, but reported an immediate image of "little men in white overalls . . . there were two . . . two men". The image suggests not merely an interesting concretization of cooks in white overalls, but also a product of clang association, "too many – two men".'[17]

Hypnagogic thinking may also contain pompous nonsense, pseudo or genuine witticism, neologisms, or symbolic meanings – all of which may, at the time, be meaningful to the subject. Here are four examples from Schjelderup-Ebbe: 'He is good as cake double'; 'The pencil holds well. To the sidewalk with Tell too'; 'Trifler, oh Brussels, bring a sail'; 'Conceit is not often being named a phantabilit'.[18] Two examples from Trömner read: 'He regally escaped into his existence', 'Yellow red and protestant means the sooner the better'. Trömner comments that 'they completely correspond to the word-salad of dementia praecox: nonsense of content but retention of linguistic structure'.[19] Archer reports the following personal example: 'A leading clerk is a great thing in my profession, as well as a Sabine footertootro', and comments, 'I had an impression on awakening that the last two words meant "feminine inspector" – that that was the idea in my mind, though I had been seized with aphasia in trying to express it.'[20] An experience very similar to that of Archer is reported by Froeschels who, on falling asleep, had the thought: 'Most important in every-day life are the littions', and on which he comments that at the time he 'was fully aware of the meaning of "littions" namely "trifles"'. Froeschels offers twenty-eight examples taken at random out of a much larger number. Here are a few of them: 'One of the most characteristic features is the acceleration of the sixteen', 'They are exposed to verbally intellection', 'Understanding is adversability to understanding', 'A Burul house schillinger to cook plate', 'Amarande es tifiercia', 'Knows how tampala sounds', 'And find that all with syphilis is immediately', 'To produce easier spice primitive of that speace (or spiece?)'.[21]

Similar examples are presented by, among others, McKellar, van Dusen and Oswald, who also give instances of hypnagogic witticism.[22] Oswald offers a choice one in doggerel verse that appeared in the *New Statesman*:

> Only God and Henry Ford
> Have no umbilical cord.

Apart from the above which are examples of hypnagogic thoughts or voices heard in one's own or in some other recognizable or unrecognizable voice, there are numerous examples of hypnagogic speech, that is, speech uttered by the subject while falling asleep or awaking, and which illustrate thought disturbances like those encountered in schizophrenic speech. The reader will recognize the following two examples which have already been reported in chapter 2 (section on 'Speech phenomena'). In the first, from McKellar, one young woman awoke to find herself murmuring 'put the pink pyjamas in the salad'. In the second, from Hollingworth, the author himself responded to his wife's 'Let's hurry and get there by ten o'clock', by saying drowsily 'Oh, that's easy, I could get there by a nickel to ten'. An example from Alexander reads, 'Our mind is not one of those (which Wesley's was) in which the relation of mind to subject is one of subject turned over and then fished up again.'[23] Schultz mentions the case of a 28-year-old woman who reported that while in hypnagogia

> [I] felt a strange compulsion to pronounce words that I did not want to say and words that did not make any sense at the time, like: wild flower, wild animal. I knew that I was saying them and I was ashamed of myself in case anyone heard, but I had to say them.[24]

Another of his subjects reported:

> ... as if in a semi-dream – I do not know how to describe this
> condition, but I know for certain that I am still awake – it seems to me
> as if someone wants to break into my house. It has happened that I
> jumped out of bed, ran, tried to escape and also took my child, only the
> locked door and the crying of the child (who is 11 years old and strong)
> brought back my consciousness and then I laid down again; ... At a
> similar occasion I shouted at my neighbour: 'what do you want with
> the night dishes?' She got up and answered that she could not
> understand me.

Schultz cites a number of cases which show in operation schizophrenic
features and phenomenology, such as: the unusual frequency of hallucinations; the bizarreness of associations; the complex character of hypnagogic
hallucinations extending to more than one sensory organ which may give a
feeling of reality; the symbolic and phantasy-like way of coping with one's
hypnagogic experiences; the attitude with which one regards these experiences,
i.e. without any trace of surprise, as something normal arising from one's
own personality; visual hallucinations serving as the basis of hypochondriac
delusions; diffused and very lively objectified physical sensations; the
complexity of the thinking process; the shifting or abolition of borders
between the Ego and the external world; the cosmic identification; the
experience that the world is ending.

An example of hypnopompic speech given by Mintz illustrates the presence
of symbolic meaning, of metaphor and analogy, 'inexact approximation', and
a state of certainty (awareness of significance) regarding the validity of the
subject's frame of reference (FR) which is not to be doubted by outsiders, i.e.
by waking, logical frames of reference (FsR):

> A 24-year-old married woman, normal, woke up one morning; her
> husband was already up. Seeing him, she said, 'Light the towel' (the
> couple was Russian; another translation of the Russian phrase is 'set the
> towel on fire'). Her husband asked her what she meant. She repeated,
> 'Light the towel'. He again indicated lack of understanding. Thereupon
> she became angry; she said that he obviously understood what she had
> meant but was pedantic enough to insist that she should express herself
> precisely. He should light the towel, that is (after a hesitation), raise the
> window shade. Subsequently, when the husband stated that he still did
> not understand why she had spoken of lighting a towel, she explained
> that lighting (or setting on fire) makes light and that a towel and a
> window shade are similar in shape.[25]

Another example, from Froeschels, reads, 'I say: "Not afterwards, but
immediately", knowing that "immediately" means "into three equal parts".'[26]

I shall dwell on these examples for a while as I believe they provide good
illustrations of a number of thought disturbances, or aspects of a core

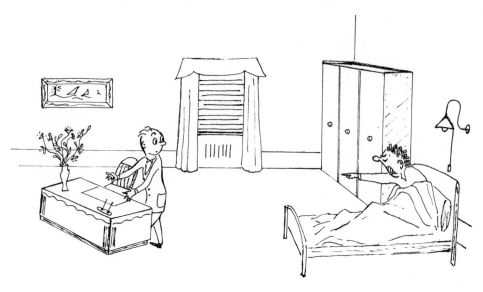

Figure 7.1 *'Light the towel. . . . You know what I mean, damn it! Raise the window shade!'*

thought anomaly, whose study and analysis may shed light on their functional presence both in hypnagogia and in schizophrenia.

To begin with, there is, as noted above, the clear presence of symbolic meaning in that the subject in Mintz's example uses the expression 'to set on fire' to stand for 'lighting' and 'towel' for 'window shade'; in Archer's example the word 'footertootro' stands for 'feminine inspector'; in Froeschel's 'littions' stands for 'trifles' and 'immediately' for 'into three equal parts'. These examples are not dissimilar to Green's 'broken' = 'consenting', 'third rail' = 'complying', and 'Uguru' = 'loneliness'. Moreover, the utterances themselves as well as both the mental attitude and explanations of the subjects strongly suggest that the latter are not only employing a frame of reference structured according to particular rules but also that perhaps the very essence of these rules is to allow the crossing of a number of FsR. The result is often an expressed identity between normally unrelated concepts. This may in fact be the cause underlying many cases of neologism, that is, neologisms may constitute the audible product of the confluence and condensation of a number of FsR and may encompass anything from known words with slight but often ungrammatical changes in their structure to completely new words that stand for simple or complex meanings. The experience-utterance of neologisms, symbolic words or sentences, and metaphors in both hypnagogia and in schizophrenia may be accompanied by a feeling of certainty regarding the truthfulness and validity of the statements made, as illustrated by the Mayer-Gross *et al.* first example in respect to schizophrenia, and the Schjelderup-Ebbe, Archer, Froeschels and Mintz examples in respect to hypnagogia.

The LEBs, hypnagogic mentation, and delusions

In analysing his own hypnagogic experiences Froeschels argues that in the transitional state between waking and sleeping

> two levels of the personality were in conflict with each other. The one was the logical thinking with its corresponding feeling of certainty – which we are accustomed to perceive while in the state of being awake; the other was an additional mental process which behaved as if it were logical and carried with it another feeling of certainty. The logic and the joined feeling of certainty as perceived in the state of being awake rejected as wrong the corresponding processes that were going on in the state of transition.[21]

It must be noted that Froeschels probably recorded his experiences from a light stage of hypnagogia in which the waking mind 'felt irritated' and 'reacted' against the emerging phenomena. Thus he distinguishes between two kinds of a feeling of certainty and considers the one accompanying hypnagogic thinking as inferior to that 'we regularly attain through the logical work of our waking mind'. Of course, had he allowed himself to progress deeper into hypnagogia, the 'corresponding' feeling of certainty in this state would most certainly have increased in proportion to the increase of his withdrawal from wakefulness and in proportion to diminishing critical attitude, thus dissolving Froeschels's distinction. Indeed, the distinction is hardly warranted in the first place. As Poincaré noted in respect to inspiration in the mathematical field, this feeling is just as vivid and convincing whether experienced in wakefulness or hypnagogia.[27]

As argued in other chapters of this book, the feeling of certainty, conviction, or sense of significance may occur on its own, unrelated to any logical activity, and its presence in the latter is merely contingent and no guarantee of the truth or validity of logical transactions.[28] Experientially, it is an accompaniment of *facts*, be these thoughts, perceptions, sensations, or hallucinations, and its degree of strength is a function of attention paid to these thoughts, perceptions, sensations or hallucinations. In the ordinary waking state this feeling is checked and controlled to a considerable extent by assumptions and generalizations of varying degrees of validity. It is important to note in this respect that in a logical activity, e.g. in carrying out a syllogism, it is the conclusion that furnishes us with a considerable degree of a feeling of certainty (or intellectual satisfaction), and that in experience in general it is the degree of absorption (closeness of subject to object) that gives rise to a corresponding degree in the feeling of certainty. In hypnagogia, especially in the deeper stages, attention is automatically absorbed thus closing the gap of intellectual reflection and diminishing the ability or tendency of the waking mind to take distinct and 'valid' steps in logical activities: for instance, it may leave out the major premise of a syllogism or appear starkly as a statement-conclusion without explicit premises, i.e. merely as a *fact*.

The differences between waking and hypnagogic mentation may be summarized thus (see also chapter 5, section on 'Sense of Reality'):

Waking mentation is based on distancing the subject from the object and the mental activity, and on employing abstract methods, e.g. the syllogism, generally considered to be valid forms of thinking, in order to draw conclusions.

Hypnagogic mentation closes the gap between subject and object blurring their differences and in many cases identifying the one with the other, and it diminishes or abolishes the gap between subject and mental activity (absence of reflection) thus leading to a kinesthetic or empathic method of knowing which 'enables' the subject to identify himself equally with any concept, resulting in the linking, overlapping or total identification of one concept with another.

Thus, the presence of the feeling of certainty often accompanying hypnagogic and schizophrenic experiences may be due to the tendency of the subject to be absorbed-withdrawn into spontaneously occurring thoughts, perceptions, images, etc. Such absorption-withdrawal would explain both the feeling of certainty (there is no room for doubt) and the tendency to relate ideas, concepts, one's ego etc., to other entities, events and so on. Clinicians and psychologists frequently complain of their inability to make contact with schizophrenic patients. Others report cases where during therapy schizophrenics have apparently communicated with them empathically on a subconscious level. It would appear that the schizophrenic, like the hypnagogist, has withdrawn his attention from the normal perceptual analytic environment and is functioning primarily in an absorbed imaginal world. Like the hypnagogist, the schizophrenic also tends to lose his *ego boundaries*. This is a feature of paramount importance as it seems to lie at the root of most experiential-cognitive phenomena encountered in both conditions. The loosening of ego boundaries (LEBs) has many ramifications and is represented, or manifests itself, at various levels of the individual's experience, encompassing body schema alterations and/or dissolution, internalization of external sensations/perceptions, identification with other egos, blurring, overlapping or assimilation of concepts, and dissociation.

We have already seen that in hypnagogia body schema alterations may take various forms, and that not infrequently the hypnagogist may lose his body schema altogether or that events outside himself are experienced 'as something happening to and around his own body'. Isakower points out two consecutive processes characteristic of sleep onset: a disintegration of the various parts and functions of the ego, and a diminution of the ego's differentiation.[29] This is in agreement with my proposition above that the

LEBs is the initial and initiating factor lying behind hypnagogic phenomena. As Isakower further notes, in the progression of hypnagogia the boundaries of the 'body. ego' (body schematization and identification) 'begin to be blurred and to become fused with the external world . . . perceptions are localized as sensations in a particular bodily region and at the same time as the processes in the external world. . . . It is natural to conjecture that the structure of the body ego in this state is comparable to that of the immediately post-natal ego.' At such a regressed state it is not unreasonable to assume that one is inundated by a 'buzzing, booming world'. This inundation, springing as it does from the LEBs, may account for the schizophrenic blurring of concepts and for the phenomenon of schizophrenic ambivalence. At the body level the loosening of body schema may account for many catatonic phenomena such as catatonic postures; the inundation may account for catatonic word-salad. Indeed, Federn proposes that the LEBs is not merely a symptom of schizophrenia but the very process responsible for it.[30]

McKellar and Simpson have drawn attention to kinesthetic hypnagogic hallucinations of body schema alterations, noting that these are similar to the sensory experiences that form the basis of psychotic delusions of bodily change.[1] Isakower further comments that

> the fully developed delusion that the world is coming to an end, as we meet with it in schizophrenia, is commonly preceded by manifestations of ego-disintegration, accompanied by a hypersensibility to external impressions and by temporal and spatial distortions of the objects perceived. . . . In such a condition the patient himself often feels that the difference between waking and sleeping has vanished.

Moreover, these manifestations described by Isakower are not singularly the prodromes and accompaniments of a specific delusion, viz. that the world is coming to an end, but are to be found with the genesis of all delusions.

In schizophrenia, Jaspers differentiated between delusional perceptions, delusional ideas and notions, and delusional awareness. In the first group of experiences the patient seems to endow an apparently normal perception with unaccountable significance. In the second, a passing thought suddenly generates unwarranted conviction. In the third, the patient suddenly feels that he is in possession of knowledge of cosmic importance, which is not related to any previous relevant thought or perception. Although the phenomena of the third group are not infrequent in hypnagogia,[31] those in the second group are much more commonly reported and appear most often as the conclusions with inadequate or missing premises spoken of above. That is, a passing thought suddenly appears pregnant with meaning, a meaning which may then become explicable to the subject as being contained in a conclusion-revelation behind which may lie the implications of a complex series of premises. In regard to delusional perceptions, these may be seen in hypnagogia as the effects of misperception, and in schizophrenia there is evidence that in some cases delusions as well as abnormal concept formation may be traced to disturbances of perception and cognition.[32] Mayer-Gross *et al.* attribute the experience of primary delusion to disturbance of symbolization.

However, whether we speak of disturbances of perception and cognition or disturbance of symbolization, it seems that the actual experience involves the seizing by the subject or patient of properties of one or more perceptions, thoughts, or concepts which properties are *felt to be essential*, i.e. as expressing the essence of the said perceptions, thoughts, or concepts. And this is the direct result of the LEBs. Now, the LEBs is to be thought of as a core event whose manifestations, as noted earlier, make their appearance on all the experiential levels of the individual. We have seen that at a particular stage of hypnagogia there is a hypersensitivity to external impressions. These are not only felt internally kinesthetically but, due to the LEBs on a higher (cognitive) level, they result in illusions or spatial distortions of physical objects as well as of images which, coupled with the accompanying fascination, acquire an, often unwarranted, significance.

In such a state, physical objects and images are merely *posited* and their strongest and most concrete features are taken to represent them, or even totally replace them. But we must also bear in mind that in this state subconscious and unconscious activities are very much to the fore, bringing forth their own 'interpretation' of what is the strongest and most representative feature of an object or image, and these features or qualities may not necessarily be the same as those thought by the waking mind to be the most important in characterizing an object or concept. This activity, then, of seizing upon essential features, takes place within a setting of LEBs whose character of diverging, 'spreading', and blurring tends to shift the importance placed by the waking mind on certain properties. Moreover, due to the LEBs, more than one FR comes into play simultaneously. Thus the subject or patient may be presented with a percept, an image, or a concept that suddenly acquires a significance which is beyond and unrelated to that normally ascribed to it.

The sense of conviction encountered in primary delusions and many hypnagogic experiences is also found to accompany hypnagogic and schizophrenic hallucinations. Its occurrence in the former has been discussed in other chapters. In regard to its presence in schizophrenic hallucinations, Mayer-Gross *et al.* note that the latter's '"unreal" appearance, even if recognized, does not reduce the patient's belief in their reality and importance. They are, in fact, frequently accepted with the same conviction as primary delusions.'[33] And, although many schizophrenic hallucinations are thought to occur in a setting of clear consciousness, this is by no means always the case. So much so that Berze attributed their appearance to reduced mental control, and Schneider, equating schizophrenia with hypnagogia, regarded hallucinations as the inevitable outcome of the general condition.[34]

Writing on Conrad's five-phase classification of schizophrenia, Fish explains that the second or apophanous phase is divided into two subphases, namely, 'apophany of external space and apophany of internal space. In the first, all external events which are experienced acquire a new significance, while in the latter internal psychic events acquire special meaning.'[35] He further proposes that

> this undue prominence of essential properties explains the misidentification of persons which is common in the apophanous phase. Unknown persons may be recognized as friends or acquaintances, while relatives and friends are not recognized as such by the patient. The emerging essential properties can be considered as causing these confusions of identity.

In hypnagogia we encountered these anomalies of recognition as the *déjà vu* and *jamais vu* phenomena, and although these may be an effect of the coming into prominence of the 'essential' properties of an object, image or concept, in their turn these properties, as argued above, are brought into prominence by the LEBs.

In respect to 'apophany of internal space', Fish says that

> once internal space is affected, there is a loosening of the coherence of the mediating processes. Memory images may lose their connection with the total field and be experienced as delusional inspirations. Thought broadcasting in which the patient's thoughts become manifest to the environment can be regarded as the reverse of delusional perception, where a new significance of a perception becomes manifest to the patient. The loss of adequate figure ground relationships in conceptual thinking naturally leads to the patient hearing his own thoughts spoken aloud, . . .

In this quotation there are a number of statements bearing directly on the state of hypnagogia and which are worth looking into more closely. First, there is the opening sentence in which Fish states that 'once internal space is affected, there is a loosening of the coherence of the mediating process'. This condition can be comfortably interpreted as the result of the LEBs. As proposed above, one of the manifestations of the LEBs is the blurring and overlapping of concepts and the relating or assimilating of concepts normally unrelated to one another. The LEBs allow for the emergence of the 'essential' properties of concepts with which the subject then identifies. We might say that the 'essence' of the subject acts as a link between the 'essential' properties of two or more concepts (objects, images, etc.). This could be interpreted as a form of withdrawal from one's immediate environment and thus account for the inability of psychiatrists to make contact with their patients.

Second, in hypnagogia as in schizophrenia, memories are often disturbed, although I would disagree with Fish in that I do not think that delusional inspirations are singularly, or even primarily, related to disturbances of memory. In hypnagogia there is a variety of memory phenomena. In keeping with the argument that in hypnagogia there is a considerable degree of regression (in a temporal sense), Kubie has demonstrated 'the recovery of repressed amnesic data'. Before him, Maury had also given examples of recovering forgotten memories.[36] The phenomena of *jamais vu* and *déjà vu* have already been noted; also, difficulty may be experienced in recalling known names and concepts, as in Archer's example in the previous section which demonstrates the phenomenon of 'thought blocking'. In *déjà vu*, it is likely that the sudden strong conviction accompanying the sense of familiarity concerning an event which is experienced as having already taken place in the past may encourage the emergence of delusions. On the other hand, the feeling of sudden discovery in the phenomenon of *jamais vu* may indeed give rise to delusional inspiration, although in the state of hypnagogia this feeling may not necessarily emerge in a climate of real paramnesia. In fact, the feeling of inspiration, in hypnagogia and elsewhere, may emerge as the effect or accompaniment of the coming together of two or more FsR in a novel relationship. Third, Fish makes reference to thought broadcasting or *echo de pensée* and, speaking in gestalt terms, he rightly attributes this to the loss of adequate figure-ground relationships. But, again, the latter is, according to my hypothesis, brought into play by the LEBs which allows for the blurring of distinctions between figure and ground.

The gradual LEBs naturally leads to the diminishing and eventual dissolution of defining distinctions between subject and object. This implies the ever-decreasing presence of self-awareness. As Maury observed, in hypnagogia the mind 'ceases to have a clear awareness of the self, and it is to a certain extent passive, absorbed in the objects which strike it; it perceives, sees, hears, but without noticing that it is perceiving, seeing, and hearing.'[37] Elsewhere Maury also suggested that for the subject in hypnagogia the sense of time and space loses its clarity or is lost altogether;[38] this compares well with Isakower's observation that in schizophrenic delusions there occur 'temporal and spatial distortions'.

Hypnagogists, madmen, and absent-minded individuals

Maury proposed that the hypnagogist, the madman, and the absent-minded person appear to behave in the same manner as a result of psychological withdrawal, and although he attempts to distinguish between the form of withdrawal present in hypnagogia on the one hand, and that present in madness and in absent-mindedness on the other, we shall presently see that the grounds for such distinction are not very strong.

First, he made the important observation that in hypnagogic speech the subject's utterance in response to a question is essentially a response to internal activity of a special kind. He writes:

it sometimes happened to me that, by a retrospective reflection, I managed to grasp a link between several of these words and what was happening in my mind. These incoherent sentences express the idea or the image that was in front of my eyes at the very moment when my interlocutor alerted my attention with his question. One talks to me, I immediately answer and I express what I was seeing at the very moment when I was questioned. One day, for example, the person who was reading asks me a question on the passage he had just read; I answer: 'There is no tobacco in this place', which had no relation in words nor sounds with the sentence addressed to me. My answer naturally provokes a noisy hilarity and my drowsiness is suddenly dispelled. I had only a vague awareness of what I had just said, but my memory still retained a few of the idea-images which had taken place in the eyes of my imagination; and I remembered then that the idea of tobacco had come to my mind in the middle of a disorderly train of a host of words and ideas linked to one another. And why that dream? My sneezing provided the explanation: a few grains of tobacco which had remained in my nose, after I had accepted some tobacco from a snuff-box, acting on my olfactory membrane conveyed to my brain the sensation which, at the time, I was not aware of.

Then, having related the above with the kind of mentation encountered in childhood, idiocy, and old age on the ground of their sharing a characteristic factor, namely, the inability to focus active attention, he further compares hypnagogic passive absorption with that of the madman and the absent-minded person noting that the *actual absorbed state* all these people find themselves in is the same although they differ in the manner in which they severally reach it, and in their ability to respond to stimuli in their immediate environment. That is to say, whereas hypnagogic absorption is the result of weakness of (active) attention, that of the madman and the absent-minded person is achieved by intense (active) attention; and whereas the latter two, although absorbed in their thoughts, can communicate verbally with their environment when interrupted, the hypnagogist 'does not have the strength to apply his attention to the object he is shown, and his talking is only an echo of the idea he is mechanically contemplating.'

A number of important points are made in Maury's observations and discussions above which deserve further examination and analysis as they relate directly to my current arguments. To begin with, Maury's example demonstrates clearly hypnagogic withdrawal and absorption: the hypnagogist is so withdrawn and absorbed in his internal (mental) environment that external stimuli can only manage to elicit what is clearly a response not to the latter but to the former, i.e. to current imaginal activity, thus throwing some light on the origins of 'irrelevant' hypnagogic utterances and showing them to be irrelevant only in an external FR. Moreover, due to the graded nature of hypnagogia, there are stages in which the hypnagogist may be able to respond to a greater or to a lesser extent to his external environment. An example of the former kind would be Hollingworth's response, 'Oh, that's easy. I could get there by a nickel to ten', showing an inability to transfer completely to an external environment and instead crossing two FsR, those of time and money. Maury's example, and that of McKellar, 'Put the pink pyjamas in the salad', among others, might serve as illustrations of the latter kind. Maury's and McKellar's examples, like those of Schjelderup-Ebbe and Archer, are also characteristically 'egocentric', that is, they are not addressed to anybody in particular.

Further, Maury's example is an illustration of how in hypnagogia a subliminal perception acting subconsciously gives rise to an image and an idea in the midst of an ongoing 'disorderly train of a host of words and ideas', which image or idea then engages the hypnagogist's absorbed attention. In Maury's case the perception, although subliminal, led to the emergence of a logically relevant idea. However, this is not always the case. In many instances the sensations, including proprioceptive ones, are transformed into symbols, as in the case of Silberer's autosymbolic phenomena. Moreover, although physiologically there is an increase of sensitivity of, for instance, auditory signals from the external environment, as hypnagogia progresses these signals tend not only to be transformed but also incorporated in ongoing imaginal activities.

Thus, at any given level the hypnagogist is presented with a gradually altering external FR which is continually transformed and incorporated into an internal space which is itself passively and absorbedly attended to and which is populated by imagery whose coherence is often based on subconscious, mediate associations. External input would reach the subject distorted or transformed in degrees in accordance with the depth of the state. It can thus be said that as hypnagogia progresses towards sleep the perceptual barriers commonly thought of as appearing in this state are not true barriers, in the sense of preventing information reaching the subject, but rather *transformers*, allowing the flow of information but changing it to fit the requirements of the prevailing internal logic, a logic which is directly the result of the LEBs. Due to the latter, the subject's normal sense of distinguishing between subject and object is relaxed and, coupled with psychological withdrawal, many phenomena occurring in this state are experienced as taking place both *internally* (external input having undergone certain transformations and been incorporated into ongoing imaginal activities) and *externally*, i.e. as being 'out there' and beyond the subject's control. The contradiction here is only apparent and is resolved when we reflect on the state of absorption the subject is in: a state of fascinated attention characterized by lack or diminution of self-awareness, especially somatic self-awareness. And this state of fascination may be brought on either by passive (receptive) or intense active attention. In this respect the hypnagogist, the madman, and the absent-minded professor may be functioning in very similar states. Moreover, and contrary to Maury's argument, (a) the madman's absorption, like that of the hypnagogist's, is brought on by passive attention, and (b) neither the madman nor the absent-minded person differ from the hypnagogist in their readiness (or rather, lack of it) to respond to signals from the external reality.

In respect to (a), there are the well-attested phenomena of schizophrenic disturbance of volition. These phenomena have been studied and analysed under headings such as 'Primary insufficiency of psychic activity' and 'Ambivalence',[39] indicating the patients' passive attitude and inability to concentrate and follow one line of thought or action without distraction from other FsR. This weakness of volition is often attributed to disturbance of the self. Indeed, as Mayer-Gross *et al.* note,

> some workers have made the weakness or loss of the self the central symptom of schizophrenia. The *passivity phenomena* in which this loss is best seen are indeed very characteristic of schizophrenia. The patient tells us that his thoughts, feelings, speech and actions are not his own.[40]

And, as in hypnagogia, 'there are all transitions from full self-identification with the abnormal behaviour to complete passivity with full insight into the strange and alien nature of the experiences.'

Significantly, and in respect to my argument about the primacy of the core phenomenon of LEBs, Mayer-Gross *et al.* further note that

> in acute schizophrenia, a loosening or *blurring of the boundaries of the self* is often experienced: the patient feels that he is part of the plants, animals, clouds, or of the whole world, and that they are parts of himself.[41]

If, together with this, we bear in mind what these authors said above, viz. that the patient speaks of his thoughts, feelings, etc., as being 'not his own', we arrive at the same apparent contradiction met with in hypnagogia and discussed above, namely, the phenomenon in which thoughts, perceptions, etc., are experienced as occurring inside the subject and yet unfold 'out there' and beyond his control or instigation.

In respect to (b), evidence again shows that both the madman and the absent-minded person are so absorbed in internal activities and withdrawn from their immediate physical environment that they either do not respond to external stimuli or else they respond erroneously, that is, their responses are inappropriate. In the case of schizophrenia the patient, who is generally thought of as being withdrawn, responds inappropriately both intellectually and emotionally. That is, his thought content and the grammatical-logical structure of his verbal responses appear incongruent with ongoing external reality and stimuli. Indeed, emotional bluntness and incongruity of affect were the phenomena responsible for giving rise to the term 'schizophrenia' coined by Bleuler. In the case of absent-mindedness one may be referred to the numerous reports – admittedly anecdotal – of the behaviour of absent-minded professors. An example from antiquity demonstrating incongruity

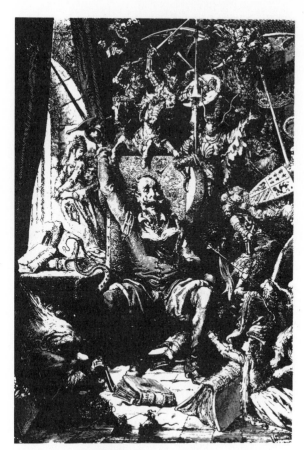

(a)

Figure 7.2 *Three examples illustrating the degree of detachment and absorption in another FR in madness, hypnagogia, and creativity: (a) Don Quixote surrounded by his hallucinations which, irrespective of whether or not he recognizes them as such, retain for him their reality and importance; (b) 'There is no tobacco in this place': drowsing during a lecture, Maury's response to the lecturer's question is irrelevant, and yet explicable and meaningful in its hypnagogic context;*

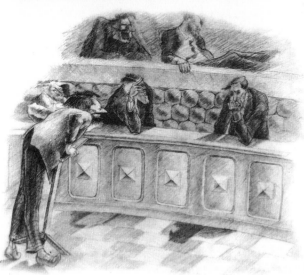

(b)

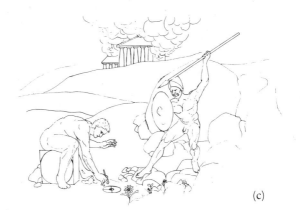

(c) 'Do not disturb my circles': absorbed in his geometrical calculations, Archimedes dismisses the invading soldier.

(c)

and flatness of affect is that of Archimedes who responded to the invading soldier about to spear him by saying 'do not disturb my circles'; his famous 'Eureka!' incident also demonstrates the degree of detachment from his physical environment and his absorption in another FR. For the sake of comparison we may remind ourselves here of one of Oswald's examples in which a drowsy subject, having bent down and kissed the EEG tape, reported, 'Leant forwards and downwards to plant a kiss upon the unmarried letters. £Coohch.'[42] As Oswald explains, this subject's mind was at the time probably occupied by the thought of his girlfriend's refusal to marry him. Concerning flatness of affect in hypnagogia, this has been noted by various workers (see chapter 3). Indeed, it has been remarked that 'some of the most hair-raising visions can be watched by the imager with surprising detachment'.[43]

In both hypnagogia and schizophrenia the subject, as noted, may not be totally withdrawn, thus retaining or re-establishing intermittent contact with his environment and having some insight into his imaginal experiences. However, even with the possession of such an insight the subject in either case is not always capable of thinking and acting entirely outside the FR created by his psychological withdrawal-absorption. Hence the phenomena of delusional interpretation, that is, the attempt by the subject to rationalize his imaginal experiences and make them fit into the intercurrent FR of the objective world. In hypnagogia this is often seen in the subjects' efforts to explain and justify their strange verbal responses. For instance, in Mintz's example the subject justifies her strange verbal expression by explaining the symbolism hidden in it. Singer, writing of his own experiences, says, 'I might actually fall asleep in midsentence, awaken abruptly and make a bizarre comment, notice the puzzled look on my friends' faces, and hastily seek to tie in the unrelated remark to the previous waking flow of conversation.'[44]

The logic involved

In Mintz's example we saw how a window shade was identified with a towel on the basis of their similarity of shape. Froeschels proposes that this tendency for identification without adequate discrimination is characteristic of hypnagogia, or 'state of transition' as he calls it.[25] He offers a number of examples to demonstrate this phenomenon, of which I quote two:

> While in the state of transition, I say: 'There is no communication between the bathroom and the hearing center'. (The previous evening I had been working on a paper concerning the hearing center and the visual center.) In the scheme of Wernicke-Lichtheim, centers are drawn in circles and are connected by lines. My living room and the bathroom are connected by a narrow passageway. The narrow, connecting passageway is common to the scheme of Wernicke-Lichtheim and the two rooms.

> Once in a transition state, I saw a piece of cloth suspended over the body of a woman. The right end of the cloth covered the body, while the remainder, approximately four-fifths of the whole, stood upright on the floor in an unknown way. The cloth is to be divided into three equal parts. I say: 'Not afterwards, but immediately,' knowing that 'immediately' means 'into three equal parts'. So space (dividing into parts) and time (immediately) are taken for one and the same.

Froeschels argues that, whereas for the waking mind the law of identity is strictly adhered to, in hypnagogia 'persons, animals, things, and functions, which seem to the waking mind entirely different or slightly similar, may be identical. *The transition state really identifies them.* They flow together into a unity.' Thus, in contrast to the waking mind which seeks to distinguish between equal and unequal, hypnagogia tends to operate on the principle of *similarity*. He further argues that this principle or category is derived from the subconscious:

> Of all the categorical terms which logic and epistemology has offered, *similarity* seems to be the one that characterizes best the basis upon which the subconscious works in the state of transition. *But this term evidently does not mean to the subconscious what it means to conscious reasoning.* The latter takes the feeling of similarity most of the time for a stepping stone on the way to thorough differentiation and identifi-cation. The subconscious on the other hand frequently considers similarity identical with identity, and does not bother with further 'research'.

According to Froeschels, then, hypnagogia tends to relate, unify and identify as opposed to differentiating and distinguishing. This is in agreement with my general proposition that hypnagogia is characterized by the LEBs resulting in the blurring of differences between one or more objects, concepts, etc. It also constitutes theoretical validation of the argument put forward earlier according to which mentation both in hypnagogia and in schizophrenia is primarily based on the subject's seizing what appear to him at the time to be essential properties of one or more objects or functions and that this is dependent on the core phenomenon of the LEBs. In chapter 3 I drew attention to the observation made by various workers that symbolization in hypnagogia tends not only to be subjective but also to unfold in imagery which carries a particular meaning *at the time of its occurrence*, i.e. the 'essential properties' of a particular image may differ on different occasions. Further, the image may hit the subject as both literal and metaphorical: the former is evidenced by the realness of the experience and the latter by the feeling of hidden significance or the actual 'knowledge' of what it means. Schultz spoke of 'the complexity of the thinking process' experienced by many subjects in this state, an observation which fits very well with my contention that both hypnagogic and schizophrenic thinking and speech express the crossing or mixing of two or more FsR.

Experiments carried out by Stransky may show at this point how hypnagogiclike-cum-schizophrenic speech may be produced in normal wakeful individuals under the influence of 'relaxed attention'. Stransky asked his subjects to say quickly, and without selecting, whatever came into their head. The result was a catatonia-like word-salad. As with hypnagogic imagery and speech, the resultant sequences appeared meaningless and irrelevant, full of alliterations, metaphors and 'a great deal of condensation, the gist of several sentences or words being merged into one sentence or word, with many resultant neologisms',[45] which, as already argued, are signs of the crossing of a number of FsR. Similar results were also obtained by Jung.[6]

A somewhat similar argument in respect to schizophrenia is put forward by Kasanin who says that 'a schizophrenic cannot abstract one principle while he neglects others. He takes all possibilities into simultaneous consideration.'[46] Angyal also proposes that although the schizophrenic is capable of comprehending relationships he fails in the apprehension of 'system-connections', that is, of sets, or FsR.[47] Thus, the schizophrenic appears to be shifting from one FR to another in a disorderly manner. Or rather, as I see it, he cuts across two or more FsR simultaneously. This often results in verbal absurdities which may sound witty or tragic.

An example from von Domarus illustrates how people, things, and functions clearly belonging to different FsR may be identified with one another in schizophrenia.[48] He cites the case of a schizophrenic who believed that Jesus, cigar boxes, and sex were identical on the basis of all three being encircled, that is, 'the head of Jesus, as of a saint, is encircled by a halo, the package of cigars by the tax band, and the woman by the sex glance of the man.' Thus the feelings experienced by this patient when he spoke of Jesus, a cigar package, or sex life were the same – an observation that may shed further light on the phenomenon of incongruity of affect and the delusional feelings and ideas experienced by both schizophrenics and hypnagogists. In this example – and in agreement with my line of argument – the accidental of 'being encircled' is seen by the patient as the essential property identifying a person, a thing, and an activity, much the same way that in Mintz's and Froeschels's hypnagogic examples the towel is identified with the window shade on the basis of their shape, and the living room and bathroom with the Wernicke-Lichtheim centres on the basis of their sharing the accidental quality of being connected by a 'passage'. In the paralogical thinking of both schizophrenia and hypnagogia, sameness or identity is concluded from identical predicates, or rather from one common predicate.[49]

As in the case of hypnagogia, von Domarus also considers schizophrenic speech to be egocentric. In this respect he says:

> In egocentric speech inner and outer speech are not yet separated. The inner speech proceeds by thinking in predicates rather than in subject-predicate sentences; . . . The paralogician expresses himself in egocentric speech habits, for his thinking is predicative and he has regressed to the egocentric speech of the child.

In such thinking, the law of contradiction is excluded since everything which lies outside the common intersection of two or more objects is irrelevant for their identification. In von Domarus's example, 'neither the nature of the "surroundings" nor that of the "surrounded" made any difference in the conclusion drawn.'

Schultz has also drawn attention to hypnagogic experiences such as 'the cosmic identification, the experience that the world is ending' which he believes to 'belong to the realm of schizophrenia' and which, together with other experiences, also to be found in hypnagogia, such as 'the complexity of the thinking process, the shifting or abolition of borders between the Ego and the external world', have been summarized by Storch as archaic-magic forms of experience.[50]

Archaic-magic features are clearly present in both hypnagogia and in schizophrenia in the paralogical process of identifying from single predicates. In primitive cultures, as well as in magical practices ancient and modern,[51] identification is effected merely on the basis of single predicates. For instance, the metal gold and the sun may be identified on the ground of both possessing the property 'yellow'. Moreover, more complex identifications may be effected on criss-cross references to other single properties. For instance, in the present example kingship may come to be identified with the sun and thus a king may come to wear gold-coloured or yellow garments and a golden crown (irrespective of the commercial value of gold). Or, the sun may be identified with life or a life-giving deity, for obvious reasons, which is then identified with the yellow flowers of certain plants, or with liquids or solids of the same colour.

This may explain to a certain degree the apparently irrelevant and illogical identifications presented in, for instance, Froeschels's example in which 'immediately' means 'into three equal parts', Archer's 'Footertootro' which means 'feminine inspector' and Green's 'third rail' meaning 'complying' and 'Uguru' meaning 'loneliness'. That is, the striking irrelevancy and illogicality of these identifications may be partly due to mediate predicate associations, i.e. to series of subconscious processes of identification based on similarities of predicates. This would mean that in the case of apparently entirely unrelated identifications, such as the above, there may be missing associating identifications. It also suggests that there are a number of FsR crowding the subject, and that the often observed syncretization or condensation is the result of bringing together these sets in a climate of openness and passivity. Not infrequently, schizophrenics engage in complex and apparently invalid explanations which clearly traverse many FsR, and yet the patients feel very confident about the validity of their conclusions and identifications. Just as often, hypnagogic subjects report apparently irrelevant thoughts and verbalizations which, as we have seen, are to them at the time meaningful identifications pregnant with a sense of significance.

Dissociation and fusion

In both hypnagogia and schizophrenia we have, due to the LEBs, the peculiar phenomenon of simultaneous dissociation and fusion. In both, one of the most important features is that of psychological withdrawal from one's external and/or social environment, which is another way of saying that a person dissociates himself from these environments. As withdrawal sets in, more and more normally associated functions, concepts, memories, logical activities, ego controls, ego schemata, etc., become dissociated. Thus dissociation is here a multifaceted affair.

But, significantly, as these aspects of experience become dissociated they recombine or fuse themselves into a different, 'wider', whole (or 'self') which typically allows them to cross boundaries and link in 'unusual', 'abnormal', or 'paranormal' ways. Within this new FR we may have, as already seen, the condensation of many images, ideas, and functions which may severally belong to different and normally unrelated FsR. Condensation of two or more words results in neologisms. Condensation of two or more ideas gives rise to complex, if faulty, systems of conceptualization where an idea is made to stand for more than it is normally meant to, such as acquiring, in addition to its normal meaning (or, unrelated to it), a symbolic one, as can be seen from examples in chapters 5 and 6. Different ideas may combine (condense) into one, again resulting in neologisms or, more significantly, in paralogically widened classifications. The latter, which are most frequently encountered in schizophrenic thinking, have been referred to by various investigators as overinclusiveness, inappropriate broadening of concepts, and openness,[52] all agreeing on the tendency of the patient to include in a given category a greater variety of objects than it is thought permissible. It has also been suggested that maladjusted persons tend to think in terms of supraordinates, or higher level abstractions[53] – a phenomenon, by the way, which is also found in the thinking of mystics who are not necessarily 'maladjusted' but who certainly view the world in a FR generally difficult to comprehend.

It is noteworthy that some writers have proposed that in normal individuals there is a basic tendency towards harmonious self-consistency, and the avoiding or getting rid of incongruence, dissonance and disparity, or, as Kelly has argued, the building of personal constructs in such a manner as to minimize incompatibilities.[54] The last author specifically proposes that the loosening of one's personal constructs is conducive to the lessening of anxiety. The same is believed by Hyman and Arieti to be effected by a blurring or imprecision in conceptualization.[55] Similarly, McReynolds, having proposed that 'the primary "cause" of schizophrenia is an extremely high quantity of unassimilated percepts', sees the reduction in the strictness of conceptualizing as a way of avoiding incongruencies and anxiety arising thereof.[11] This is in agreement with observations and theories presented by other investigators who argue that schizophrenic symptoms first appear at the peak of a crisis in the life of an individual and that they are the result of such a crisis.

If such theories are correct, then the paralogical widening of classifications as a schizophrenic symptom which reduces the patient's anxiety can be found in full swing in hypnagogia, in addition to its presence as a 'disturbance' of thought. Indeed, reduction of anxiety, or relaxation, is, as we know, a constituent of the hypnagogic syndrome. We know that hypnagogic experiences take place against a background of increasing relaxation and receptivity and that tension or anxiety is apt to bring hypnagogia to an end. One effect that the hypnagogic deepening of relaxation has on the subject's mentation is the transformation and incorporation into imaginal experiences of stimuli from his physical, social, and psychological environments. This reduces and eliminates any need to attend actively to such stimuli, which attendance would have given rise to anxiety, as can be seen from sleep deprivation experiments.

Relevant to the present discussion is Payne's suggestion that the phenomenon of overinclusiveness is the result of a breakdown in a hypothetical filter mechanism which normally screens out those stimuli, both internal and external, which are irrelevant to a task in hand, to allow the most efficient processing of incoming information.[10] Such breakdown, according to West's theory of hallucinations and dreams, may arise from either an extreme decrease or increase of stimuli.[56] Whereas the former is the case with hypnagogia, the latter may be true of schizophrenia. That is, in schizophrenia we may have a 'jamming of the circuits' as the result of a crisis which is characterized by extreme anxiety brought on by either a gradual or a sudden and very considerable increase in unassimilated stimuli. As already observed, many mystics, too, are reported to have had their mystical experiences at the peak of similar crises, an observation suggestive of not so much a breakdown as a switch to a different and wider FR, an important difference between the schizophrenic and the mystic perhaps lying in the general constitution and ability of the latter to cope with the flooding of 'irrelevant' information – although the line is not always easy to draw, seeing that in both there is a fusion of the realm of 'reality' with that of 'imagination', and that in many cases of both there is the belief that the unity of the personality – the new FR – consists of a number of what might be called sub-selfs.

Hypnagogic experiences and pathogenesis

In 1846 Baillarger referred to hypnagogia as a 'passing delirium' and argued (presenting some evidence to this effect) that hypnagogic hallucinations are found extensively both in individuals predisposed to insanity and in insane patients, especially at the beginning of their illness.[57] The first group, viz. those predisposed to insanity, comprised mental patients whose record showed that for years prior to the onset of the illness they had frequent (mostly unpleasant) hypnagogic experiences encompassing the whole sensorium. Most of these individuals were genetically predisposed to mental illness. Their hallucinations occurred initially only at sleep onset or on awakening but eventually extended to the waking state. A typical case illustrating the course of this development is the case of a woman whose most frequent hypnagogic hallucination was the seeing and hearing of soldiers beating their drums. At the beginning, this experience only frightened her but gradually she came to see some intention in it: it was clearly sent to annoy and disturb her. Later, the sight of soldiers in the streets or the sound of drums during the day upset her greatly. Eventually she became paranoid. It was pointed out by Baillarger that at the beginning of the course of their hypnagogic experiences these people had a clear insight of the situation – i.e. they knew that these experiences were imaginal – which, however, they eventually lost.

In respect to the second group, which comprised the current experiences of mental patients, Baillarger argued that, first, the hallucinations of many of these individuals were restricted to those occurring at sleep onset, and second, in many cases of wakeful hallucinations these were noticeably pronounced at bedtime. Indeed, the mere lying down and/or closing the eyes tended to exaggerate these hallucinations. He cited cases where the course of the illness began with hypnagogic hallucinations which, as the illness worsened, turned into wakeful hallucinations, then back into merely hypnagogic ones as the patient began to recover, eventually disappearing with full recovery. Thus, naturally, Baillarger considered hypnagogic hallucinations to be important prognostic factors as he believed they formed part of a predisposition to insanity. Similar arguments suggesting that prolonged and persistent hypnopompic experiences lead to insanity were put forward by de Manacéine.[58]

Earlier in this century, Schultz proposed that hypnagogic experiences share the same psychological, and probably physiological, mechanisms with dreams and schizophrenia. This view is also shared by Vogel *et al.* who, having drawn parallels between dreaming and schizophrenia, noted 'shared regressivity' components between REM sleep and hypnagogia and suggested that sleep onset may provide the physiological basis required to test the hypothesis that dreaming and schizophrenic mentation share the same physiological correlates.[59]

Schultz appears to suggest that we are all latent schizophrenics, and that for many people the experiences of hypnagogia are indistinguishable from those of schizophrenia. Further, and in agreement with Baillarger, he argues that for a great many schizophrenics the only kind of hallucination they experience is the hypnagogic type which, nonetheless, is indistinguishable from so-called 'proper' hallucinations in terms of intensity and realness – 'proper' hallucinations experienced by schizophrenics in hypnagogia being rare by comparison with quasihallucinations which are numerous. More recently, McKellar and Simpson have remarked that 'a psychotic might readily interpret a hypnagogic image in terms of his delusions' and that hypnagogic imagery might 'enrich the content of a pre-existing psychosis'.[1]

However, although, in what has been examined, hypnagogic and schizophrenic experiences may at times be indistinguishable phenomenologically, there is no statistical evidence to show that their frequent occurrence indeed predisposes the normal individual to mental illness. As we shall see in the next chapter, the opposite is in fact the case.

Finally, in closing this chapter I should like to address myself to a possible objection to my relating hypnagogia to schizophrenia, namely that hypnagogia, as a state characterized by relaxation, cannot accommodate the common clinical picture of an acute schizophrenic who is terrified, with widely dilated pupils, and experiencing hallucinatory voices of people threatening to torture and kill him.

Now, as I pointed out at the opening of this chapter, my intention is not to argue that *all* forms and aspects of schizophrenia are to be found in hypnagogia – although, again, it may be the case that schizophrenic experiences are initiated in a hypnagogic climate, as Baillarger and Schultz appear to argue. It will also be remembered from previous chapters that hypnagogia can fairly easily be diverted from its original setting as a pre- or postsleep state and turn instead into a psi/mystical experience or a waking dream. It may be that, unprepared, and without being asleep, the schizophrenic finds himself in such a state of wakeful dreaming. This may partly explain why some schizophrenics, unlike most hypnagogists, find themselves locked in terrifying 'nightmares', that is, they find themselves in waking dream situations in which either the initial stages of a hypnagogic setting are missing or their presence has not been recognized by the patient due to the overwhelming prevalence of his psychological set, i.e. his preoccupations, worries, etc.

Here, once more, hypnagogia may shed light on the situation through the study of those cases of otherwise normal people who, at sleep onset, experience inexplicable and unreasonable anxieties and fears 'such as the insane have at times',[60] or awake in the middle of the night or in the morning possessed by 'a sense of presence', i.e. a feeling that someone is in the room with them, and who, unable to shake off these feelings and impressions, resort to getting out of bed and leaving their room to get away from them.[61] As in many cases of schizophrenia, these people may have an insight of their situation but, although conscious and ashamed of their unreasonable thoughts and actions, they feel incapable of controlling them (see also Schultz's examples in the second section of this chapter).

Besides providing us with cases which, taken in isolation, are indistinguishable from many cases of schizophrenia, hypnagogia is here presenting us with a typical feature of its unique character, namely the lifting of 'critical fetters' and the relaxing of constraints and inhibitions as a result of which all manner of unconscious and nonrational thoughts, feelings and attitudes are let loose. Thus, in the hypnagogic cases under discussion, as in certain cases of schizophrenia, we are probably dealing with 'arrested' dreamy mental states in which the people concerned are suddenly overwhelmed by anxieties and fears that they normally either keep in check or are mostly unaware of but of which there is a continuous build-up (possible cerebral 'causes' will be considered in chapter 10).

8 · Creativity

It might sound paradoxical at first to hear that halfsleep states could have anything to do with creativity, and yet few people would deny having had occasional flashes of inspiration while drifting off to sleep or awaking. Indeed, in the literature on the subject there exists a whole spectrum of references, ranging from mere suggestions to evidential reports, relating hypnagogia to creativity. A brief, impressionistic collection of remarks speaks of hypnagogia as a state in which there is a lifting of all the mental faculties 'into a higher range of freedom', where there is 'a general heightening of faculty', a 'spontaneous generation of ideas', 'an immense amount of high creative work'.[1] 'Hypnagogic mentation has been referred to as 'an entirely new way of thinking', and compared to 'the flights of genius' or even identified as such: 'To dream and altogether not to dream. This synthesis is the operation of genius, by which both activities are mutually reinforced.'[2]

Poems, ideas for novels, and novels in their entirety have been conceived in hypnagogia,[3] and many famous authors and artists are known to have used hypnagogic imagery as source material.[4] Brahms, Puccini, Wagner and Goethe described hypnagogic-like trances as states in which they had created some of their best-known compositions,[5] and Keats probably had similar experiences judging by the wording of his 'Ode to a Nightingale'. Again, various scientists and mathematicians have reported having had answers to difficult problems, or even having conceived their most original contributions to their respective disciplines, in hypnagogia.[6] Edison, for one, is said to have made extensive use of hypnagogia as a means of arriving at new ideas:

> Edison used to work very hard in his research – at beta, the faster brain wave frequencies. Then when he would reach a 'sticking point' he would take one of his famous 'cat naps'. He would doze off in his favourite chair, holding steel balls in the palms of his hands. As he would fall asleep – drifting into alpha – his arms would relax and lower, letting the balls fall into pans on the floor. The noise would wake Edison and very often he would awaken with an idea to continue with his project.[7]

Some recent studies have drawn attention to the likely existence, as the above quotation suggests, of a positive link between alpha-theta brainwaves, hypnagogic imagery, and creativity.[8]

With this potpourri of reports and comments acting as an introduction, I should like now to examine briefly the general concept of creativity and what are thought to be the necessary and sufficient conditions of creative activity. Next, I shall present cases of inspiration and creativity occurring in hypnagogia and argue that the latter contains some, and sometimes all, of the necessary and sufficient conditions of creativity, and that these conditions are

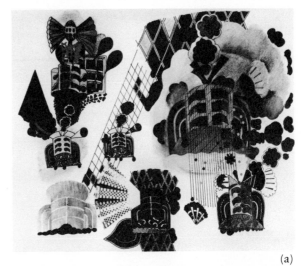

Figure 8.1*(a) and (b)   Two examples of hypnagogic imagery used as source material by artists.*

(a)

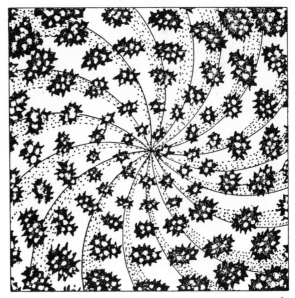

(b)

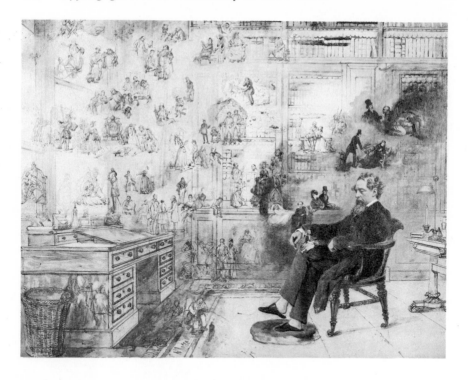

Figure 8.2   Dickens is said to have conceived many of his stories and characters in hypnagogia.

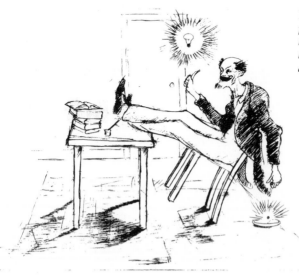

Figure 8.3   Edison dropping his balls. He is said to have made extensive use of hypnagogia as a means of arriving at new ideas.

functions of the LEBs which is a defining feature of hypnagogia. I shall also relate madness to creativity and propose that the state of hypnagogia is their natural meeting place.

In itself, the subject of creativity covers a wide range of aspects and research orientations the most relevant to the present study being those concerned with the creative process *per se*, the identification of personality traits, abilities and attitudes in creative individuals, and the possibility of training for the acquisition of such characteristics. Taking the area as a whole, Hallman has identified five criteria which he considers to be the necessary and sufficient conditions of creativity, and which, with certain qualifications in respect to the last one, are found to be fully present in hypnagogia. These are: connectedness, nonrationality, originality, openness, and self-actualization.[9] Among the first four of these criteria there is, as we shall see, a considerable degree of overlap and mutual implication so that although, for analytical purposes, they are examined individually under separate headings each instance of creativity discussed in the light of one of them can be seen also to contain the others. This, of course, flows partly from the definition of creativity whose definiens is expressed by these features, but it is of particular importance to bear these remarks in mind as we examine the *process* of creativity and compare it with hypnagogia, and especially in viewing both processes within the frameworks of three widely acknowledged sets of theories of creativity, viz. the 'chronological stages' (preparation, incubation, illumination, verification), the 'vertical layers' interchange (conscious ↔ unconscious), and the 'types of thinking' (creative vs. non-creative) theories. Because of the particular stress they place on the unconscious-nonrational activities in the creative process, I decided to discuss these theories in the section after next, but all that is said in respect to connectedness in the next section should also be viewed in their light.

Connectedness and 'actualized' metaphors

The criterion of connectedness has been described variously as combinatorial activity, fusion, unexpected connections resulting from unconscious symbolic activity, compositional activity whose outcome is a new object, experience or image, and new configurations.[10] Hallman explains that

> connectedness comprises relationships which are neither symmetrical nor transitive; that is, the newly created connections as wholes are not equivalent to the parts being connected. Neither side of the equation validly implies the other, for the relationship is neither inferential nor causal; rather, it is metaphoric and transformational.

In respect to hypnagogia, this feature is encountered both as the fusion of relatively relevant components to form a composite, as in Galton's and Katz's[11] photographs, and as the fusion of apparently disparate elements belonging to entirely different matrices. The mechanisms of this activity may be present in the waking state as 'contrary imaginations' or divergent thinking,[12] but the quality of fusions in hypnagogia is considered unique.[13] In regard to the first kind of fusion, there are the numerous reports of hypnagogic experiences which contain unrecognizable images whose parts are, nonetheless, recognized as belonging to past perceptual or imaginal experiences, as being 'like' something already experienced but with added dimensions; that is, in agreement with Hallman, 'the newly created connections as wholes are not equivalent to the parts being connected.'

A case in point here is that of Miller in which the author relates how one night she experienced and wrote a hypnagogic drama she called 'Chiwantopel'.[14] Lying in bed with closed eyes, she writes, '[I] had the sensation that I was waiting for something to happen. Then I felt a great relaxation and I remained as impassive as possible.' There followed the familiar hypnagogic mosaic of 'lines, sparks and spirals of light ... [and] ... a kaleidoscopic and fragmented review of recent trivial events. Then came the impression that something was about to be communicated to me.' There suddenly appeared the figure of an Inca, complete with headdress, who bore the name of 'Chi-wan-to-pel', which Miller heard spelled out syllable by syllable. Round this character raged a battle and the cries of 'wa-ma, wa-ma' were heard. Other scenes followed and the little drama ended with Chiwantopel's dying monologue that was delivered in English except for the last words which were: 'Ja-ni-wa-ma, Ja-ni-wa-ma' and stood for 'You will understand'.

Miller attempts to explain her experiences by reference to previous wakeful ones which she believes probably provided the various elements that eventually came together (fused, combined) in hypnagogia and unfolded as a new, self-contained drama. Although she does not attempt to explain the genesis of the Inca-like neologisms 'wa-ma' and 'Ja-ni-wa-ma', she suggests that 'Chi-wan-to-pel' may have been subconsciously constructed along the lines of 'Po-po-cat-a-petl', a central American volcano whose name she was familiar with. Other elements were also condensed and rearranged unconsciously before emerging in their new form during her hypnagogic experience. But, more important, she explains that during the days before this experience she 'had been searching for inspiration, for an original idea', and that this 'mosaic' was the outcome of distant and recent experiences brought together by this need. She recounts a number of other hypnagogic experiences, some of which were 'hypnagogic poems', and which she explains in a similar manner.

Koestler suggests that Coleridge's 'Kubla Khan' originated 'in an intense day-dream or hypnagogic state ... some intermediary kind of "waking dream"'.[15] Coleridge himself noted that prior to having the Kubla Khan experience 'in which all the images rose up before him as *things*', he had been reading *Purcha's Pilgrimage* where Khan Kubla's palace and stately garden were described.[16]

An experience similar to Miller's and Coleridge's, but occurring at the hypnopompic end, is described by one of Prince's subjects. She writes,

> I woke suddenly some time between three and four in the morning. I was perfectly wide awake and conscious of my surroundings but for a short time – perhaps two or three minutes – I could not move, and I saw this vision which I recognized as such.[17]

The vision, which was 'extraordinarily clear', depicted a tender love scene that unfolded against 'a sort of rosy atmosphere'. The subject notes that she did not experience any emotion at the moment of seeing the vision and that she wrote it down, in verse, at once. In the next morning she read over what she had written and 'was amazed at the language and the rhythm'. Again, as in Miller's case, the subject notes that for two or three days previously she had been trying to write some verses and that she had been reading a good deal of poetry and thinking in rhythm.

Einstein's basic insight into the relativity of Time, which came to him early one morning as he got out of bed, had been preceded by ten years of contemplation on the subject. Likewise, Hadamard's long and intense thinking on a particular subject culminated in a hypnopompic illumination. He writes:

> One phenomenon is certain and I can vouch for its absolute certainty: the sudden and immediate appearance of a solution at the very moment of sudden awakening. On being very abruptly awakened by an external noise, a solution long searched for appeared to me at once without the slightest instant of reflection on my part – the fact was remarkable enough to have struck me unforgettably – and in quite a different direction from any of those which I had previously tried to follow.[18]

In a similar manner, Lamberton achieved the solution to a problem that had 'bogged' him after two weeks of intense thinking over it. Having put aside the problem for a week, he woke up one morning with its solution projected in front of him. He wrote:

> On opening my eyes on the morning in question, I saw projected upon this blackboard surface a complete figure, containing not only the lines given by the problem, but also a number of auxiliary lines, and just such lines as without further thought solved the problem at once . . . the solution was entirely geometrical, whereas I had been labouring for it analytically without ever drawing or attempting to draw a single figure.[19]

Cocteau saw hypnopompically what he later turned into his play *The Knights of the Round Table*. He reports:

> One morning, after having slept poorly, I woke with a start and

witnessed, as from a seat in a theater, three acts which brought to life an epoch and characters about which I had no documentary information and which I regarded moreover as forbidding.[20]

The plot of Mary Leader's novel *Triad* came to her complete, and without previous preparation, one afternoon as she lay down for a nap. She recounts:

I settled myself in a contour chair and prepared to doze off – but I didn't sleep. Instead I drifted into a peculiar state of consciousness, neither asleep nor awake. Then this – thing – began happening.

I felt I was in another world, a twilight world in which I wandered, as if in a forest. Never before had I felt like this. It was as though it were a film – the entire panorama of my novel reeled off before me, its theme, its plot, even details. . . .

I don't remember how long I was gone, but when I broke out of it, it was all there.[21]

Poincaré relates how one night, when he was unable to sleep because he had drunk black coffee, 'ideas rose in crowds' and he 'felt them collide until pairs interlocked, so to speak, making a stable combination'. This resulted in his establishing the existence of a class of Fuchsian functions, contrary to his earlier intense efforts to prove that there could be no such functions.[22]

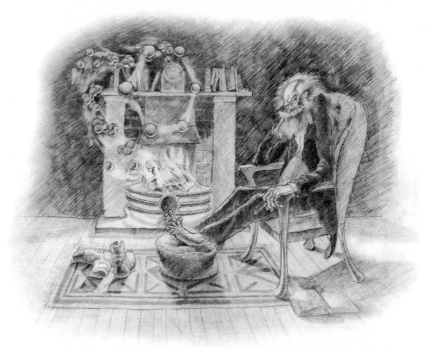

Figure 8.4 *Kekulé's discovery of the benzene molecule while dozing in front of a fire is held to be the most brilliant piece of prediction in organic chemistry.*

But perhaps the most celebrated case of creativity in hypnagogia, one that led to a discovery which has been called 'the most brilliant piece of prediction to be found in the whole range of organic chemistry', is that reported to the German Chemical Society in 1890 by Kekulé. He recounts how one evening he dozed on a London bus and saw atoms gambolling before his eyes and spent part of that night making sketches of these forms. Some years later, a similar event led to the discovery of the ring of the benzene molecule. He relates:

> I was sitting, writing at my text-book; but the work did not progress; my thoughts were elsewhere. I turned my chair to the fire and dozed. Again the atoms were gambolling before my eyes. This time the smaller groups kept modestly in the background. My mental eyes, rendered more acute by repeated visions of the kind, could now distinguish larger structures, of manifold conformation: long rows, sometimes more closely fitted together; all twining and twisting in snakelike motion. But look! What was that? One of the snakes had seized hold of its own tail, and the form whirled mockingly before my eyes. As if by a flash of lightning I awoke; and this time also I spent the rest of the night working out the consequences of the hypothesis.[23]

As McKellar rightly points out, the illumination occurred in Kekulé's hypnagogic mental life '*because* his mind was stored with the relevant facts from past perceptual experience'.[24] But it is just as important to note that it was under the special conditions prevailing in hypnagogia that a number of perceptual experiences came together and became relevant within a particular framework. Moreover, the facts from past experiences emerged in the hypnagogic vision in a symbolic form, that is, the snake-like formations *represented* molecular structures. Interestingly, in this type of example can be seen in operation a mechanism rather opposite to that observed by Silberer in his autosymbolic phenomena. That is, instead of conceptual activity becoming symbolically represented in visual imagery, the emergence of the latter gives rise to a concept, viz. that some organic compounds, such as the benzene molecule, are closed chains or rings.

This character of transferring the concept to imagery and vice versa is, in fact, an aspect of a wider feature of hypnagogia that encompasses synesthetic activity where imagery of one sense modality transforms itself into, or gives rise to, imagery of another sense modality. It can also be seen as a transfer from one conceptual FR to another. Indeed, synesthetic transformations are themselves transferences across FsR.

This form of activity is referred to in papers on creativity as the subject's employment of metaphor, and it is significant in this light that metaphors have been called 'synaesthetic descriptions'.[25] The creative use of metaphor is thought to enhance, or present in a new light, a certain state of affairs. Aristotle, writing on the use of language in his *Poetics*, stated that 'by far the greatest thing is to be a master of metaphor' and that such mastery is 'an indication of genius, since the ability to forge a good metaphor shows that the poet has an intuitive perception of the similarity in dissimilars', i.e. that the poet is capable of shifting imagery and concepts across FsR. He also argued that it is a great thing for a creative poet to use unusual word order, 'as well as compounds and strange words, in the proper way'.[26] It might, of course, be objected that the crossing of FsR and the employment of unusual word order, compounds and strange words in hypnagogia are not executed 'in the proper way', that they occur out of context and are irrelevant. But, as I have already argued, and shall presently augment that argument, this is not always the case. Moreover, given the appropriate attention to the hypnagogic imagery, it may never be the case.

Although, in hypnagogia, as in everyday life and in the arts and sciences, metaphors can be seen by the waking mind as such, they are often *experienced* as *actualities*, that is, they are taken on their face value. This is strongly reminiscent of Nietzsche's description of the creative process in which 'one loses all perception of what is imagery and simile',[27] and Coleridge's Kubla Khan experience 'in which all the images rose up before him as *things*'. It is only by oscillating in and out of hypnagogia, thus allowing the waking mind some room for judgment, or by learning to remain passive-receptive in hypnagogia, that one can come to appreciate the metaphoric aspect of the imagery in this state. But these metaphor-actualities occurring as they do in hypnagogia render the state unique in acting as the general condition wherein artistic and scientific creativity, as well as schizophrenic and primitive-regressive mentation, emerge. Thus, we find Kretschmer writing on artistic creativity:

> Such creative products of the artistic imagination tend to emerge from a psychic twilight, a state of lessened consciousness and diminished attentivity to external stimuli. Further, the condition is one of 'absent-mindedness' with hypnoidal over-concentration on a single focus, providing an entirely passive experience, frequently of a visual character, divorced from the categories of space and time, and reason and will.[28]

Under the same or very similar conditions, a schizophrenic patient of Kretschmer's related to him how, whilst in a transitional phase between normality and abnormality, 'he passively experiences the outcropping of a mass of images which arise from abstract concepts, or which appear to exist in concrete objects', a type of mentation comparable to the language of primitives which is 'like the unfolding of a picture strip, where each word expresses a pictorial image, regardless as to whether the picture signifies an object, an action, or a quality'.

And yet it is this primitive and regressive type of mentation that very often creative individuals resort to in order to experience (perceive-conceive) and understand their own ideas. Einstein, for instance, said that 'the psychical entities which seem to serve as elements in thought are certain signs and more or less clear images', Bartlett stated that the 'image method remains the method of brilliant discovery', Richardson linked vivid imagery in adults with creativity, Paivio suggested that the stage of illumination or discovery is characterized by concrete imagery, McClelland remarked that 'scientists . . . still live to a moderate degree in the world of witches, gnomes, fairies and ogres', and Schaefer concluded from the study of various reports that in creativity 'there is at least a partially controlled lowering of ego controls so that fantastic and primitive associations arise to the consciousness'.[29]

Einstein's statement does not seem to me at all dissimilar either to those by Kretschmer describing primitive and schizophrenic thinking or to reports by hypnagogists whose experiences may constitute quasiperceptual representations of abstract concepts, functions, actions, relationships, etc. Moreover, Schaefer's remark fits exactly a deliberately induced-sustained hypnagogia. In this respect, Green and his co-workers have spoken of 'hypnagogic-like imagery' as the 'sine qua non of creativity for many outstanding people', explaining the use of the qualifying term 'hypnagogic-like' 'because our subjects were trying to remain awake rather than go to sleep'.[30] But, as I have already argued, hypnagogia can be prolonged, and its imagery, to a certain extent, manipulated, if the subject learns to poise himself in a passive-receptive mode and enter into a conversational-empathic relationship with the imagery. In such cases, where the imagery is fascinatedly attended to, there is often also an accompaniment of a sense of significance. It is of interest to compare this with what Wallas says about the stage of illumination in the creative process:

> I find it convenient to use the term 'intimation' for that moment in the illumination stage when our fringe consciousness of an association train is in the stage of rising consciousness which indicates that the fully conscious flash of success is coming. . . . If this feeling of intimation lasts for an appreciable time, and is either sufficiently conscious or can by effort of attention be made sufficiently conscious, it is obvious that our will can be brought directly to bear on it. We can at least attempt to inhibit, or prolong or divert the brain acitivity which intimation shows to be going on. And, if intimation accompanies a rising train of association which the brain accepts, so to speak, as plausible, but would not without the effort of attention automatically push to the 'flash' of conscious success, we can attempt to hold on to such a train on the chance that it may succeed.[31]

Wallas's state of intimation will become clearer, and its relationship to the hypnagogic 'fringe' consciousness more obvious, if we bear in mind what has been said earlier, namely that both in hypnagogia and in creativity there is present what might be called an activity of *imaginal perception*, that is, an experience of vivid, lifelike imagery. Walkup has noted that 'creative individuals appear to have stumbled onto and then developed to a high degree of perfection an unusual ability to visualize mentally – almost hallucinate – in the areas in which they are creative'.[32] He uses the word 'visualize' 'to include the mental synthesizing of many sensory experiences, not just ocular experiences'. In analysing the nature of this sense of 'seeing' in the field of scientific creativity, he writes:

> It is almost a *feeling like* the object being visualized. One can *feel* the pressure of contacting objects or the erosion of material by friction, or the flow of heat from one point to another, or the swing of the oscillating electrical circuit, or the bending of light as it passes from one medium to another, or the appropriateness of a well-designed structure to hold a maximum load, with every part equally strained in the process, or the eternal bouncing about of the molecules of gas, or the almost physical transfer of energy from the gasoline, through the motor, transmission, and to the driving wheels of the automobile. It is as though one's kinesthetic sensing mechanisms were associated with the physical object and that he thus sensed directly what was going on in the external system.

Figure 8.5 *As in hypnagogia, creative 'regression' may bring to light features of nature that are not so much metaphoric as actual, such as Faraday's electromagnetic lines which can be seen here (a and b) in an electrophotograph of a magnet and in a Kirlian photograph of the apparent interaction between a magnet and a human finger; in (c) is shown the electron density map of benzene which is practically identical with Kekulé's hypnagogic vision-concept.*

(c)

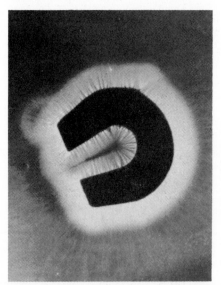

(a)

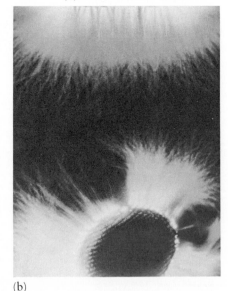

(b)

Similarly, Faraday 'saw' electromagnetic lines of force, and Einstein, referring to the 'elements in thought' mentioned above, says that in his case these were 'of visual and some of muscular type' and that 'the play with the mentioned elements is aimed to be analogous to certain logical connections one is searching for'. Thus, even logical connections may be experienced as forms of imagery, and it is sometimes argued that meanings, too, depend on images.[33] I shall have more to say on this below. My aim at this point is to put into relief the paradox that highly intellectual individuals engaged in abstract mental activities resort to 'primitive' imagery to solve their problems, and to further my argument that most, if not all, of the conditions of creativity are present in hypnagogia.

The paradox referred to above might not be thought of as being present in hypnagogia since the state is considered in general to be regressive anyway and so the occurrence in it of concrete and vivid imagery might not be regarded as contradictory. However, if Kretschmer's 'psychic twilight', Walkup's 'visualization' and Wallas's 'intimation' in the creative process mean anything, these conditions are not dissimilar to those obtained in hypnagogia. This does not only imply that at least some essential aspects of creativity are necessarily regressive in character, but also shows that hypnagogia possesses the very conditions that give rise to the creative 'flash'.

Moreover, hypnagogia may render more obvious certain important mental processes, such as the presently discussed use of concept-images in scientific creative activity, and the structure and employment of concepts in general. When, in the ordinary waking state, we think of a generic or abstract concept, we usually engage in some form of imaging in which the relevant concept is but vaguely represented and is typically impressionistic.[34] However, when we try to become more clear and precise in our conceptualization we find that the concept begins to display unique spatio-imaginal qualities which go beyond the sum total of the particular cases it may represent, and that we concurrently engage in internal kinesthetic activities in relation to the concept – as if we are mentally giving birth, sculpturing, or moulding inside ourselves in a pliant medium: in a specific sense, the concept becomes 'subjectified'. (It might be of some interest to note that the Greek words for *understanding* – καταλαμβάνω, ἀντιλαμβάνομαι – literally mean to seize, occupy, take possession, make one's own.)

Now, we have already seen that this is in fact the case with hypnagogic imagery, that is, the latter, due to the subject's absorption and LEBs, becomes 'subjectified', linked empathically and kinesthetically to the subject. We have also seen that some images *look like* objects perceived during the day or on earlier occasions, and that they are not exact reproductions of actual perceptions but rather 'idealized' images of them. It can thus be argued that some hypnagogic images are no less than generic concepts and that these, and probably all, concepts, are not only representable in imagery types but also, in the last analysis, they must be experienced as such. This contention is further supported by the fact that even mathematical and philosophical thinking is expressed in some kind of shifting inner tension, i.e. in kinesthetic activity.

In this way hypnagogia may throw light on the mechanism of a normal mental activity and suggest an explanation, and perhaps a resolution, of the apparent paradox of the use of primitive types of imagery (visuo-kinesthetic) in intellectual tasks. This is essentially achieved by virtue of the specific state of consciousness the hypnagogist finds himself in, a state which in many respects resembles the one an individual enters when engaged in an act of creation. But, although 'idealization', or the process of arriving at a generic concept, is a normal and ordinary process, the indication afforded by hypnagogia of both how it is arrived at and how it looks and feels points to a much wider underlying process of *fusion* and *condensation* that stems out of the root phenomenon of the LEBs of the subject in both hypnagogia and the creative act.

We have seen in earlier chapters how the LEBs shows itself at one level of hypnagogia as the facilitation of overinclusiveness in conceptualization and the fusing of a number of apparently unrelated FsR. It is significant that similar observations have also been made about the nature of creativity. We saw earlier that creativity consists mainly in the making of combinations of elements that have not been made before. It is further said that 'among chosen combinations the most fertile will often be those formed of elements drawn from domains which are far apart', that 'creative individuals must have access to improbable associative responses', or, as Cropley put it:

> the more a person treats data which look to have nothing to do with each other as though they are related, the more likely he is to make data combinations which are unusual (i.e. to think creatively). The kind of person who codes in this broad way is referred to as a wide categorizer, . . . Creative thinking thus looks to be related to width of categorizing.[35]

Similarly, it has been pointed out that 'in science the process of discovery and invention consists of freeing the tendency to "note identity in difference"'.[36] (See also section on 'Originality', this chapter).

The actual state of consciousness in which such relationships and identities are effected is, as already argued, the same as that in which metaphors and analogies are experienced as actualities. Indeed, if we consider an analogy in itself as a concept, then the experiencing of such a concept as an actual event or thing, and not as something analogous to something else, becomes the same as experiencing the original idea about which the analogy is made. This is clearly the case in hypnagogia, as pointed out earlier: metaphors and analogies are experienced as actualities. It might be countered that this is not the case in creativity, that in the latter analogies are seen as such and nothing more. However, this is debatable. Apart from Cropley's and my own argument above there are numerous introspective reports which strongly suggest that creative persons often experience analogies and metaphors *as things*, i.e. as actualities.

Significantly, such imaginal events may move in either of two different directions and bring together FsR which are not obviously related. Thus, in Silberer's autosymbolic phenomena an abstract concept belonging to its own particular FR is first transformed into imagery and experienced as such, i.e. as a new thing in a different FR, and then it is identified with the concept it represents. In Kekulé's example the procedure is reversed: there is first the vision of the snake biting its tail, in itself an imaginal actuality, then comes the transfer to a different matrix, viz. that of chemistry. In an earlier example (chapter 6) we saw how Slight, while in a hypnopompic state, thought of a particular woman he knew who represented a certain character type and who then *turned into* another woman he also knew. While still in the hypnopompic state he then realized that the identification of these two women resulted from the analogy afforded by certain character traits shared by both. But he did not immediately see the *resemblance*; on the contrary, he began by identifying the one with the other. The same is often the case with creativity, as can be seen from Wallas's, Kretschmer's and Walkup's quotations above. From these quotations it is clear that the metaphors 'seen' by many creative people are not only literally seen and felt but sometimes also turn out to be identical with what they are supposed to be metaphors of – for instance, Faraday's electromagnetic fields composed of lines of force are precisely that, as can be seen in Kirlian photographs. Incidentally, such observations have important epistemological implications as they tend to suggest that a great deal of mental 'seeing' is more of a literal experience than a metaphor taken from visual perception, as some writers seem to believe.[37]

The imaginally actualized metaphors constitute only one side of the balancing act which leads to the culmination of the creative process, the other side being the recognition that the metaphor brings together two or more FsR. In the case of Kekulé, for instance, the hypnagogic vision of a snake biting its tail would not have acquired the importance attached to it had not Kekulé seen it as an analogy within the framework of organic chemistry. Hypnagogia is replete with such metaphors and symbols, and most likely with unrecognized solutions to problems. The recognition of these solutions is partly dependent on the degree of problem saturation a person subjects himself to and his readiness to appreciate symbols and metaphors encountered in hypnagogia. A main difficulty in appreciating the hypnagogic 'language' in this respect is the fact that it is often expressed in oblique or condensed forms of metaphor and not in overt and explicit analogies. Moreover, hypnagogia operates most often *multisociatively*, that is, it brings together (and condenses) a number of FsR. These associations and condensations, as suggested in chapter 6, are effected unconsciously via mediate types of association thus resulting in imagery which is considered simply strange or irrelevant – which is not to say that the hypnagogist could not come to appreciate the symbolic nature of the imagery should he adopt the appropriate stance towards it.

The unconscious-nonrational

Our discussion of the manner in which hypnagogia and creativity 'actualize' and 'connect' has already involved Hallman's second criterion of creativity, namely, that of nonrationality according to which the fusing of images into new creations is effected by certain unconscious-nonrational mental processes. It is important in this respect that multisociation is clearly uncharacteristic of the logic employed in the conscious waking state. It is of some relevance, too, that the language which gave to the western world the word *logic* also contains the word φρήν = 'mind' (logical mind, reason) whose derivative φρένον means 'brake' or 'damper', thus suggesting that to be logical is to put the dampers on, to control and constrain oneself. It also implies a narrowing and converging type of mentation which reflects a deeper and far-reaching condition of tightening of ego boundaries, of sharply outlining an 'outer', objective world clearly defined and differentiated from one's ego schema, i.e. from what constitutes one's sense of self as a separate and individual entity. By contrast, the LEBs occurring in hypnagogia flouts the laws of logic, it raises the dampers and facilitates ego 'fluidity' and multisociation, conferring on a person the ability to internalize and subjectify diverse matrices and thus identify them with one another: it is widening and diverging as opposed to narrowing and converging. In this sense, it is also regressive, primitive and paralogical (see chapter 7 where waking and hypnagogic mentation were also contrasted).

The significant point here is that identical remarks have been made about creativity. For example, Barron stated that 'at the very heart of the creative process is this ability to shatter the rule of law and regularity of the mind'; Popper suggested that 'there is no such thing as a logical method of having new ideas' and that 'every discovery contains "an irrational element"'; Koestler pointed out that the creative act 'presupposes a relaxing of the controls and regression to modes of ideation which are indifferent to the rules of verbal logic, unperturbed by contradiction, untouched by the dogmas and taboos of so-called common sense' and that 'at the decisive stage of discovery the codes of disciplined reasoning are suspended'; Hallman remarked that 'during the experience all boundary lines fade, distinctions blur, and the artist experiences himself as one with his materials and his vision'; Nietzsche spoke of 'a feeling of being completely beside yourself', and Jung commented that in such a state 'consciousness only plays the role of slave to the daemon of the unconscious' which 'inundates it with alien ideas'.[38] Hallman further proposes that nonrationality is both a condition of novelty and a cause:

> The relationship between such process as condensation, symbolization, displacement, and neologisms and the production of new connections is a causal one. . . . In every case it is the nonrational, the autistic, the metaphoric, the internally oriented, the spontaneous and involuntary,

the integrating, unbound energies which are active in producing new connections. . . . These nonrational processes account for the seeming effortlessness and the spontaneity of creative activity; they explain the autonomy, the quality of 'otherness', of being visited by a daemon or a voice.

Here belongs a discussion of hypnagogic experiences in relation to the three conceptual schemes referred to at the beginning of this chapter and identified by Hallman as agreeing on the major point that the segment or level of the creative process which is invariably associated with the creation of novelty is both nonrational and unconscious. The first framework considers creativity as a series of four stages, viz. preparation, incubation, illumination, and verification. The second explains creativity as the interplay and collaboration between free and bound energies, gestalt-free and articulating tendencies, unconscious processes and conscious deliberation: the creative fusion itself transpires in the unconscious and it is then projected into consciousness where, at the rational level, enter elaboration, testing and socially derived approvals. The third framework views creativity as a type of thinking distinct from non-creative types: it is distinguished from the latter by its being relational, combinatorial and fusing, and by the fact that its activities are not bound by rationality.

In relating hypnagogia to the four-stage theory of creativity, the second and third stages are of the greatest relevance. Indeed, hypnagogic experiences are characterized by the very features describing these two stages. Significantly, Hallman remarks that

> The second and third stages actually produce the new connections, the novel relationships, and these transpire in the form of nonrational operations. The incubation stage, for example, consists of spontaneous, uncontrollable events which cluster themselves seemingly in accordance with their own autonomous laws. It involves the relaxation of conscious thinking operations and the inhibition of logical control.

He refers to Maslow's voluntary regression, Ehrenzweig's surrender of the ego, and Rogers's openness to experience, in this respect.

Now, it will be recalled that in the previous section were presented cases of creativity in hypnagogia some of which were entirely unsolicited and others preceded by lengthy and/or intense preparation. In the former type of case, the unconscious-nonrational element is clearly present in the very fact of the occurrence of the experience which was unsolicited, spontaneous and uncontrollable. In the latter kind of case, its presence is again obvious in the fact that the sought for solutions appeared in unexpected or even contrary directions and forms.

We have seen that the experiencing, controlling and remembering of hypnagogic events is highly dependent on the hypnagogist's degree of awareness, that is, on his natural or acquired disposition to stay relaxed and withdrawn without either falling asleep or becoming fully awake. Again, similar observations have been made regarding the stages of incubation and illumination. Wallas says that if the psychological process involved in these stages is to enter the subject's consciousness and be controlled,

> it is necessary that that process should not only last for an appreciable time, but should also be, during that time, sufficiently conscious for the thinker to be at least aware that something is happening to him. On this point, the evidence seems to show that both the unsuccessful trains of association, which might have led to the 'flash' of success, and the final and successful train are normally either unconscious, or take place (with 'risings' and 'fallings' of consciousness as success seems to approach or retire), in that periphery or 'fringe' of consciousness which surrounds our 'focal' consciousness as the sun's 'corona' surrounds the disk in full luminosity. This 'fringe consciousness' may last up to the 'flash' instant, may accompany it, and in some cases may continue beyond it. But, just as it is very difficult to see the sun's corona unless the disk is hidden by a total eclipse, so it is very difficult to observe our 'fringe consciousness' at the instant of full illumination, or to remember the preceding 'fringe' after full illumination has taken place. As William James says: 'when the conclusion is there, we have always forgotten most of the steps preceding its attainment'.[31]

Let us take a closer look at this quotation as it contains a number of relevant points. If we begin with the last one, the quotation from James could easily have been describing the statement-conclusions encountered in hypnagogia. These, as we have seen, may appear as statements 'heard' or spoken by the subject and carrying with them a feeling of concluding, that is, a feeling that a certain associative or logical activity has taken place below the threshold of consciousness and that the statement constitutes the conclusion of such activity. They are forms of condensation, examples of 'collapsed logic' in both senses of the word 'collapse', i.e. both in the sense of falling together, condensing, and in the sense of falling down, disintegrating. However, these two processes are not necessarily consequent on each other but may take place concurrently, in which case aspects or constituents of one image or concept may merge with constituents of another (or others) to form a new one in the midst of an ongoing process of disintegration. Thus there may appear 'irrelevant' associations, logical jumps, conclusions without (obvious) premises, intuitions. Such phenomena often look and feel like solutions without problems, and should they turn out to be true intuitions they may present us with the difficulty of justifying them, of finding both their origins and the intermediate steps that led to them. They are reminiscent of Gauss's statement, 'I have had my solutions for a long time, but I do not know how I am to arrive at them.'[39]

Wallas's description of the fringe consciousness and the stage of illumination in the creative process fits hypnagogia like a glove. We can easily recognize in the 'fallings' and 'risings' of consciousness the 'oscillations' of hypnagogia. The latter, due to its abolition of constraints and to its LEBs, provides the general milieu conducive to the occurrence of the 'flash': it precedes the flash, accompanies it, and may last beyond it, although usually the excitement generated by the flash tends to terminate the state. However, unlike Wallas's description in which the 'fringe consciousness' becomes unobservable at the moment of illumination, in many cases where the latter occurs in hypnagogia one can both be aware of the 'fringe' and remember the phenomena preceding the flash. Indeed, it is by the special, and yet natural, character of maintaining a form of awareness, of being preconscious, of constituting an intermediary state between the full waking consciousness and the unconscious, that hypnagogia not only makes it possible for material which might never reach consciousness directly to do so but also furnishes us with clues concerning the workings of the creative process and enables us to become aware of the epistemological changes that occur during the emergence of creative insights. I say 'epistemological changes' because the creative process in itself clearly contains forms of mentation which although foreign to the logic of wakefulness yet lead to new knowledge. In this regard, we have also seen (chapter 6) that some writers have suggested the use of hypnagogia as a means of entering, without losing consciousness (and without contradiction), the realms of the unconscious. Pinard, writing on the nature of 'spontaneous images', spoke of them as apparently 'creative not only of themselves but of a non-sensory world which has its own structural and developmental laws';[40] identical remarks, as we remember, were made earlier by Hallman concerning the events that take place during incubation. But if such laws exist, their knowledge, or the individual's functioning within them, clearly requires subjective internal changes, that is, changes in the mode of experiencing and knowing. Such changes are, as already proposed, facilitated by the LEBs occurring in hypnagogia. Moreover, although it is well argued by many workers that the creative linkages are effected in the unconscious, and, as we have seen, also in preconscious hypnagogia, in some cases the latter may further *re*-present to consciousness activities that have already transpired in the unconscious.

Let me substantiate these claims by referring to the case of Prince's subject mentioned earlier in this chapter. It will be recalled that this subject had a hypnopompic vision of a tender love scene which she recorded immediately in the form of a poem. In discussing the case Prince noted that:

> The script was written automatically. . . . The 'thoughts' of the verse were in her 'subconscious mind' [Prince explains in a footnote that 'by this is meant "thoughts" of which she was not aware']. These 'thoughts' (also described as 'words') were not logically arranged or as written in the verse, but 'sort of tumbled together – mixed up a little'. 'They were not like the thoughts one thinks in *composing* a verse.' There did not seem to be any attempt at selection from the thoughts or words. No

> evidence could be elicited to show that the composing was done here. . . . In other words all happened *as if* there was a deeper underlying process which did the composing and from this process certain thoughts without logical order emerged to form a subconscious stream and after the composing was done the words of the verse emerged as coconscious images as they were to be written. This underlying process then 'automatically' did the writing and the composing.[17]

In her report, the subject recorded that although the thoughts expressed in the poem were the thoughts she experienced at the time of seeing the vision, 'the language was entirely different from anything I had thought and the writing expressed the emotion which I had not consciously experienced in seeing the vision.'

The important sequel to the case is that Prince, having hypnotized his subject, discovered that the hypnopompic vision was in fact an accurate re-presentation of a dream experienced immediately prior to waking up. Furthermore, he noted that the vision 'expresses the mental attitude, sentiments and emotions experienced in the dream but not at the time of the vision' and that 'the script gives of the vision an interpretation which was not consciously in mind at the moment of writing'.

Now, if we assume that unrecalled dreams constitute unconscious mental events, then we are here presented with a case in which the subject re-experiences hypnopompically such events and transfers them to conscious memory. This is not to argue that dreams are not recalled in other circumstances, but that in hypnagogia these may be *re-experienced*. What is more, even when such events are re-experienced in apparently different circumstances, it is found that the actual mental state of the subject is hypnagogic-like (dreamy, twilight). It is important to note, however, that although this subject did not re-experience the dream in all its details – the mental attitude, sentiments and emotions were not present – these were given accurately in the poem which, moreover, was composed and written 'automatically', i.e. in a state of dissociation. In the dream the subject was a participant, in the hypnagogic vision she was a spectator, in the poem the dream's added dimension, another FR, was revealed; but had she not been hypnotized this added dimension might not have been uncovered. This suggests, once more, that many hypnagogic phenomena that appear puzzling – strange, irrelevant, illogical, crazy – may do so because of hidden FsR, and that they may be considered original or creative when these FsR are suddenly made known. The condition of dissociation may also provide 'the quality of "otherness", of being visited by a daemon or a voice' that Hallman noted in respect to creativity.

That the preconscious character of hypnagogia renders it ideal for the emergence of nonrational and otherwise unconscious mental processes culminating in creative insights is further supported by the claims of various writers to the effect that creativity requires precisely such a character in order to manifest itself. Thus, Gowan proposes that 'creativity involves the "gentling of the preconscious", since it allows the conscious mind to gain insights from, and to establish an intuitive relationship with the preconscious', and that Silberer's autosymbolic phenomena 'correspond closely to what has often been described as the work of intuitive insight or creative insight'.[41] And, to quote Koestler once more: 'The capacity to regress, more or less at will, to the games of the underground, without losing contact with the surface, seems to be the essence of the poetic, and of any other form of creativity.'[42]

It is, of course, not totally true, as seen from the evidence adduced, that regression in the creative act always takes place 'without losing contact with the surface'. Much creative activity may transpire unconsciously during sleep and the creative insight flash up in the subject's consciousness at the moment of awakening (see also 'informational' cases in chapter 6). Some individuals have even learned to communicate to their unconscious their desires for solutions to certain problems, which solutions are arrived at or 'given' in a state of hypnagogia. Garrett, for instance, says, 'I give my consciousness the task of finding the answer while I sleep, and in the morning at the threshold of awakening, I find the information I sought.' Similarly, Walter Scott wrote to a friend saying, 'It was always when I first opened my eyes that the desired ideas thronged upon me.' It is also said that 'Brindley, the great engineer, when up against a difficult problem, would go to bed for several days till it was solved'.[43] It is noteworthy that in a great many cases of this kind we find the subject thinking about the problem as he falls asleep, thus transferring his desire for a solution to his unconscious via the hypnagogic fringe consciousness, and receiving an answer at the preconscious hypnopompic end – at the beginning of this chapter reference was also made to Edison's use of hypnagogia to arrive at new inventions.

Originality: creativity and madness

When the operation of unconscious or preconscious processes achieves a connection between widely separate matrices, the result is undeniably original: it may appear, or be considered, crazy but we can hardly deny that it is original. Simple though it may seem, this criterion of creativity is said to comprise four qualities, viz. novelty, unpredictability, uniqueness, and surprise. Novelty is expressed in the finding of new connections, relationships, compositions, insights, organizations of experience, and constellations of meanings.[44] Some writers see creativity on the whole as the fusion of perceptual experiences in novel ways, or as remoteness of association and unusual response.[45] Unpredictability, Hallman explains, asserts that 'creativity produces qualities which never existed before and which could never have been predicted on the basis of prior configurations of events'. Likewise, uniqueness asserts that 'original creations are incomparable, for there is no class of objects to which they can be compared. They are untranslatable, unexampled.' Surprise 'refers to the psychological effect of novel combinations upon the beholder.'

The criterion of originality, so essential to the concept of creativity, has been reported by many hypnagogic subjects, as can be seen from the numerous examples cited throughout this book. The quality of novelty has been partly discussed in reference to 'connectedness' where we saw how different perceptual and conceptual FsR fuse or combine in hypnagogia resulting in strange imagery and statement-conclusions. We have also seen that hypnagogia abounds in neologisms, strange combinations of images, words or ideas, visual images viewed from unusual angles, fusions of images or ideas belonging to widely different matrices.

Similarly, unpredictability is a regular feature of hypnagogia. Many subjects have spoken not only of the irrelevancy of hypnagogic images to concurrent trains of thought but also of their irrelevancy to each other and their often unpredictable and apparently disconnected sequences that led to their being compared to a mixed-up collection of lantern slides belonging to a number of different lectures.[46]

Referring back to Part One, again we come across reports in which hypnagogic imagery is described as something never experienced before, as unique, as unparalleled in beauty or ugliness and incomparable to any perceptual experience. This has led some subjects to place it in a supernatural or spiritual world. Also, the unpredictable fusion of unrelated matrices of imagery or thought, which are typical of hypnagogia, have contributed to the production of unique, if peculiar, ideas. We shall see more of this below.

The quality of surprise as the subject's reaction to the novelty, unpredictability, and uniqueness of his imagery and thought is also encountered in hypnagogia. Many people have remarked that their hypnagogic images often 'surprise and delight by their beauty and originality'. And although hypnagogia is, on the whole, characterized by a lack of affect, there have been many cases where the subject was startled back to the full waking state by the unpredictability and strangeness of the imagery. The magnitude of the subject's reaction (surprise), however, seems to be partly dependent on the stage, that is, the lighter the stage the greater the surprise.

As noted, originality is often defined as the production of unusual, far-fetched, or remote 'responses', and, in this sense hypnagogia is teeming with original products. It has also been suggested that 'the essence of discovery is that unlikely marriage of cabbages and kings', the relating of disparate FsR which will solve the previously insoluble problem.[47] Although solutions to posed problems are not infrequent in hypnagogia, the latter is, of course, better known for its unsolicited responses which, consisting as they do of very peculiar marriages, convey a certain air of poetry. This is most apparent in visual and auditory hypnagogic imagery and speech and has led to comparisons with surrealist products.

Indeed, the comparison with surrealism is most fitting. As Brèton wrote in his manifesto,

> surrealism is sheer psychological automatism, by means of which it is intended to express verbally, in writing, or in any other way, the actual function of thought. Thought's dictation in the absence of all control exercised by reason and outside all aesthetic or moral prejudice.[48]

Automatism, which, as Brèton explains, is a monologue uttered as rapidly as possible, thus eliminating control and criticism, is reminiscent of Jung's and Stransky's experiments of the same nature which invited parallels with schizophrenic thinking and states of inattention, and which I have related to hypnagogia in the previous chapter.

In surrealist artistic creations, as in hypnagogic imagery and mentation, well-known objects are presented in a fantastic manner, 'they are freely linked in a way unheard-of in our conscious, wakeful, purposeful, reality . . . things penetrate each other and give birth to new beings no longer "after their kind".'[49] Thus, it is hardly surprising that Max Ernst's 'oneiric' collages, for example, are strongly reminiscent of hypnagogic imagery. Ernst himself reported painting from his own hypnagogic imagery, of 'being present as a spectator, indifferent or impassioned' at the birth of his own work. Indeed, he explains that he owes his discovery of *frottage* to 'one of those dreams between sleeping and waking'.[50]

Another painter whose works and method can be most closely related to hypnagogia is Salvador Dali. Not only has this artist made use of hypnagogic material in his own paintings whose contents, like the hypnagogic imagery itself, are sharply and minutely detailed, but also the development of some of his themes as well as the method he employs to conceive of his images are relevant to our discussion. Dali speaks of a

> spontaneous method of irrational knowledge based upon the interpretive-critical association of delirious phenomena. . . . By this method paranoiac-critical activity discovers new and objective 'significance' in the irrational; it makes the world of delirium pass tangibly on to the plane of reality.[51]

In this method, by deliberately suspending the wakeful, critical activities of the mind, Dali would allow the emergence of unconscious and irrational elements and then seize upon them and utilize them. This is not unlike my description of hypnagogia as a preconscious state in which material from the unconscious comes to the surface. We saw that this material appears in forms that flout the laws of logic, such as crossing or fusing together unrelated FsR, assimilating unrelated objects or mental processes, allowing objects to have added meanings and significances unwarranted by waking logic, allowing objects to be themselves and yet something else. Dali's paintings contain all of these paralogical manifestations. One of the most striking effects in his employment of the paranoiac-critical method is the creation of the double or

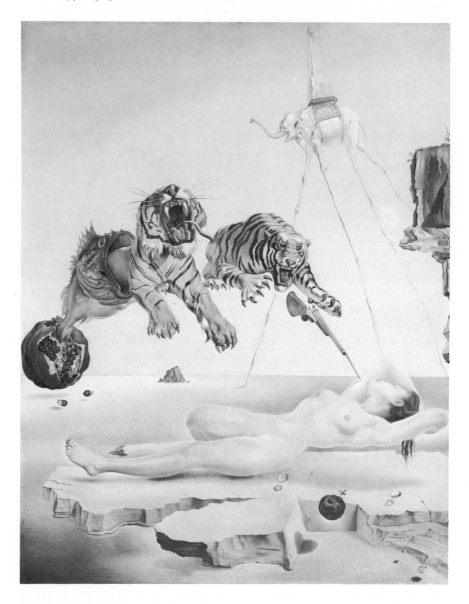

Figure 8.6 *Dali's* Dream Caused by the Flight of a Bee Around a Pomegranate One Second Before Waking Up.

'paranoiac' image which he describes as 'the image of an object which, without the least figurative or anatomical modification can at the same time represent another, absolutely different object'.[52]

The two best-known paintings in which this effect appears are the 'Swans Reflecting Elephants' and the 'Metamorphosis of Narcissus'. The former, as

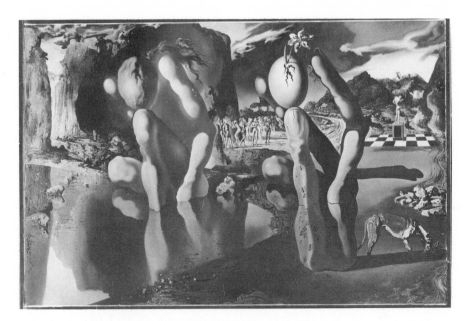

Figure 8.7 *Dali's* Metamorphosis of Narcissus.

the title suggests, depicts four swans in a lake whose reflections are strikingly represented by four elephants. The latter carries a much greater significance not only because of its profound theme but also because a book by Dali of the same title provides us with a clue as to its origin and a glimpse of the workings of Dali's paranoiac-critical method. In the book, two fishermen of Port-Lligat are talking about a slightly demented person from their village:

> *First fisherman:* 'What's the matter with that chap staring at himself in a mirror all day?'
> *Second fisherman:* 'If you really want to know he's got a bulb in his head.'

Dali explains, '"A bulb in the head" in Catalan corresponds exactly with the psychoanalytic notion of "complex". If a man had a bulb in his head it might break into flower at any moment, Narcissus!'[53] As Wilson comments, 'Dali's instant association of the mirror with the Greek myth followed by the mental jump of his transformation of the Catalan phrase into the image of the flower sprouting from Narcissus' head, vividly evoke the dynamic processes of paranoiac thought.'[54] Dali is also said to have trained himself to doze in a chair with his chin resting on a spoon which was held in one hand, propped by his elbow which rested on a table; in this position, when his muscles relaxed and he was on the verge of falling asleep, his chin would drop and he would wake, often in the middle of a hypnagogic dream or vision which he would then proceed to paint.

Comparable to Dali's 'Metamorphosis of Narcissus' is one of Leroy's reports (cited in chapter 3) in which the hypnagogic vision of a carpet being shaken from a window brought to the subject's mind the thought of a tooth which led to the carpet's turning into a molar tooth whose roots represented (turned into) the legs of the person who was shaking the carpet! Two other examples of obvious surrealistic nature, given by McKellar, are the image of a crab smoking a cigar and the vision of an eye sitting in a glass of water which splits into two to reveal inside it a metal sphere with tiny people moving around it.[55]

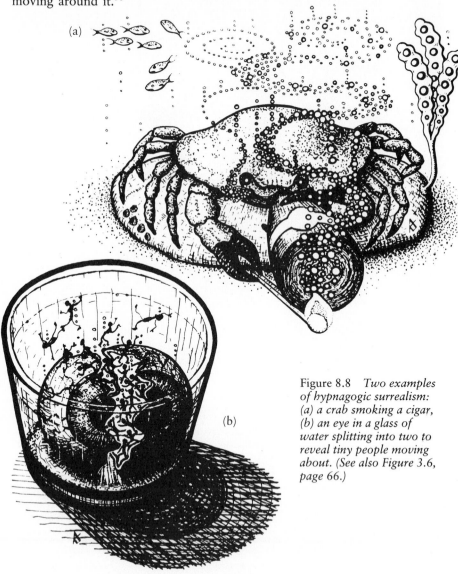

(a)

(b)

Figure 8.8 *Two examples of hypnagogic surrealism: (a) a crab smoking a cigar, (b) an eye in a glass of water splitting into two to reveal tiny people moving about. (See also Figure 3.6, page 66.)*

Figure 8.9 *(a) Blake's* The
Ghost of a Flea, *(b)* The
Man Who Taught Blake
Painting in his Dreams.
*Visual hypnagogic images
of horrible faces have been
compared (e.g. by
Greenwood in the last
century) to some of Blake's
paintings and in particular
to his 'ghost'. Blake is said
to have reported that his
depiction of the ghost was
the result of an absorbing
conversation he had had
with a flea which revealed
to him that fleas were in-
habited by the souls of evil
men. He was also thought
to have been taught painting
by a teacher who appeared
to him in his dreams. Some
writers believe that Blake's
paintings in general contain
clear elements of psychotic
ideation.*

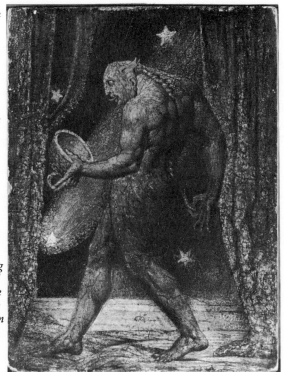

(a)

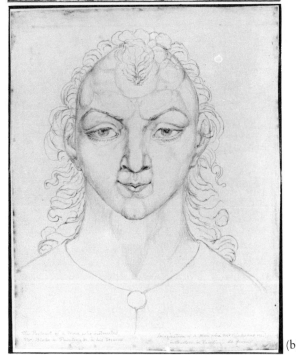

(b)

To an extent, the paranoid patient who systematically relates normally unrelated events, thoughts and situations to his delusion resembles the creative individual who produces unusual, remote and far-fetched associations. The resemblance is often too strong to be ignored. It generalizes into one's behaviour. As Guilford remarked, 'the highly creative person's behaviour is sometimes eccentric. This has sometimes branded him as being abnormal and even pathological.'[56] Dali encapsulated the problem in his classical retort, 'The only difference between me and a madman is that I am not mad.' On the other hand, Einstein's jingle reads:

> A thought that sometimes makes me hazy:
> Am I – or are the others crazy?

Referring to Kekulé's hypnagogic vision, Koestler remarks, 'the whirling, giddy vision reminds me of the hallucinations of schizophrenics, as painted or described by them'; Faraday's visions resemble 'the stable delusional systems of paranoia'.[57] Thus, the resemblance sinks deeper than Dali's witticism. In some cases it is more than resemblance: it is the employment of identical mental processes. These latter, as already seen, are clearly revealed in hypnagogia which thus brings together on to a common ground the genius and the madman.

The production of unusual and unique associations viewed as partaking of the criterion of originality in creativity, but also found in madness and in hypnagogia, can, further, be seen as the creation of 'actualized' metaphors or analogies in all three conditions. This can be seen in examining and comparing the following four cases: (a) von Domarus's patient who, as we saw in the previous chapter, identified with each other a saint, a box of cigars, and sex on the basis of their all being encircled, (b) Kepler's comparison of the sun, the stars or planets, and the space between them to God the Father, the Son, and the Holy Ghost, (c) Kekulé's vision of the snakes as an analogy with the benzene molecule, and (d) Silberer's autosymbolic hypnagogic phenomena.

To begin with, in all four cases the associations are indeed unusual. It might be objected to that in the case of von Domarus's patient the identification is not only unusual but entirely unjustified, indeed crazy. But the madness is not so much in the remoteness of the associations as in the fact that a metaphor has been taken literally, it has been 'actualized', in the mind of the patient a cigar box *is* a saint. In Kepler's case I suspect a similar process. On one occasion he specifically stressed that 'it is by no means permissible to treat this analogy as an empty comparison; it should be considered by its Platonic form and archetypal quality as one of the primary causes'.[58] The interesting point here is that the image of the holy trinity as an analogy was superimposed on the solar system much in the way a paranoid relates phenomena to fit his central belief. Kepler's comparison of the planets to the Son is not merely unusual but entirely irrelevant: there is neither external similarity (the Son is one, the planets are many) nor an internal one (the Son does not 'revolve' round the Father). Kekulé's and Silberer's examples have already been discussed.

Poetry, like all other forms of art, makes perhaps an easier comparison with hypnagogic mentation and speech than scientific invention. It also makes an easier comparison with madness. In science one may apply the criterion of usefulness, no matter how relative the latter might be; one can also apply sheer logic and rational analysis to scientific products. But with poetry such criteria may not be merely inadequate but altogether inappropriate. Housman speaks of poetry as essentially devoid of meaning, and regards Blake as 'the most poetical of all poets' and 'more poetical than Shakespeare' primarily because 'Blake's meaning is often unimportant or virtually non-existent, so that we can listen with all our hearing to his celestial tune'.[59] He further notes that 'the production of poetry, in its first stage, is less an active than a passive and involuntary process', and quotes Plato who said:

> He who without the Muses' madness in his soul comes knocking at the
> door of poetry and thinks that art will make him anything fit to be
> called a poet, finds that the poetry which he indites in his sober senses
> is beaten hollow by the poetry of madmen.[60]

In this transient state of madness the creative poet brings together images from distant FsR and produces unusual associations and, as Aristotle noted, compounds and strange words, or, as Freud believed, condensations of several meanings or allusions into a phrase or word.[61] (In German, to 'write poetry' is to 'condense': '*dichten*'). As already pointed out by many writers, the more remote these elements the more fertile or creative the process. Thus Mednick, for instance, quotes as an illustration a line from Marianne Moore's poem 'The Monkey Puzzle' which reads, 'The lion's ferocious chrysanthemum head'.[62] Compare this with Green's schizophrenic 'Heat-craze my teeth in bitterest anger' and 'there was a gear all teeth, two at least world-caught. And now nothing engages the world!' And compare both with the hypnagogic sentence reported by one of Trömner's subjects: 'He regally escaped into his existence.' Many other hypnagogic examples comparable to the above have been given in chapter 7 and throughout this book.

Housman's statement in respect to the first stage of poetic creation being passive and involuntary, and his reference to Plato's view of poetic inspiration, introduce into the present discussion certain terms which are often used in relation to creativity and sometimes as its synonyms, namely, 'intuition', 'insight' and 'inspiration'. I consider it a good place to discuss them here as they relate not only to creativity but also to madness and hypnagogia, both through their nonrational-unconscious character and through their originality as represented by the qualities of novelty, unpredictability, uniqueness and surprise.

Further to his comments above, Housman offers a personal example illustrating the process of inspiration. Having drunk a pint of beer at luncheon, he says, he went for a walk during which, thinking of nothing in particular, would flow into his mind unexpectedly,

> sometimes a line or two of verse, sometimes a whole stanza at once, accompanied, not preceded by a vague notion of the poem which they were destined to form a part of. Then there would usually be a lull of an hour or so, then perhaps the spring would bubble up again. I say bubble up, because, so far as I could make out, the source of the suggestions thus proffered to the brain was an abyss which I have already had occasion to mention, the pit of the stomach.

Earlier on he calls this process 'a secretion'.

There are two points in this excerpt I consider relevant to my discussion. The first concerns Housman's noting that his conceiving a line or two of verse or a whole stanza is accompanied by a vague notion of the whole poem. This is very much like the feeling of significance encountered in hypnagogia. In most cases of course it remains just a feeling, undirected and unattached. Sometimes it is the beginning of a flash of insight, as in Kekulé's case. And yet on other occasions it constitutes an intimation of an impending poetic inspiration, as in Miller's case (see also her hypnagogic poem 'The Moth to the Sun' reported in the same paper).

The second point is his reference to inspiration as a secretion and as having its source in the pit of the stomach, i.e. as being 'visceral'. Similarly Williams, speaking of the phenomena of intuition, said that 'the primitive, the visceral, the unconscious mind gives information to the conscious, and like the experienced judge, it announces its conclusions but withholds its reasons'.[63] Koestler said of intuitions that they 'give the appearance of miraculous flashes, of short-circuits of reasoning'.[64] Hutchinson noted that 'insight . . . is often accompanied by a flood of ideas, alternative hypotheses appearing at the same time, many of which are difficult to make explicit owing to the crowded rapidity of their appearance'. He also drew attention to 'the almost hallucinatory vividness of the ideas appearing in connection with any sense department – visual, auditory, kinaesthetic' in this experience.[65] Berne remarked that 'directed participation of the perceptive ego interfered with intuition' and that 'when the perceptive ego was not directed the activity of some other function could be "felt"'.[66] Kris pointed out that in their purest form states of inspiration are found in primitive societies: 'They are mostly connected with a partial loss of consciousness' and 'may be described as phenomena of regression.'[67]

Although it is not to be argued that hypnagogia is always and in all respects a state of inspiration, it must be noted that the features described by these authors as constituting this latter state are also characteristic of the former: the spontaneity, vividness, autonomy, rapidity of change and multitude of imagery and ideation, the 'underground' fusion whose results appear strange, 'miraculous' or irrational, the dissociated or semi-dissociated state, the diminution or dissolution of self-consciousness and logical controls, the regression or functional reorientation, these are all known features of hypnagogia.

Inspiration can also be understood as both 'bubbling' *and* 'babbling' of the unconscious: as the primitive, kinesthetic-visceral feeling of welling up, often with a sense of being filled up and oozing out or overflowing, and as the irrepressible tendency to let go of all conscious controls over thought, movement, speech, and so forth, resulting, for instance, in talking seeming nonsense. It is encountered in hypnagogia in both of these senses. In the form of 'poetical nonsense', as Housman might have said, it is found, for instance, in neologisms, alliterations, assonance, sound associations, verbal-auditory and visual punning, strange verbal constructions with intimations and undertones of mysticism, philosophy, religion, and poetic grandeur.

Openness

We have seen that to be creative one must be able to lift one's logical 'dampers', thereby disinhibiting the free flow of mental life and allowing the rising to consciousness of unconscious-nonrational and original combinations of associative elements, and we have also seen that this happens naturally in hypnagogia. This is almost the same as saying that one must be 'open'. Rogers explains that openness is

> the opposite of psychological defensiveness, when to protect the organization of self, certain experiences are prevented from coming into awareness except in disturbed fashion. . . . It means lack of rigidity and permeability of boundaries in concepts, beliefs, perceptions and hypotheses.[68]

Like originality, openness encompasses four features, viz. sensitivity, tolerance of ambiguity, self-acceptance, and spontaneity. Although these are seen by some psychologists as character traits, they are not necessarily inherited but mostly acquired. Sensitivity, Hallman tells us, refers to 'a state of being aware of things as they really are rather than according to some predetermined set', and of being receptive to 'unconscious impulses'. Tolerance of ambiguity refers to the ability 'to tolerate inconsistencies and contradictions, to accept the unknown, to be comfortable with the ambiguous, approximate, uncertain'. Out of sensitivity and tolerance of ambiguity come flexibility, one implication of which is the ability 'to perceive meaning in irrelevancies', and self-acceptance, since 'the creative person . . . needs to rely upon his own sensitivity for guidance'. Finally, spontaneity 'gives the creative act the feeling of being free, autonomous, undetermined.'

In a factorial analysis of the personality of creative scientists, technologists and inventors, Guilford found the following eight traits (not all of which, however, are applicable to all forms of creativity): sensitivity to problems, fluency (i.e. the ability to produce 'a large number of ideas per unit of time'), novelty, flexibility of mind ('the ease with which one changes set'), analysing ability (as a complement to organizing ability), reorganization or redefinition of organized wholes ('transformation of an existing object into one of different design, function or use'), complexity or intricacy of conceptual structure ('how many interrelated ideas can a person manipulate at the same time'), evaluation.[69] On the other hand McKellar, equating the concept of creativity with that of originality, points out that 'an individual may exhibit high originality on one occasion and remarkably little on others', and suggests that 'it may often be more fruitful to regard the term like "originality" as descriptive of instances of behaviour rather than underlying personality traits'.[70]

However the case may be, most of the conditions referred to above are to be found, in one form or another, in hypnagogia. This is not to say that hypnagogists are necessarily endowed with these traits but that the state of hypnagogia is conducive to their emergence, i.e. hypnagogia may represent one of McKellar's 'instances of behaviour' characterized by creativeness. We have already seen that the hypnagogist is open to preconscious elements, and that, similarly, the creative person is sensitive to 'unconscious impulses', among other things. (A wider view of openness in hypnagogia was discussed in chapter 3.) Throughout this book we saw that the hypnagogist is sensitive to internal activity, e.g. imagery, ideas, impulses, intuitions; that boundaries of the self and of concepts are fluid and permeable; that psychological openness as opposed to defensiveness is the *sine qua non* of hypnagogic induction and progression. In hypnagogia the subject accepts approximations, ambiguities, and contradictions. He may be thought of as 'fluent' in the sense of producing a large number of images which are characterized by spontaneity and autonomy, 'flexible' in terms of 'the ease with which he changes set' and the variety and changeability of his imagery. In respect to the latter, it is interesting to note Hudson's remark that persons whose imagery is overly flexible are like nomads in regard to their inner and outer world, that their ego boundaries are poorly maintained and they tend to differentiate neither between their own inner and outer life nor between themselves and other people[71] – observations pointing, once again, to the LEBs. Further, the hypnagogist reorganizes or redefines in the sense of transforming an existing object into one of different design or function, and his conceptualization is often complex, consisting of intricate crossings of FsR.

In respect to self-acceptance, the hypnagogist may be said to be in a state of 'forced self-acceptance', that is, he is placed, by the very nature of hypnagogia which requires relaxation and abandonment, in a position of allowing normally constrained or simply unconscious mentation to come freely to the fore. It is true that this form of self-acceptance does not entirely coincide with that proposed by Hallman; also, hypnagogic imagery and thought are generally characterized by the feature of 'externality', of transpiring 'outside' the subject, and thus the hypnagogist might be thought of as transferring reliance on to something outside himself. However, we have only to reflect on cases like those of Kekulé, Poincaré and Hadamard to understand that acceptance of spontaneous and autonomous thoughts and images which have the appearance of externality does not necessarily imply reliance on factors lying outside the subject – such reliance, as already seen, is related to set and setting.

Again, tolerance of ambiguity in hypnagogia is both 'forced' and necessary. It is 'forced' in the sense that it occurs irrespective of the personality of the subject, and necessary because there must be no sense of unacceptable ambiguity in the mind of the subject as he enters the state: there must be relaxation, and a diffuse feeling of certainty that ambiguities, incongruities and contradictions will either be resolved in due course or they are just what they are and should be taken in one's stride.

Self-actualization

The features discussed above can easily be seen as constituting some of the conditions required for achieving psychological growth and health. Further, creativity is often equated with psychological health, and the latter with the self-actualizing process.[72] Self-actualization is also linked with strength of motivation which acts as the energy source for change and growth. Thus, it is proposed that 'all instances of personality growth are possible grounds for creativeness, and that 'unless significant transformation occurs in personality during an activity, that activity will fall short of the creative'.[9]

Now in hypnagogia, though there are many changes, these are mostly fleeting and transient. However, various investigators have pointed to the therapeutic value of hypnagogia, either directly[73] or in relating it to the creative process[74] (through which it is again related to 'therapeutic' mystical experience due to their common connection with preconscious mentation[75]).

If the *process* of self-actualization is seen as a *progressive integration* of the personality wherein the individual comes to strike a balance between the conscious and the unconscious, the rational and the nonrational, then hypnagogia may play a twofold major role in the achievement of such a goal: first, it may contribute directly to the realization of the target, and second, it may point to an underlying aetiology and provide the framework for understanding the presence of the particular traits characterizing the self-actualized person.

In regard to its first role, hypnagogia may indeed constitute instances of personality growth which are possible grounds for creativeness in the sense of facilitating self-acceptance and personality balance characterized by practically all of the features of Maslow's creative personality, viz. spontaneity and effortlessness, expressiveness and innocence, lack of fear for the uncertain, ambiguous or unknown, ability to tolerate bipolarity and ability to bring together and integrate opposites.[76] Moreover, because of its character of bringing to the surface unconscious material, hypnagogia may act as a diagnostic screen against which are projected both the physiological and psychological states of the individual. Evidence from various sources indeed shows that somatic, psychosomatic, and psychological states are reflected in the contents of the subject's hypnagogic imagery.[77]

Significantly, on the psychological level it has been variously shown that hypnagogia is a most fertile period for the emergence of symbols, and for symbol interpretation.[78] What is more, Silberer's idea of 'functional' symbolism in hypnagogia argues both for a type of 'dream' symbolism which is independent of repression or censorship, and for 'anagogic' interpretation, i.e. for states or processes to be realized in the future, thus relating present preoccupations with problems and their possible future resolution.[79] In addition, hypnagogic symbolism appears to contain Freudian references to the outside world as well as integrative Jungian representations in which aspects of the subject's personality are symbolically manifested. More important, the Foulkes et al. study showed that good hypnagogists reflect personalities with positive characteristics.[80] Green and Green have also noted that

> on the one hand, many outstanding creative people have reported their greatest insights . . . were associated with reverie and hypnagogic imagery, and, on the other hand, the imagery and insights reported by college students in the theta training project involved changes in their personal lives. . . . These are also amenable to insight, intuition and creativity.[81]

It has, thus, been suggested, for instance, that hypnagogia may be used to advantage by training less positive people to become more tolerant of others, less dogmatic, and better able to express their feelings – simply by training them to enter and remain in this state for increasing intervals. Personality changes and treatment for depression and obesity, *inter alia*, are also said to be facilitated by the use of suggestopedic programmes utilizing hypnagogia[82] (see chapter 3). The light stages of this state alone may be utilized for their beneficial effects of psychophysical relaxation, especially when combined with autogenic practices. Thus, hypnagogia may indeed contribute directly to the process of self-actualization both by facilitating the emergence of unconscious material and by aiding in the acceptance and integration of such material into an expanding personality, either by simply allowing the material to surface or by utilizing the receptivity of the state to suggest positive personality changes.

Finally, Maslow's features of the self-actualized personality listed above are typically psychological aspects of the root phenomenon of the LEBs which characterizes hypnagogia. Thus, the latter's central feature of the LEBs may account for the presence or emergence-development of the traits characteristic of self-actualized, creative individuals. In this sense, hypnagogia plays another important role in the area of creativity, by revealing a possible underlying aetiological factor out of which emerge the character symptoms ascribed to the creative personality.

9 · *Other relevant areas of experience*

Under this heading I shall discuss very briefly a number of other mental states, processes, and experiences which share various phenomenological features with hypnagogia. The brevity of the treatment is partly due to lack of space but also to lack of time for more detailed research. Some of these phenomena certainly warrant more attention, and it is hoped that this brief outline can provide impetus for further investigation.

Hypnosis

William James thought it probable that we go through a hypnotic state as we fall asleep, and de Manacéine and Arnold-Forster drew attention to the naturally occurring hypnosis at both ends of hypnagogia.[1] The induction of both hypnagogia and classical hypnosis centres on progressive psychophysical relaxation, and in both cases the subject's attention is gradually withdrawn from his environment, becoming increasingly internalized. In hypnosis, as in hypnagogia, the subject feels passive, and experiences body schema alterations, floating and drifting or spinning. Some reports read: 'My body began to swell up, until it broke off in great chunks, and there was nothing left but my mind', 'I had an odd sensation as though I was immense in size – maybe three or four miles high – sitting on earth – each movement covering a great distance – as if I had some new conception of distance and size'.[2] As Gill and Brenman noted, in hypnosis

> we see a significant departure from normal, *waking* modes of thought: instead of relatively stable, logical kinds of thought – which for the most part employs words as its material – we see the emergence of fluid, archaic forms which often employ visual images and symbols as material, forms which do not follow the ordinary rules of logic, and which moreover are not bound to realistic limitations of time and space.[3]

Hilgard has isolated seven important features of hypnosis (the seventh not being altogether essential), namely: passivity, diffuse and redistributed attention, availability of memories and heightened ability for fantasy production, reduction of reality testing and tolerance of reality distortion, increased suggestibility, role behaviour, and posthypnotic amnesia.[2] The reduction of reality testing and the readiness of the subject to accept nonrational and bizarre phenomena as nothing unusual has led Orne to speak of *trance logic*.[4] These observations and remarks make, of course, exceedingly good comparisons with hypnagogia.

In hypnosis, a distinction is usually drawn between the induction or hypnotic process and the hypnotic state itself. The former can be achieved by a variety of techniques all of which have in common 'a withdrawal from usual environmental relationships through relaxation, contemplation of sleep, free play of imagination, or concentration upon a small target or some part of the body and upon the hypnotist's voice'.[5] Kubie and Margolin point out that hypnotic induction is generally characterized by immobilization and monotony, that is, by restricting the subject's sensorimotor relationships and causing him to listen to the hypnotist's monotonous or rhythmical voice.[6] This has the effect of putting a person in a state of 'partial sleep' in which a 'dissolution of Ego boundaries' takes place, so that 'the incoming stimuli become indistinguishable from the self, seemingly as endogenous as the subject's own thoughts and feelings'. There is a psychological fusion between subject and hypnotist and the latter's voice is experienced as part of the subject's own psychic process – a condition analogous to the sensorimotor state assumed to be present in infancy. It is proposed that the observed suggestibility of the subject arises out of the restriction of sensorimotor relationships and 'the lessened opportunity to make comparisons with actual concurrent sensations', which also accounts for the 'undiluted intensity' of imagery and memories that flow through the subject's mind during the resultant hypnagogic state. In the fully developed hypnotic state there is a partial re-establishment of the subject's ego boundaries along with an incorporation of a fragmentary image of the hypnotist who 'becomes something which the subject carries around inside of him'.

Discussing the emotional factors in the induction of the hypnotic state, Kubie and Margolin suggest that the state of alertness necessary for response to exteroceptive signals is dependent on a number of factors and experiences in the life of an organism. 'Thus, if an animal is satiated, or if the "promise" is never fulfilled, or if pain finally cannot be overcome or avoided, the reaction may become reversed and the same signal will induce drowsiness' instead of the expected alertness. In this way, attentiveness to exteroceptive stimuli comes to have a complex significance in all animal life. 'To withdraw attention from such stimuli implies either a state of satiation, or a retreat from painful tension, or else a sense of security that reaches to the deepest unconscious layers of the personality. The latter state is the goal of the hypnotist' – it is also the *sine qua non* condition for the induction of hypnagogia which can never take place in the absence of a sense of security. These remarks may also be helpful in shedding some light on two other situations, namely, schizophrenia and the 'confusion technique' in hypnosis. In regard to schizophrenia, we saw that this may be the result of the crowding of unassimilated percepts leading to a 'jamming of the circuits', which is another way of describing 'a retreat from painful tension' or from a state of frustration which is the result of numerous unfulfilled 'promises'.[7]

The 'confusion technique' was originated and perfected by Milton Erickson[8] who also employed successfully many other techniques, including the multilevel use of anecdotes. Basically, in the confusion technique the subject, who may believe himself unhypnotizable and not even know that an attempt is to be made to hypnotize him, listens to the hypnotist who, in complete earnestness, says or does something puzzling. While the subject is trying to 'puzzle out' the verbal expression or behaviour of the hypnotist, the latter continues with another sentence or bit of communication which, although perfectly sensible in itself, is irrelevant to what has preceded it. And so on: all items of communication in this exercise are by themselves sound and sensible but, taken in context, they are confusing, distracting and inhibiting. Erickson explains that

> As this procedure is continued for hypnotic purposes, there often arises
> an intolerable state of bewilderment, confusion and a compelling,
> growing need for the subject of this procedure to make some kind of
> response to relieve his increasing tension and he readily seizes upon the
> first clear-cut easily comprehended communication offered to him.[8]

In this way, the need to dissipate the created confusion results in the subject's relinquishing of resistances, and often leads to a state of trance. As one subject reported while under hypnosis, 'as soon as I experienced the slightest feeling of confusion, I just dropped into a deep trance.'

Another method used by Erickson to induce hypnosis is the employment of anecdotes. These are in fact used for a number of purposes, one of which is to forge an empathic link with the subject or patient (usually on an unconscious level), but they are also often used to induce hypnosis by virtue of their character of 'engaging', and of decreasing resistance, causing distraction, assisting in the reframing and redefining of problems and desensitizing from fears, promoting dissociation, and breaching one's defences indirectly. Because, when listening to an anecdote, one is kept off balance, Erickson used anecdotes to create confusion and promote hypnotic responsiveness. Anecdotes can be confusing because they are ambiguous, and may have multiple meanings. 'Anecdotes can "set up" an induction by distracting and depotentiating the conscious set. Thereby, the subject can become more open and more responsive to concurrent and subsequent suggestions.'[9] In other words, they are conducive to the subject's LEBs.

Hypnotic induction may be seen as the disruption of our usual, wakeful, state of consciousness and the repatterning of a new (hypnotic) state.[10] The hypnotic or trance state itself is, as already noted, characterized by the elimination of waking patterns of behaviour.[11] In regard to drawing comparisons between hypnagogia and the hypnotic state it is noteworthy that most of the latter's indicators of trance development are the already familiar hypnagogic markers, e.g. spontaneous, autonomous, 'objective' ideation, comfort and relaxation, pupillary changes and eye closure, facial features ironed out, feeling distant, lack of body movement, lack of startle response, retardation and loss of reflexes, literalism, response attentiveness, sensory muscular and body changes, slowing of pulse and respiration, time distortion and time lag in motor and conceptual behaviour, regression, amnesia, paresthesia, and catalepsy.[12]

'Response attentiveness' is seen by many workers in this area as a most important marker in the initiation of hypnosis. So much so that Erickson has called it the 'everyday trance' and noted that it occurs in everyday life whenever we become absorbed – hence his extensive use of anecdotes to engage and absorb the subject's attention and create what is known as a 'yes set'. Absorption, monoideism, and centring of attention are related concepts, all implying a capacity for dissociation, the latter often being assigned a central role in explanations of hypnosis.[13] We have, of course, already discussed the relationship of these features to hypnagogia and their presence in other states closely related to it. Needless to remind ourselves that response attentiveness in hypnagogia is not to be understood as referring to centring of attention in something external but to absorption in intrapsychic activities.

In the previous chapter we had occasion to see how a dream, of which there was no memory, was *re-presented* in the hypnopompic state, and how under hypnosis the subject of this experience (or some psychic part of her) was able to 'fill in' items of the dream which were missing from the subject's hypnopompic re-presentation. It is interesting in this respect that the neodissociationist theory of hypnosis speaks of a 'hidden observer' who registers 'experiences' that the hypnotized person bypasses.[14] For instance, a person who is hypnotized and told not to feel any pain when he puts his hand in ice cold water may respond appropriately by reporting absence of pain, but when he is further told that on being tapped on the shoulder a hidden part of himself will tell what it remembers of the experience, the tapping is indeed followed by a report that the experience was painful. We have seen that this 'unconscious' registering of experiences can be made conscious through the preconscious nature of hypnagogia. Moreover, the observer function in hypnosis, as in hypnagogia, may not always be so 'hidden', as witnessed by the reports of subjects who speak of observing detachedly, impersonally, and objectively what takes place during the experience. This sometimes gives the impression to the subject in either state that he is not hypnotized (or falling asleep, as the case may be). This phenomenon in hypnosis is very similar to the experience of double-consciousness in hypnagogia whereby a person is aware simultaneously of two environments.

We have also seen that in the deep stages of hypnagogia subjects may have mystical expriences. Similar phenomena, such as the feeling that one's mind is separate from one's body, a feeling of being one with the universe, a sense of gaining 'incommunicable' knowledge, are reported as occurring in deep hypnotic trances.[15] It must be noted, however, that, in contrast to hypnagogia, in hypnosis trances may be produced which are characterized by hyperalertness and tension.

Perceptual isolation and sensory deprivation

At first sight the evidence for positive relationships between hypnagogic and sensory deprivation experiences is conflicting. Whereas some workers have found that hypnagogic imagery is clearly present in sensory deprivation experiments,[16] others have argued that visual phenomena occurring under these conditions – so-called 'reported visual sensations' (RVSs) – are found both in wakefulness and drowsiness, or, even, only in wakefulness.[17]

The confusion as to what exactly RVSs are plays an important part in the interpretation of these phenomena.[18] Moreover, the term 'sensory deprivation' describing experimental conditions of absence or marked reduction of sensory stimulation is loosely exchangeable with the term 'perceptual isolation' which stands for invariant or monotonous experimental settings.[19] But relative invariance of stimulation is one of the necessary components of the hypnagogic syndrome, and so is marked reduction of stimulation. It is a well-known fact that monotony, for instance, is conducive to sleep, i.e. it is hypnagogic, and that 'limitation of voluntary activity, limitation of the field of consciousness and inhibition all help to a greater monotony'.[20] Immobilization was also seen in the previous section to have the effect of putting a person in a state of 'partial sleep'.

It has been argued that if hypnagogic and sensory deprivation phenomena are the same then persons who doze and sleep frequently during isolation should have both more RVSs and of a more complex variety than persons who remain alert, which, as evidence shows, is not the case.[21] Now, the first of these arguments is unsound in that it assumes that incidence of drowsy episodes and sleep should correlate with RVSs. But, people in non-experimental situations who feel drowsy and fall asleep more often than others do not necessarily have more *visual* hypnagogic hallucinations than the latter: besides individual differences that may show predilection for some other sense modality (especially kinesthetic and somesthetic[22]), the actual *attentional state* of the individual is of great importance as it may not only influence the latency in the emergence of the phenomena but also the type of visual experience (e.g. complex, meaningful) and the modality involved – *attentional shift* is also of importance. Further, in sensory deprivation the results and their interpretations are subject to other interacting conditions, such as kind and duration of confinement, and criteria for the classification of the experiences.

These objections will also apply to the second argument. In addition, attention must be drawn to the observation that RVSs, just like visual hypnagogic experiences, appear gradually and in degrees of complexity, stretching from dots and lights to lines and simple geometric patterns, 'wallpaper' patterns, isolated objects, and integrated scenes.[23] Thus, conclusions to the effect that the majority of reported visual and auditory sensations in sensory deprivation experiments were 'unstructured'[24] may only point to the possibility that the majority of subjects in these experiments either never relaxed enough or fell asleep too quickly, whereas descriptions by subjects who remained 'alert' may simply refer to the effects of their efforts to think while drowsing lightly, i.e. the reference may be to complex autosymbolic phenomena. The parameter of effort to think while drowsing was, unfortunately, not considered in these studies.

Some investigators have found significant positive correlations between prior history of hypnagogic images and sensory deprivation imagery,[25] and in perceptual isolation studies where the Block's MMPI scale for neurotic under-control was applied negative correlations with imagery frequency were obtained – which were interpreted as 'reflections of the *intellectual flexibility* and *emotional freedom* clusters' forming part of an 'adaptive reaction',[26] reminiscent of the Foulkes *et al.* personality findings in respect to hypnagogia.[27]

Further, neither the argument that to refer to all sensory deprivation phenomena as hypnagogic is an oversimplification, nor the contention that sensory deprivation phenomena are a potpourri of daydreams, fantasies, hypnagogic images, and dreams,[28] is properly justified. Reviewing the literature one cannot help but be struck by the phenomenological richness of hypnagogia within whose boundaries are encountered all of those phenomena that occur in sensory deprivation. Moreover, a careful examination of the conditions of hypnagogia reveals that both the spontaneous and the experimental induction of the state is clearly achieved, as noted earlier, by a considerable degree of perceptual isolation.

Photic, pulse current, and direct electrical stimulation

Experiments in photic stimulation with a stroboscope, excitation of the brain by means of externally attached temporal electrodes, and direct electrical stimulation of the visual cortex[29] have all yielded phenomena identical with those encountered in hypnagogia.

Further, (a) subjects that experience a great amount of imagery during photic stimulation fall into the same category as those people who experience freely hypnagogic imagery, and are characterized by the possession of an artistic, sensitive and creative self-concept which is found to relate to a syndrome that includes imagery;[30] (b) prior history of naturally occurring hypnagogic imagery is found to be related to the incidence of visual imagery experienced in rhythmic photic stimulation;[31] (c) the external conditions of photic and pulse current stimulation are similar to those under which hypnagogic imagery occurs, i.e. lying on a bed with closed eyes in a quiet room; and (d) electrical stimulation 'induces a state of consciousness which makes it more probable that primary-process modes of functioning will prevail'.[32]

Sleep deprivation

Sleep deprivation may be considered as a condition in which the need for sleep and the effort to stay awake place the subject in a vacillating intermediate state not unlike the naturally occurring hypnagogia. Hypnagogic experiences in sleep deprivation have been noted by various workers,[33] many of whom have observed that even slightly sleep-deprived persons fall into lapses of inattention or take catnaps while standing, sometimes not being aware of falling asleep and often having 'the sensation of floating in and out of consciousness with their eyes open'.[34] Some investigators have grouped together 'the visions of hypnagogic states, dreams, and sleep deprivation' on the grounds that they 'have in common the elements of semi somnolence and altered electroencephalographic activity'.[35]

The motor behaviour of sleep deprived subjects is erratic: they appear as if drunk, and they mumble and ramble and slur their speech, mispronounce, repeat, use jargon, change topics for no apparent reason, avoid any task that requires effort or attention, and have experiences that involve, or consist of, body-schema and weight alterations, time and space distortion, macropsias and micropsias, tactile hallucinations, visual hallucinations such as seeing smoke rising from the floor or people standing in the room, and auditory hallucinations.[36] For instance, it will be remembered from chapter 7 that one of Oswald's subjects bent forward and kissed the EEG paper in the laboratory while having 'dream-like thoughts about his girlfriend' and recorded his experience by writing 'Leant forward and downwards to plant a kiss upon the unmarried letters'. Another subject wrote what he considered to be a 'profound statement' whose ending was the irrelevant comment 'Owes $8.00'.[37]

Dream scintillations

Various workers have observed what have come to be called 'dream scintillations' or 'flickering images', that is, 'a rapid succession of images which intrude upon awareness and are difficult to remember'.[38] One investigator noted that these experiences may last up to half an hour, and described them thus:

> One feels as though he has just had a dream which he is trying hard to recall. He keeps trying to recall it, but while thus striving in vain, that which he is trying to recall seems to change. Then the realization dawns

that this effort to grasp the dream is itself part of a dream state, a dream state which goes on like a real dream, shiftingly and distractingly, but while one is fully awake and in full command of his behaviour and feelings so that no one else could observe or suspect anything unusual unless it is a slight distraction.[39]

Dream scintillations often appear after physical exertion but in the absence of drowsiness.

Forbes, another experient of such phenomena, having drawn a distinction between three types of dream, one of which was that occurring 'at the onset of sleep or during transient dozing in the day', pointed out that '"dream scintillations" were striking examples' of this latter type.[40] The contents of these visual experiences were mostly fragments of recent or long forgotten dreams and bits of actual events. Throughout these occurrences, Forbes recounts, 'I experienced a strange dreamy feeling, but at no time did I actually doze. . . . They were like the first dream figures of ordinary dozing and they kept on coming in a rapid-fire sequence.' He noted that during the time he had this 'strange dreamy feeling' his memory was confused: he had difficulty in deciding what day it was, and previously familiar names and words were either impossible to recall or looked unfamiliar. On one occasion he reported:

About 12.30, when dream flashes were about maximum, I dictated a fairly long letter to a friend. At 4 p.m., reading over before signing, I noted that much of it seemed strange and unfamiliar. The letter said what I wanted to say, but I didn't recall using some of its phrases. I was surprised at reading what I had dictated.

The phenomenological similarities between dream scintillations and hypnagogic imagery need no stressing. Moreover, as Forbes pointed out, the former are 'striking examples' of the latter. Horowitz suggested the replacing of the term 'dream scintillations' with that of 'flickering images' on the grounds that these experiences take place when the person is not asleep and 'because the event could be a transient change in consciousness due to a minor variant of temporal lobe epilepsy or migraine'.[41] The term 'flickering images', however, falls short of conveying the mental state of the subject, viz. a *dreamy* 'transient change in consciousness', which is more accurately conveyed by the older term.

Hallucinogenic-drug-induced phenomena

In 1895 Prentiss and Morgan initiated the systematic investigation of the hallucinogenic properties of mescalin, and in the following year Mitchell drew attention for the first time to the similarities of mescalin and hypnagogic experiences, and in particular to the autonomous nature of both and to the tendency of the former to become intensified during sleep onset.[42] Other workers since have confirmed Mitchell's observations and exposed additional similarities.[43]

Klüver identified 'form constants' that occur in both, viz. (a) grating, lattice, fretwork, filigree, honeycomb, chessboard-design, (b) cobweb figure, (c) tunnel, funnel, alley, vessel, (d) spiral.[44] In addition, he noted that mescaline visions, like those of hypnagogia, are characterized by a large variety of colours, intense brightness, unusual saturation of colour, sourceless illumination, lack of 'an exact egocentric localization', microscopic clarity of detail, autonomy, continuous and rapid change. The size of the objects seen can be 'gigantic' or 'lilliputian' (macropsia and micropsia), although Klüver's personal experiences were solely of the latter kind. Images of objects sometimes appear distorted (dysmorphopsia) and in multiples of themselves (polyopsia). In most cases when a subject tries to visualize a particular image, a similar or related one appears.

A very interesting mescaline phenomenon is what Klüver called the *presque vu-experience*, that is, the experience of a feeling of *incompleteness* as one views a vision, accompanied by a sense of hidden significance often of cosmic dimensions – frequently the result of minute and apparently irrelevant details acquiring central importance. Voices are sometimes hallucinated, and so are tactile or haptic sensations, e.g. sensations of hot or cold in various parts of the body. There are also olfactory and kinesthetic 'hallucinations' and body-schema distortions, e.g. shortening or lengthening of limbs, swelling, shrinking or melting away of the whole body; 'irregular muscular contractions may take place in different parts of the body, yet the subject may doubt that the muscles belong to his body'; synesthesias are also reported, e.g. the hearing of rhythmically presented sounds accompanied by the seeing of small grey circles. In some cases the drug may cause such a 'marked depression of the muscular system' as to render the subject unable to stand up. The ability to think and to organize and abstract material diminishes dramatically. Although consciousness appears to narrow down to the experience of sensory and imaginal details, these details expand and the subject becomes identified with the object of his experience. As with hypnagogic experiences, there is here also a progression from simple to complex phenomena, from clouds of colours and sparkles of light to geometric figures and patterns to landscapes, faces, and complex scenes.[45] Klüver concluded that mescaline and hypnagogic experiences involved the same processes.[46] An identical conclusion was reached by Ardis and McKellar who also confirmed the phenomenological similarities of the two states emphasized earlier by Klüver.[47]

Another hallucinogen that shares features with hypnagogia is marihuana, which when taken in fairly strong doses first stimulates the user and then puts him to sleep. As with LSD, there are reports of OBEs, of feeling childlike, being open to experience, and believing that one can communicate telepathically.[48] Under the influence of hallucinogens, as in some hypnagogic experiences, the user may also have mystical visions, feel omniscient, and conceive of or compose music and poetry and other artistic and scientific works all of which may seem magnificent at the time but are not always so when viewed more critically after the effects of the drug have worn off.

Richardson hypothesized that previous experience of hypnagogic imagery should facilitate the experiencing of meaningful hallucinogenic-drug imagery.[49] Although this hypothesis has not yet been tested, Holt found a zero correlation between the intensity of LSD imagery and previous experience of hypnagogic imagery.[50] On the other hand, as noted, hallucinogenic-drug and hypnagogic experiences are found to summate.

Eidetic imagery

A close look at the literature on eidetic imagery reveals some striking similarities with hypnagogic images, such as clearness and richness in detail, three-dimensionality, colouration, externality of localization with eyes open or shut, relatively clear distinction from after-imagery and memory, involvement of all sensory modalities, gradation in 'degrees of strength' or vividness, and autonomy.[51] Functionally, they are both thought to subserve an earlier, easier, concrete, percept-like type of cognizing.

Until very recently, the concept of eidetic imagery was a rather narrow one consisting entirely of what is known as 'typographic' imagery, i.e. imagery which is mainly induced by an immediately preceding stimulus (and sometimes linked with so-called 'photographic' memory). Ahsen,[52] and Marks and McKellar have broadened this concept to include a 'structural' kind of imagery which 'is evoked purely by exercising the imagination',[53] e.g. by staring into a blank circle, a 'crystal' or one's closed eyelids. The latter authors define eidetic imagery as 'any mental image projected into the sensory environment which cannot be attributed to a material change in sensory input and which is known to the imager to be subjective'. They include in this definition what they call 'formation' eidetic imagery, i.e. 'the perception of any meaningful form of stimuli which are purely random', such as seeing forms in clouds and inkblots and hearing music or voices in white noise.

If we go by this definition, then practically all the eidetic phenomena are encountered in hypnagogia. Indeed, in some cultures hypnagogia is made use of for the purpose of recalling and 'scanning' (eidetic) images of the day's activities.[54] Examples of structural and formation imagery are to be found throughout this book, the latter kind being richly illustrated by cases of hypnagogic 'illusions' and visions that acquire particular shapes and meanings in accordance with the subject's autosuggestion. The typographic sort, very rare in general, can be found in hypnagogia in the form of 'absolute reproductions' (see chapter 2) – differing from the traditional type in that it may not be preceded immediately by the relevant stimulus (though, again, some people experience hypnagogic replays of films they have been watching on TV just prior to going to bed).

The criterion of lucidity or reality testing ability included in the above definition does not, of course, disqualify hypnagogia since many phenomena in this state are 'known to the imager to be subjective' at the time of their occurrence. Moreover, Marks and McKellar's describing of scrying and the seeing of ghosts, spirits and apparitions as 'essentially eidetic' calls the validity of this criterion into question since some of the authorities they cite in suport of their arguments (e.g. Rawcliffe, Sidgwick) refer to these phenomena as 'hallucinations' and 'illusions "in which some real object is perceived, but misinterpreted as something else"' (see also chapters 4 and 11 for my arguments regarding the status of the concept 'reality testing'). Two other possible objections to relating eidetic to hypnagogic imagery, namely that the former, unlike the latter, is realistic (as opposed to bizarre) and can be scanned, are disposed of on the grounds that hypnagogic imagery appears in 'a vast range of styles – realistic, painted, drawn, cartoon, super-realism',[53] and that 'you can zoom in on any detail you want to see more clearly'.[55]

Oswald suggests that no sharp distinction can be drawn between eidetic, hypnagogic, and sensory deprivation imagery.[56] As with the latter two, eidetic imagery has also been associated with good health and normality.[52]

Epilepsy

In his 1895 Cavendish lecture, Crichton-Browne drew attention to the observation that epileptic attacks are particularly prone to show themselves 'during the invasion of sleep', and that even when, in some patients, the fits wear off in adult life, the last vestiges of them are experienced while the patient is drowsy and just falling asleep.[57] In general, epileptic attacks occur 'almost invariably in solitude' and when the patient is in a 'meditative mood', whereas they are prevented when in company and when attention is engaged actively.

Like hypnagogia, epilepsy contains a wide spectrum of alterations of consciousness ranging from minor disorientations and quasihallucinations to full hallucinations and loss of personal identity and consciousness. The hypnagogic and hypnagogic-like quasiperceptual elements that often precede and/or accompany an epileptic fit – known collectively as 'intellectual aurae'[58] – take on a number of forms and appear in all the sensory modalities. For instance, there are flashes of light that sometimes develop into complete scenes that appear as a comic strip.[59] Likewise, 'cartoon-like' pictures may be seen with open or closed eyes and appear external and beyond the patient's control.[60] 'Interpretative illusions' also occur, i.e. distorted auditory and visual perceptions (palyopsias),[61] as well as macropsias and micropsias. As in hypnagogia, epileptics often hear their names being called and may, likewise, hear nonsensical comments, have delusions, and even manifest all the symptoms of schizophrenia;[62] they also hear and see religious visions, create neologisms,[63] have feelings of expectancy or a sense of significance about their experiences, have thoughts and speech in which punctuation is almost entirely absent,[64] experience thoughts and words that succeed each other in the manner that hypnagogic visions do, incorporate and internalize their environment,[65] experience fear or fright very much like that experienced by normal hypnagogists, and their myoclonic spasms have clear parallels in the common hypnagogic jerks.[66] Although, on the whole, epileptic experiences are said to occur against a background of clouded consciousness, some epileptics experience a 'sense of power and control' and have a 'clearer head and a clearer understanding' during their attacks; on occasion, they also experience OBEs and autoscopic phenomena.[64]

An interesting phenomenon that occurs in epilepsy, and is also linked with hypnagogia, is the *déjà vu* experience, i.e. the feeling of 'having lived through this before'. Buck and Geers reported significant positive correlations between the incidence of hypnagogic imagery and visual and auditory *déjà vu*.[67] Earlier, Ellis had claimed that the *déjà vu* is a common experience in hypnagogia, and linked the two with 'the prodromal stage of the epileptic fit' and sleepdream consciousness.[68] From a psychoanalytic viewpoint, Isakower related the similarity of feeling between the *déjà vu* and 'oral cathexis' in hypnagogia, and noted that in hypnagogia, in the epileptic aura, and in the experience of *déjà vu* 'the subject knows, or thinks he knows, exactly what is going to happen'.[69]

Summary and conclusions of Part Two

In this part I examined the relationship of hypnagogia to a number of states, processes and experiences, and further expanded my analysis of hypnagogic phenomena. In relating hypnagogia to sleepdreams it was found that the former contains experiences indistinguishable from the latter, that in hypnagogia a subject may watch his fragmentary images turn into full-blown dreams, that this state encompasses a wide variety of types of dream some of which are experienced in the absence of sleep, and that it is the perfect state for observing and experimentally investigating dreams. Further, the fact that the hypnagogist may retain awareness of his environment and/or awareness of being awake in a dream argues against the contention that dreams are not experiences and that statements about them are mere inferences about experiences that did not take place.

In respect to the relationship between meditation and hypnagogia, it was, again, found that these share the same psychophysical factors of induction, viz. relaxation, shift to parasympathetic predominance and hypometabolic processes, lowering of EEG to the theta range, psychological withdrawal, ego abandonment, receptive attention leading to absorption-fascination. Non-analytic 'regressive-primitive' organization of perception and thought was found to characterize both states, as were the presence of unusual sensations, the feeling of intense realness, the feeling of being 'chemically' linked with the world, the inability to describe some of these experiences, and the sense of temporal immediacy. It was also found that meditation tends to lead to hypnagogia and that the latter sometimes breaks out into a state of satori or mystical enlightenment.

Some psi states and processes, viz. telepathy, clairvoyance, clairaudience, psychometry, ecsomatosis and some forms of trance have also been found to be closely related to hypnagogia in their psychophysical induction and phenomenology. Further, hypnagogia was found to be highly conducive to psi activities while psi states were clearly seen to be hypnagogic in nature, i.e. they tend to lead to sleep. Furthermore, the mentation encountered in psi states, like that of hypnagogia, is typically non-analytic and regressive. Indeed, a close examination of physiological and psychological parameters shows that the above mentioned psi states and processes are only

231

distinguishable from hypnagogia by the subject's set of beliefs and/or the setting in which they take place.

Hypnagogic mentation was further found to contain most of the features that characterize schizophrenic disturbances such as the loosening in the association of ideas, dissociated thinking, overinclusiveness in conceptualization, thoughts spoken aloud, hallucinations, delusions, and body schema alterations. These phenomena, it is argued, are the direct result of the LEBs which facilitates the breakdown of the filter mechanism operating in the normal, waking state. This leads to a loss of figure-ground relationships and allows the simultaneous emergence and crossing of a number of FsR which often results in neologisms, punning, poetic or funny remarks and the identification with each other of concepts on the basis of apparently tenuous similarities. Schizophrenics, like hypnagogists and absent-minded individuals, appear to be responding primarily to an internal, imaginal FR.

Hypnagogia was also found to be conducive to creativity, constituting an essential part of the creative process and often containing the act of creation itself. Specifically, the creative act is characterized by LEBs and regression to earlier modes of mentation in which emerging imagery is accompanied by a sense of reality, and concepts from apparently unrelated FsR are connected, combined, or fused. Much of this is effected at an unconscious-nonrational level which, however, can be made conscious through the preconscious character of hypnagogia. Both hypnagogia and creativity are further characterized by their subjects' openness, sensitivity, tolerance of ambiguity, self-acceptance, and loosening of ego strictness. Moreover, since both creative thinking and schizophrenic mentation are encountered in hypnagogia, this analysis of the latter clearly reveals common dynamics and facilitates understanding of both schizophrenia and creativity.

In relating hypnagogia to hypnosis it was seen that the former is a natural autohypnotic state – a point already noted in chapter 3. In particular it was pointed out that hypnagogia and classical hypnosis resemble each other both in their psychophysical induction and experiential aspects. That is, they are both dependent on relative immobilization and monotony or regularity of low intensity stimuli that induce in the subject relaxation and secure expectancy, thus freeing him from distracting affects. Further, they are both characterized by absorbed and fascinated attention, LEBs and regression to prelogical ideational processes typified by the tendency to experience the environment as part of oneself, dissolution of time barriers so that, for instance, everything (including memories) appears to be endowed with the immediacy of the present.

In regard to the relationship between hypnagogia and epilepsy, the former was found to be conducive to the occurrence of epileptic attacks during which many hypnagogic phenomena, known as 'intellectual aurae', are also present, e.g. loss of personal identity, loss of orientation, visual, auditory, olfactory, gustatory and other quasiperceptual experiences, thought disturbances, and *déjà vu* phenomena. Hypnagogic phenomena are also found in sensory deprivation or perceptual isolation experiments which are conducted under conditions very similar to those present in the naturally occurring hypnagogia, i.e. reduction and relative invariance of stimulation. Further, hallucinogenic-drug-induced states are populated with quasiperceptual and cognitive phenomena and features which are very similar to those encountered in hypnagogia – indeed, it has been suggested that both conditions involve the same processes. Photic, pulse current, and direct electrical stimulation experiments have also yielded hypnagogic-like states and phenomena. In addition, eidetic imagery displays strong similarities with hypnagogic imagery such as clarity of detail, externality of localization and three-dimensionality. Sleep deprivation is conducive to the occurrence of hypnagogic experiences, and dream scintillations are considered as striking examples of hypnagogic imagery.

In concluding this part of the book, two general observations can be made. First, all of the above states, processes, and experiences possess a measure of hypnagogia, that is, they begin with, lead into, or contain strong features of, hypnagogia. Indeed, some are indistinguishable from hypnagogic experiences both in their phenomenology and physiology. In respect to the latter, the shift to theta rhythms in the EEG and to a parasympathetic predominance have been especially noted. In regard to the phenomenology, the similarities were striking both in the quasiperceptual and the cognitive-affective spheres. Even in the weakest of cases, a degree of 'dreaminess', psychological withdrawal, and primacy of an internal FR were clearly present. This observation contains at least two important implications: first, that hypnagogia might comprise the psychophysical mechanisms by which these states and processes are produced, and second, that the study of the nature and function of hypnagogia should shed light on the nature and function of the above states and processes. These studies constitute, of course, the major aim of this book. The study of the former, i.e. the nature of hypnagogia, has now almost been completed. I say *almost*, because an analysis of the phenomenon of LEBs, which I consider to be a highly important aspect of the nature of hypnagogia, has not yet been offered. This will be undertaken in Part Three which deals with the brain mechanisms and function of the state. The reason for this is that the LEBs partakes both of the nature and function of hypnagogia, that is, it both constitutes an aspect of its phenomenology (hypnagogia is characterized by its presence) and lies at the centre of its evolutionary role.

The second general observation rising out of the discussions in Part Two concerns the interrelationships existing among the various states and processes. For instance, eidetikers are good hypnotic subjects, and epileptics may display all the phenomena of schizophrenia. On the other hand, some well-known creative individuals have been epileptics whereas others have been categorized as schizophrenic. Meditative moods have been found to be conducive to the onset of epileptic fits. The factors of 'intellectual flexibility' and 'emotional freedom', characteristic of creative individuals, have been found in subjects most susceptible to the emergence of hallucinatory phenomena in sensory deprivation and photic stimulation experiments, and in good eidetikers. Hallucinogenic-drug-induced states have been related to psi, creativity, mysticism and schizophrenia: these last four have also been related to one another. Since these states and processes are, severally, strongly related to hypnagogia, their interrelationships strengthen the view that they all share of the nature and function of one central state or process, namely hypnagogia – a conclusion that takes us back to the significance of hypnagogia as a state whose nature and function underpins some very important aspects of mental life.

Part III

Brain mechanisms and function of hypnagogia

Introduction

In the preceding two parts I examined the nature of hypnagogia and its relationship to other states and processes mainly from a phenomenological perspective. In this part I shall look into the possible brain substrate-correlates of these phenomena, and examine the function of hypnagogia in a wider, evolutionary, scheme.

These three areas of investigation – phenomenology, brain correlates and function – are, I believe, so intimately connected that at our present stage of knowledge any attempt to identify a clear-cut, one-way causation from one of them to any of the others without qualifications, riders or reservations would most certainly be considered a gross oversimplification. One can, however, as a tentative first step, draw inferences from psychological phenomena to possible brain correlates and then seek empirical confirmation or confutation of such inferences, e.g. by comparing with reports on electrical brain stimulation. At the same time, verbal reports of subjects can be recorded together with measurements of concurrent brain activity (see Appendix II). The combined results of phenomenology and brain activity would then be used as indicators of the functions of the state.

One of the main benefits accruing from discovering brain correlates is that they, in combination with reports of concurrent experiences, can suggest not only ontogenetic but also phylogenetic dimensions, and thus offer a view of hypnagogia in an evolutionary perspective. Another advantage of this method is, as noted above, the indicating of functions. Whether, however, the latter are to be regarded as the chance outcome of evolution – psychological phenomena and brain correlates giving rise fortuitously to a state of affairs that then imposes itself as a 'need' – or whether they are, as a matter of fact, signifiers of deeper, longer-lasting, 'natural necessities' which can be thought of as causes of the observed psychological and physiological phenomena, is a question that no amount of brain research, with its current methodology, can hope to answer. Perhaps such an answer can only be ultimately found, if it can be found at all, 'extraphysically' although not *super*naturally.

10 · The old versus the new brain

Various theories, ranging from religious and parapsychological to neuro-physiological and psychological, have been propounded to account for the genesis, nature, and function of hypnagogic phenomena. The category of religious explanations is represented by authors who ascribe supernatural significance to such experiences.[1] In particular, Tappeiner, as we saw in chapter 6, argued that even though the act of religious prophesying has a spiritual genesis it registers and expresses itself through the psychological mechanisms operating in hypnagogia. Then there are parapsychological theories which argue that a full explanation of hypnagogic events requires the postulation of either paranormal faculties or a disembodied agent.[2] The more orthodox psychological explanations include psychoanalytic-regressive theories which stress alterations in ego functioning during hypnagogia,[3] unconscious-dissociative theories which emphasize that visions, sounds, and other hypnagogic experiences appear to be external to the subject's personality,[4] accounts which argue that simple sensory data experienced during the onset of sleep are elaborated by the imagination into objects, scenes, and so on.[5] This latter kind of theory tends to overlap with neurophysiological explanations which implicate somatosensory conditions and stimuli such as internal and external sensations, muscular relaxation, physiological and chemical changes,[6] electrical currents and phosphoric acid in the body, inadequate blood circulation, cerebral blood congestion, increased carbon dioxide in the blood.[7] In connection with the visual phenomena, there are a number of accounts each severally arguing that such images are entoptic in origin or formation, i.e. they rise out of the physiology and chemistry of the eye and/or the excitation of the optic nerve and the visual cortex.[8] Such claims are based either on observing complex visual hypnagogic imagery forming out of the ideoretinal light or dissolving into it.

Clearly, none of the above theories alone can account for all of the hypnagogic phenomena and at the same time get away with its own unaccountable basic assumptions, even though each one may contribute explanations that can hold good for a group of phenomena at a certain level. Indeed, most of them are not exclusive of each other, and a number of workers have held more than one at the same time. My own attitude is to view at least certain of these theories as descriptive of conducive conditions, triggers, sluices or correlates that provide individually some of the circumstances that 'make it possible'.

Accordingly, in what follows I shall, first, examine some of these theories (or, rather, arguments pertaining to such theories as I consider relevant), and then substantiate with specific data and arguments my own claims that the activities of certain subcortical structures constitute the neurophysiological substrates of hypnagogic experiences.

Hypnagogic visions are not generated in the eyes

In contrast to the contention that hypnagogic visions may form out of entoptic lights and patterns, various workers have argued that these are essentially centrally initiated and that oculoretinal participation is of secondary importance or even entirely inessential. As Alexander put it, these visions 'are *externalizations*, or, to use the word in its common-speech sense, *materializations* of mental facts; that is, they end rather than begin in sensation, acquiring a kind of phantasmal reality.'[9] More specifically, it has been suggested that entoptic lights and hypnagogic visions may have nothing in common except for the fact that they tend to appear more prominently under the same conditions, and that the nature of the former leaves them short of accounting for the appearance of the majority of these visions. The latter may appear suddenly, complete, and not be immediately recognizable,

(a)

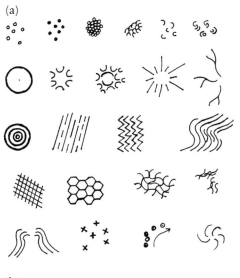

Figure 10.1 *(a) Redundant elements in hallucination and visual imagery, (b) hypothesized patterns of special retinal receptivity (after Horowitz 1978). These shapes and forms appear in hypnagogia, and various other conditions besides, and seem entoptic in origin. However, they fall short of accounting for the majority of hypnagogic visions and dreams which contain faces, figures, scenes, and other complex features.*

(b)

i.e. they do not seem to form by a play of imagination on entoptic spots. Further, they may develop into, or be replaced by, other images which are not visually related to them and thus, again, reveal no entoptic links.[10] Furthermore, ocular movements do not necessarily imply essential or active participation of the eyes in the perception of hypnagogic visions: they may simply appear in response to our natural habit of moving our eyes in pursuance of a moving object. Even the fact that they appear in front of us might only be 'because we are used to always seeing objects in the line of vision',[11] i.e. in front of us, whereas hypnagogic visions can in fact be placed anywhere as they are not truly related to our optical space: there is no need to turn left, right, up or down, no need for an effort to focus our eyes, no eye convergence, no nose shadow, no blinking (see also other relevant arguments in chapter 5).

Some support for the above contentions comes from arguments in respect of functional similarities of imaging and perceiving, according to which visual images acting as centrifugal impulses from the brain may stimulate the oculoretinal complex which, in turn, may involve the whole or part of the visual pathway through movement feedback mechanisms.[12] In this view, 'mental images can be functionally equivalent to physical objects and events at many levels of the visual system',[13] thus themselves causing the activation of the visual mechanism, as opposed to being its product, resulting in the sensation of their being seen as if they were physical objects.

A triple source of evidence supporting the hypothesis that visual hypnagogic images are primarily centrally initiated and that their 'projection' may secondarily activate or involve peripheral receptors are reports of the occurrence of both positive and negative after-images from hypnagogic-hypnopompic imagery,[14] deliberate conscious visualizations,[15] and visualizations suggested to subjects under hypnosis.[16] Also supporting the theory of 'central initiation' of visual imagery in general are the results of a number of experiments in direct electrical stimulation of the visual cortex and excitation of the brain by means of temporal electrodes (see relevant section in chapter 9).

The implication of subcortical structures in hypnagogic vision

However, although electrical stimulation of cortical areas has elicited visual imagery it does not necessarily follow that these areas are directly responsible for the occurrence of such phenomena. It has been noted, for instance, that the surgical removal of those cortical areas which yielded specific memories when electrically stimulated produced no detectable loss of memory.[17] Moreover, there is a considerable accumulation of evidence arguing that the destruction of the visual cortex does not lead to total blindness, and that, in some such cases, human subjects and experimental animals may behave as if still fully sighted.[18] Indeed, in lower animals, such as birds and reptiles, 'vision' appears to be achieved by the relatively more powerful subcortical structures.[19]

Another source of information lessening the importance of the visual cortex, this time in respect to hallucinations, comes from Schatzman's experiments with an unusual subject.[20] Ruth, Schatzman's subject, would sit with eyes open in front of a television screen which displayed changing checkerboard patterns that elicited normal visual evoked response. Then, by producing an apparition of her daughter and placing it in front of her – thus imaginally blocking the screen from her visual field – she would cause her visual evoked response to completely disappear. Electroretinographic recordings showed that her retinas responded normally to external stimuli from light while she was engaged in the production of the apparition. This would suggest that stimuli entering her eyes were blocked before they reached the visual cortex. One is forced to conclude that Ruth's imaginal, and yet in a sense very real, activities must have involved visual pathways in subcortical structures.

Now, in view of the facts that in the production of visions neither the eyes nor the visual cortex need be involved at all, and bearing in mind the remarks of hypnagogic subjects that they cannot mix their more vivid hallucination-like hypnagogic visions with ordinary memory images and visualizations, I would propose that fully formed hypnagogic visions (as opposed to ideoretinal lights and phosphenes) are neither retinal nor cortical in nature. They may rise, of course, initially at any level of the visual system, that is, they may be instigated at a retinal, cortical, or subcortical level, but they are subcortical *in nature*. The retinal components, when present, are incidental: they do not develop any further in the absence of absorption and psychological withdrawal. Likewise, in the absence of these two features, visions initiated in the visual cortex will remain faint visualizations – and will become hypnagogic and/or hallucinatory when these features are strongly present.

Added strength to my claim comes from observations in respect to the nature of alpha rhythm and states of attention. In contrast to earlier arguments which associated the alpha rhythm with absence of both sensory stimulation of the visual system and the formation of visual imagery,[21] Oswald found that 'subjects could experience changing or static visual images without any blocking of the alpha rhythm *providing that difficulty was not experienced in perceiving the images*'[22] (my italics). Similarly, Jasper[23] had found that Einstein displayed a fairly continuous alpha rhythm while engaged in complicated mathematical operations which, as we saw in chapter 8, involved a high degree of absorption in visuokinesthetic imagery. Conscious, effortful visualization, then, may indeed be initiated at the visual cortex and thus cause suppression of alpha. But with absorption setting in, the role of the visual cortex diminishes and the imagery becomes intensified, taking on a life of its own as it becomes increasingly dissociated from the cortex.

It will be recalled that in chapters 2, 6 and 8 reports were presented describing how concentration on a mental image would result in the latter becoming vivified and either leading to sleep or to the subject's becoming 'fascinated', absorbed, and kinesthetically involved in the character of the image. These phenomena might be better understood if related to the activities of subcortical structures which become functionally severed from retina and visual cortex, the latter being primarily concerned with locating one's body in *external* space. This functional severance might also explain the hallucinatory character of the phenomena of a deep hypnagogic stage as well as the fact that, in general, hypnagogic visions are seen in sharp detail and yet possess depth and perspective.

One other area of research that may be brought in at this point of the discussion is that encompassing theories of 'paroptic vision' or 'eyeless sight',[22] 'eyeless vision',[23] and 'dermo-optic sense'[24] developed to account for the phenomena of 'seeing' by means of one's skin. In these phenomena, as with cortically blind subjects, visual perception is 'felt', colours are perceived as 'smooth', 'sticky', or 'rough'.[24] It is said that paroptic vision is circular, or

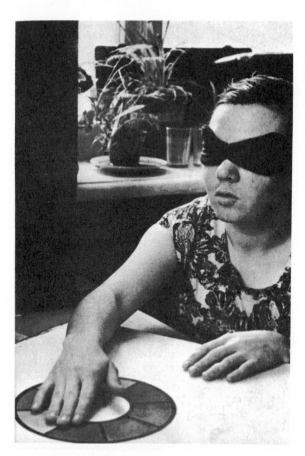

Figure 10.2 *Eyeless vision: the Russian Kuleshova 'seeing' with her fingers. She is reputed to be able to tell colours by simply passing her fingers over or lightly touching them. Such vision is thought to be non-directional, and is typically kinosynesthetic.*

even spherical, that is, by means of it one could see in all directions, it does not involve the eyes although there is an acquired 'cerebro-visual attitude of accommodation', its colour perception is wider on the ultraviolet side, it posesses the same characters as clairvoyant vision.[22] Although I will refrain from discussing the details of these theories I would make a point of drawing attention to the fact that the experiences they seek to explain, even though purportedly visual, are characteristically synesthetic and kinesthetic phenomena which, I shall argue, typically characterize the activities of subcortical structures.

Concerning synesthesia, it is widely argued that there is an evolutionary ascent 'from a synesthetic stage to a stage of differentiated configurations which give the impression of a world containing constant objects'.[25] Thus perceptions, which are a later evolutionary acquisition, and characterize higher animals and especially humans, are 'localized' on the cortex, which is of recent evolutionary development, and are concerned with 'stabilizing' and 'objectifying' sensations. By contrast, the synesthetic stage, which is evolutionarily older, should be found in its strongest form in lower animals and thus in the activities of the oldbrain. Schiller demonstrated this in a series of experiments with fish in which the latter, having learned to discriminate between a bright and a dark chamber, synesthetically related brightness with a 'bright' odour and darkness with a 'dark' odour.[25] Commenting on his results, Schiller stated that in these phenomena 'there is a transfer of training between different senses'. In the case of subjects who were trained to 'see' with their skin I would paraphrase Schiller's comment and propose that in such experiences there is a training of transfer between the senses, or perhaps even a learning of sensing through one nuclear sense out of which developed and differentiated sensations and perceptions. As we know, in hypnagogia, due mainly to the LEBs, such transfers occur spontaneously. Moreover, the experiences are *felt* kinesthetically, thus strengthening both the view that hypnagogic imagery is correlated with activities of subcortical structures and pointing to the possibility that, evolutionarily, a nuclear sense, primarily tactile in character, existed before distant receptors were developed. Ontogenetically, this may still be witnessed in the way infants presumably perceive the world inside and outside them. I shall return to this point in the following sections and in the final chapter.

Subcortical involvement in other hypnagogic phenomena

It has been commented by a number of investigators that the 'floating' sensation experienced in hypnagogia seems to involve a depression of cortical activity, and that the occurrence of hypnagogic hallucinations and the 4–7 cps theta rhythms recorded from the parietotemporal regions and characteristic of hypnagogia are associated with cortico-subcortical perturbations.[26] Such observations and remarks accord well with my general proposition that the occurrence of hypnagogia is closely related to subcortical activities which have gained the upper hand, so to speak, in their synergetic relationship with the cortex. Indeed, there is sufficient evidence in this respect to show that facilitation of slow rhythms, including alpha, and suppression or total abolition of cortical activity is achieved through specific manipulations of subcortical structures.[27] In a wider context, various researchers have presented evidence and argued to the effect that, from a developmental and functional point of view, the cortex is to be regarded as a dependency of the thalamus, the latter being the mediator to which all stimuli congregate and become modified and distributed to subcortical centres and being generally concerned with the regulation of the brain's electrical activity.[28]

Significantly, and in respect to my relating epileptic aura phenomena to hypnagogia, it has been remarked that the focal epileptiform discharges observed in the cortex may be simply 'evoked potentials or secondary epileptic activation of the cortex in response to intense bombardment over specific projection pathways from subcortical structures', and that 'if the thalamic discharge is sufficiently prolonged and intense, a self-sustained cortical discharge develops which continues after the thalamic discharge has ceased'.[29] Indeed, it has been shown that electrical stimulation of the mesial portion of the thalamus of cats and monkeys produces not only the electrographic picture but also the clinical form of both *petit mal* and *grand mal* epilepsy.[30]

On the other hand, stimulation of the deep structures in the limbic system of epileptic patients has elicited experiences very similar to those reported in the hypnagogia of normal subjects. For instance, on stimulating the left posterior hippocampus of a patient, Horowitz reports that the subject 'seemed to comprehend some of the meaning of the questions, but his verbal contents and tonal inflections resembled those found in aphasia, sleep-talking,

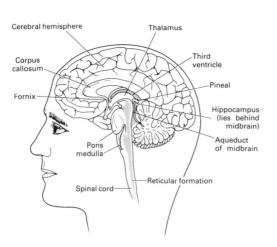

Figure 10.3 *Diagram of the brain showing areas relevant to the discussions in this chapter. The hippocampus and related structures of the limbic system, except for part of the fornix, are not in view (see Figure 10.4).*

or hypnagogic speech'.[31] The stimulations, Horowitz notes, tended to produce an altered state of consciousness in which lexical cognition was reduced and image formation was enhanced or disinhibited, and increased influence of primary process prevailed. The contents of the experiences ranged from sparks, lights and geometric figures to complete scenes with animals and humans. Some of the latter constituted memories and others were condensed pictorializations of the patient's current ideas and motives. And yet others were images and hallucinations probably 'never actually seen in prior experience. Sometimes the self was seen in a way in which would not be possible by self-perception.'

Drawing on his own findings and on those of McLean and co-workers,[32] Horowitz suggests that either 'there are visual pathways to the posterior hippocampal gyrus or this area is, in some way, involved in the regulation of image formation'. A review of the literature on the function of the hippocampus in man indicates that this structure is concerned with the maintenance of a distinction between images arriving from actual perceptions and internal imagery.[33] In view of findings that the cortex fires into the posterior hippocampal gyrus which in turn fires into the hippocampus,[34] it might be conjectured that at sleep onset when general cortical activity is considerably reduced the cortico-hippocampal firing would also diminish. But, if at this time of diminution of cortical firing into the hippocampal gyrus a certain minimal arousal is maintained, or even deliberately initiated, in the brainstem, then the function of the hippocampus as a regulator of imagery may be severely upset. Internal imagery may take on the character of external perception. A certain minimum degree of arousal without active thinking ('passive alertness') is, of course, what investigators and experients of hypnagogia indicate as one of the most important characters of the state.

My relating schizophrenia to hypnagogia may also gain extra support here by the findings of various investigators indicating disturbances of the reticular system, thalamic nuclei, mesencephalon, diencephalon and brainstem of patients.[35] Indeed, the complexity, plasticity of structural organization, sophistication in modes of activity, and centrality of the reticular brainstem core – it appears to be the only system that can be demonstrated to be involved anatomically and physiologically at each or all levels of neural activity – have led some workers to suggest that this subcortical structure may be implicated in the production of non-object-bound, i.e. hallucinatory, phenomena in general.[36]

The control exerted by the brainstem on respiration, body-posture, spinal reflexes, and even cortically induced movements, may shed light on, among other things, some hypnagogically induced psi phenomena, such as OBEs. We saw in chapter 6 that some subjects learned to make use of both ordinary and cataplexic hypnagogic-hypnopompic states to achieve exteriorizations. Fox makes specific mention of a 'pull' he felt at the region of the medulla oblongata during the initial stages of his projections.[37] Muldoon reports that conscious ecsomatosis may be preceded by the feeling of 'a tremendous pressure being exerted in the back of the head, in the *medulla oblongata* region'.[38] This pressure causes, or results in, a rhythmical shaking or pulsating of the body accompanied by a 'pandemonium of bizarre sensations – floating, vibratory, zigzagging and head-pulling' followed by the hearing of 'somewhat familiar and seemingly far-distant sounds'. Psychics, practitioners of the occult, mystics and meditators speak of employing patterned breathing to achieve paranormal effects. And it is a well-known fact that in the medulla oblongata are to be found certain nerves that control respiration, and that disturbance of this structure can affect both breathing and consciousness.

The phenomena described by Muldoon, which occur spontaneously in hypnagogia, are sometimes preceded and accompanied by the sheer awareness that one exists but is unable to locate oneself. Later in life Muldoon learned to induce these phenomena, followed by ecsomatosis, by means of a deliberately produced hypnagogia. He connects them with epilepsy and reports the case of a woman who 'became gifted with unusual clairvoyant powers about the same time when she became a victim of epilepsy'.[39]

The arguments for the involvement of subcortical structures suggested by the above may be further strengthened by reports that psychics tend to function better when they are 'turned on' by their sitters.[40] Further, Garrett, as already mentioned, noted that 'in the telepathic experiment the senses of taste and smell were serving me as keen agents in knowing that a telepathic state was functioning'[41] – smell being the most 'visceral' of the senses, as Koestler rightly remarked, the limbic system being known as the 'visceral brain'. Warcollier remarks that 'in its most primitive form telepathy may produce coenesthetic disturbances, that is, sensations arising within the vital organs, including sensations of a depressing type; it may give rise to fits of weeping, vague presentiments or premonitions, confusions or disorientations'.[42]

Supporting my relating hypnagogia to subcortical activities and to states of psi, there are reports to the effect that 'psi in animals has seemed more consistent than in humans',[43] suggesting that in humans there may be interference by cognitive elaboration and distortion from higher centres in the brain. Moreover, some of these results have been obtained from precorticate animals.[44]

The data and arguments presented in earlier chapters in regard to the regressive nature of hypnagogia are here also supported by the current arguments, by the fact that in childhood the 4–7 cps theta waves are predominant, and by suggestions that growing babies pass through a state of consciousness which takes place without participation of the cerebral cortex.[45] In addition, it has been shown that when an adult subject is given the appropriate dose of chloral hydrate, and the cortex is put into an inhibitory state, he responds to words by *sound* association (as opposed to *sense* association)[46] – a punning phenomenon common both in hypnagogia and in childhood. Similar results are, conversely, obtainable by manipulating subcortical areas, as in the phenomenon known as 'Förster's syndrome' originally elicited by Förster when, operating on a patient, he manipulated a tumour in the third ventricle – a small cavity in the midbrain. This threw the (conscious) patient into a flight of speech quoting passages from Latin, Greek and Hebrew:

> He exhibited typical sound associations, and with every word of the operator broke into a flight of ideas. Thus, on hearing the operator ask for a *Tupfer* [tampon] he burst into '*Tupfer . . . Tupfer, Hupfer, Hüpfer, hüpfen Sie mal. . . .* ' [Tampon, jumper, go and jump into the air]. On hearing the word *Messer*, he burst into '*Messer, messer, Metzer, Sie sind ein Metzel, das ist ja ein Gemetzel, metzeln Sie doch nicht so messen Sie doch Sie messen ja nicht Herr Professor, profiteor, professus sum, profiteri*'. [Knife, butcher, you are a butcher in a butchery, truly this is a massacre, don't go butchering take measurements why don't you measure professor, profiteor, professus sum, profiteri].[47]

In placing primary importance on subcortical structures in the 'production' of hallucinatory phenomena I do not wish to ignore the fact that some of these phenomena can be elicited at the cortical level. However, even in these cases, subcortical structures may still be directly or indirectly involved given the data on their wealth and structural organization. Cairns points out that 'destruction of both frontal lobes can result in profound disturbances of will, reason and emotion'. But he also notes that 'destruction of the thalami can do the same thing and, in addition, may be followed by the most profound loss of memorizing or by loss of crude consciousness'.[48] It has been known for some time now that sleep and wakefulness are controlled by subcortical 'centres' and that, as we have seen, consciousness can be disturbed by lesions or excitation at any level of the brainstem and thalamus. It is also known that, although they normally work in harness, there is a fair degree of independence between cortex and thalamus. It is this independence which is probably declared, 'irrationally', by the thalamus and other subcortical structures during hypnagogia. It is not here claimed that complete independence is ever achieved in this state, or that it is desirable, but that brain predominance becomes clearly subcortical.

After a brief discussion of hemispheric lateralization views, I propose to further expand on this theme making use of data and arguments relating to epilepsy and the functional dichotomy between the old and the new brain. In so doing, I shall also return to certain points made in earlier chapters both in connection with the nature of hypnagogia and in reference to the latter's relationship with meditation, mysticism, schizophrenia, and creativity.

Concerning hemispheric lateralization

Some evidence for hemispheric lateralization (HL)[49] might appear to argue that the psychological features ascribed to hypnagogia, and to hallucinatory phenomena in general, are exactly those claimed to be correlated with right hemisphere (or non-dominant brain side) activities. I have the following points to make in regard to such claims. In the first place, such features and attitudes as creativity, holistic approach (as opposed to sequential, linear, analytic), artistic activity (e.g. spatial, musical), unconscious processes, are not clearly shown to be properties of the non-dominant hemisphere as opposed to being related to activities of subcortical structures. For instance, in experiments in connection with HL, Galin reported 'relatively higher alpha amplitude (a measure of idling) over the right hemisphere during the verbal tasks, and relatively more alpha over the left hemisphere during the spatial tasks. In other words, the hemisphere expected to be less engaged in the task has more of the idling rhythm.'[50] This conclusion is hard to reconcile with data showing bilateral continuous alpha during intricate mathematical operations.[29] Workers in the hypnagogic area have often spoken of switching to an easier cognitive mode requiring the expenditure of less energy. This accords well with the general passive-receptive state of the person at sleep onset. Are we to suppose that, on the whole, the non-dominant hemisphere expends less energy than the dominant one? How can this be explained physiologically and evolutionarily? By contrast, we know that such states of lessened expenditure of energy (trophotropic states) are brought on by the activities of subcortical structures controlling sleep and wakefulness.

The features ascribed to the non-dominant hemisphere are clearly ontogenetically and phylogenetically older than those ascribed to the dominant one. If the HL arguments were correct, should there not be anatomical correlations showing the temporal development of these two sets of features, such as the existence of animals having a 'right' hemisphere only out of which a 'left' hemisphere grew through evolution? On the other hand, decorticate humans, such as anencephalic and hydrocephalic monsters, are known to display 'pleasure, in a babyish way, when being sung to'.[51] Clearly, here we do not have non-dominant hemispheric appreciation of music.

The problem with HL theories lies not so much in the data as in their interpretation. The general approach has been to dichotomize functions and relegate them to one or the other hemisphere. But such dichotomies are obviously gross oversimplifications of diverse functions, and have the added disadvantage of sometimes contradicting each other as well as militating against psychological and physiological evidence. For instance, some writers have offered left-right dichotomies such as symbolic or propositional vs. visual or imaginative, symbolic vs. visuospatial, verbal vs. visuospatial, verbal vs. perceptual or non-verbal, linguistic vs. visual or kinesthetic. Now, it is known that damage in early childhood to the Wernicke's area on the left hemisphere (this area being involved in the understanding of the written and spoken language) does not result in the non-acquisition of the ability to understand the written and spoken language but merely in the developing of the relevant speech mechanisms on the right hemisphere instead. In other words, the above dichotomies in their unmodified form appear to ignore the well-established facts of the plasticity of function and redundancy of structure in the brain. What is more, the same anatomical asymmetry in Wernicke's area (it is bigger on the left hemisphere) is also present in the brains of chimpanzees and gorillas, and yet verbal-propositional language, as commonly understood, is not a capacity readily associated with these animals. On the other hand, the latter are known to communicate among themselves by means of elaborate displays involving some (visual-auditory) or all of their sensory modalities. These displays are generally thought to be 'symbolic'. But in such a case, the purported distinctions between the opposite terms in the above dichotomies not only become blurred but turn out to be identical, perceptual symbolism and propositional symbolism being presumably subserved by the same brain structure.

Other problems arise from allocating 'expression', 'audio-articulation', and 'propositionizing' to the left, and 'perception', 'retino-ocular' activities, and 'visual imagery' to the right hemisphere.[52] One of the problems here is that artists are, on the whole, thought to be right-brain creatures, and yet nobody would deny that they are also 'expressive', if nothing else. The situation is particularly difficult with musical ability which appears to be mediated by both hemispheres, as is also the case with the deployment of various aspects of mental imagery during wakefulness.[53] And, in respect to speech, the problems are multiplied. For example, left hemispherectomy does not always leave the patient incapable of articulating and understanding speech; indeed, it may be followed by either partial reappearance of the propositional function in the right hemisphere or by no obvious diminution in the patient's intellectual capacity. Moreover, in the case of congenital cerebral hemiatrophy it is clear that one hemisphere does the work of both.[54]

It is sometimes claimed that in splitbrain animals and patients the two hemispheres are capable of solving problems simultaneously and independently of one another. Be that as it may, such observations also show that the two hemispheres handle information at very much the same level and in a similar manner. For instance, in the experiments carried out by Gazzaniga and his co-workers splitbrain monkeys could handle nearly twice as much visual information as intact monkeys. But such results show that the animals' left hemispheres were just as capable of handling *visual* information as their right hemispheres were capable of *comprehending* what was required of them.

Careful review of the literature on HL shows that the non-dominant hemisphere is not entirely devoid of intellectualization: it does not deal so much with space as with spatial thinking or comprehension. Lesions in this part of the brain lead to impairment of intellectualization of space, i.e. to impairment of relationships between the subject and his body or between his body and the surrounding space[55] – disturbances known as apraxias. To be sure, in the majority of cases the non-dominant half of the brain is less verbal than its opposite (in fact, women and left-handed men are found to be less lateralized), but it is still tied down to the 3D concept of space. Like the major hemisphere, the so-called minor is concerned with particularization of space and time. Thus, the usual propositional vs. spatial dichotomy of functions drawn between left and right hemispheres is more appropriately seen (in so far as there is such a dichotomy) as the 'propositional logic' vs. '3D space logic'.

Conversely, the paralogical, primitive, regressive, dreamy, dereistic, holistic, intuitive, etc. features encountered in hypnagogic experiences are hardly ascribable to either of the cerebral hemispheres. Moreover, the various spontaneous physiological phenomena appearing during hypnagogia, such as decrease of respiration, dizziness, floating, and myoclonic spasms, are all controlled at the brainstem level, thus suggesting, in a general way, the direction of brain predominance in this state. In particular, the phenomena of dizziness, floating, disorientation and LEBs argue strongly against any spatial control by the 3D logic of the non-dominant hemisphere. The alpha rhythm, observed in the light stages of hypnagogia, is thought to be characteristic of 'decorticate' states.[56] More significantly, the upper brainstem has been found to have equal functional relationships with the two hemispheres,[57] which implies that if HL is a fact then this fact looks like a development out of an initial subcortical lateralization (a point to be discussed further in the next section).

The inarticulate brain

Writing on epilepsy, McLean says:

> From animal experimentation on limbic epilepsy (induced by electrical stimulation) it has become evident that seizure-discharges induced in the limbic lobe tend in their spread to be confined to the limbic system. . . . Such experiments provide the most striking evidence available of a dichotomy of function (or what has been called a 'schizophysiology' of the limbic and neocortical systems). Patients with smouldering limbic epilepsy may manifest all the symptoms of schizophrenia: the schizophysiology in question is possibly relevant to the pathogenesis of this disease. . . . From the standpoint of the patient lying on the couch, the schizophysiology under consideration is significant because it indicates that the lower mammalian brain is able to some degree to function independently, to make up its own mind. The primitive, crude screen provided by the limbic cortex might be imagined as portraying a confused picture of the inside and the outside world.[58]

In the above quotation McLean makes a number of important remarks, at least three of which are highly relevant to my current discussion. I shall point them out and devote most of the rest of this chapter to discussing them in relation to both the experiential features of hypnagogia and adjacent states and to my view regarding the brain substrates of hypnagogia expressed in the preceding sections. Indeed, I shall expand on the latter to include considerations as to the genesis and nature of consciousness. Earlier, I used the self-explicit term 'subcortical structures' to stand for all brain structures below the cortical level. Another term bearing the same meaning is that of 'oldbrain' which I shall be using both as a convenient term and because of its phylogenetic connotations: it is collectively older than the cerebral cortex which is a mammalian acquisition.

McLean's relevant remarks are: first, limbic epileptic discharges tend to confine themselves to the limbic system; second, the oldbrain tends to confuse the inside and the outside world; third, there is a dichotomy of function between limbic and neocortical systems, the former being capable of functioning and deciding to a certain degree independently of the neocortex.

In discussing McLean's first observation, we must bear in mind that not all oldbrain discharges confine themselves to the subcortical level. As we saw earlier in this chapter, electrical stimulation of oldbrain areas may reflect clearly on various parts of the cortex, accompanied by the occurrence of related subjective experiences. Indeed, McLean is careful to qualify his remark by saying that limbic discharges *tend* to be confined to the limbic system. However, in limbic epilepsy there is a spread of the discharge within the limbic system indicating that a number of emotional and cognitive states may result. This is supported by the results of experiments in electrical stimulation of various loci in the oldbrain of animals which show that there is a spillover effect resulting in 'abnormalities' of experience and behaviour, e.g. aggressive behaviour may combine with sex or oral activity. (Interestingly, in a wider context, and under normal circumstances, babies and dogs are observed to have erections during feeding.) Conversely, surgical ablations in which certain parts of the limbic lobe are excised lead to an abolition of fear and anger, inability to avoid painful situations, loss or perversion of instinctual feeding, mating, and parental habits.[59] It is possible that in those cases of epilepsy where fear precedes the seizure, the experienced emotion of fear is a mere concomitant of the excitation of a particular limbic area; it may be related to an instinctive cognition (at the level of the oldbrain) that the seizure may terminate the organism's life or incapacitate it in the event of having to defend itself against a predator during the fit. On the other hand, mystical experience may correlate with the defunctionalization (akin to surgical ablation) of certain parts of the oldbrain and stimulation of others (in addition to a suppression of higher cortical centres). Both of these conditions – inexplicable fear and indescribable bliss – are, of course, occasionally met with in hypnagogia where the former always leaves the subject in a state of puzzlement and bewilderment.

As we saw in chapter 5, the meditator seeks to do away with emotions, desires, and external and internal noise, and achieve maximum psychological withdrawal (stages 1 to 5 of meditation). Two of the first emotions to go are those of fear and anger: they are conquered partly by the physiological switch to the parasympathetic system and receptive mode, a process that leads to the near elimination of all characteristic sympathetic-adrenal features. Painful situations, likewise, are not avoided: they are ignored (e.g. pain from cross-legged positions is simply ignored, attention being directed elsewhere). Also instincts are supplanted in meditation exercises: feeding and mating instincts are often denied 'normal' expression and are sought to be sublimated in ascetic abstinence. Interestingly enough, reports of mystical experiences are replete with expressions such as 'divine marriage', 'divine union', 'becoming one with the Absolute', 'becoming one with the Cosmos', 'realizing the Cosmos within oneself', 'expanding and embracing the World'. It is not at all difficult to see how such expressions stand as symbols representing sublimated oldbrain instincts. It is tempting to argue that the mystic, unlike the ablated animal, has the choice of returning to the pre-mystical (pre-ablated) reality. However, the issue is debatable. The long and persistent meditation and other exercises practised by mystics are unlikely not to have created permanent 'conditions' in their nervous system. This 'physiological' argument is supported by the experiential reports of mystics who declare that their experiences carry with them a form of permanent mutation. An important symbol in mysticism is that of the *ouroboros*, the snake that bites its own tail, symbolizing the return to the unconscious (and perhaps to autosexuality). The return to the unconscious or the union with the Absolute suggests an abolition or weakening of boundaries that distinguish the internal from the external, the 'I' from the 'It'. These, as we have seen, are characteristic features of hypnagogia. They are also to be found in epilepsy.

In regard to his observation that the oldbrain tends to confuse the inside with the outside world, McLean says that the clinical impression gained is that

> [these patients] show an exaggerated tendency to regard the external world as though it were part of themselves. In other words, internal feelings are blended with what is seen, heard or otherwise sensed in such a way that the outside world is experienced as though it were inside. In this respect there is a resemblance to children and primitive peoples.[60]

The suggestion of ontogenetic regression is quite clear. The characteristics of internalization and incorporability we observed in hypnagogia, and through it in other states, are also present. An example quoted by Koestler of an epileptic girl who, as a child, walked into the sunlight and reported the experience of having 'a funny taste in my mouth of the sun',[61] shows not only internalization of the environment but also a crossover or translation of one group of perceptual data into another – just as in hypnagogia auditory, kinesthetic, tactile, and other sensations turn into visual images, and visual imagery often carries with it tactile, kinesthetic, and other sensations. This crossover from one sense modality into another is, as noted, another form of boundary dissolution: information input in one modality is shared by another.

McLean's suggestion that there is a dichotomy of function between the limbic system and the neocortex may further strengthen the possibility of a switch to oldbrain predominance during hypnagogia and related states. We already know that the oldbrain occupies a strategically central position for correlating internal sensations with perceptions from the outside world, and for initiating appropriate action according to its own lights, i.e. it has its own mental process: it emotes and *thinks* – though not in verbal concepts,[62] but rather in a non-verbal type of symbolism. This, McLean remarks, would have significant implications in so far as symbolism affects the emotional life of the individual:

> One might imagine, for example, that though the visceral brain could never aspire to conceive of the colour red in terms of a three-letter word or as a specific wave-length of light, it could associate the colour symbolically with such diverse things as blood, fainting, fighting, flowers, etc., – correlations leading to phobias, obsessive-compulsive behaviour, etc. Lacking the help and control of the neocortex, its impressions would be discharged without modification into the hypothalamus and lower centres of affective behaviour. Considered in the light of Freudian psychology, the old brain would have many of the attributes of the unconscious *id*. One might argue, however, *that the visceral brain is not at all unconscious (possibly not even in certain stages of sleep), but rather eludes the grasp of the intellect because its animalistic and primitive structure makes it impossible to communicate in verbal terms.*[63]

We have already seen that in hypnagogia mentation is 'paralogical'. In particular, it has been observed that the notion of similarity is often totally replaced by the notion of sameness both on the quasiperceptual level of imagery and on the conceptual level. This is not necessarily a matter of weakening of consciousness – implying a mere reduction of higher cerebral activity – but more of a shift to oldbrain activity. An extreme shift of functioning to the oldbrain may lead to one or the other (or even, in really extreme pathological cases, to both) of two polarized groups of activities: (a) destruction, and (b) preservation, or, to use Koestler's terms, self-assertive tendencies and integrative tendencies, which may be linked physiologically to the sympathetic and parasympathetic systems respectively. In either case, however, when the shift is considerable the resulting logic is peculiar to the locus of excitation. For instance, in many epileptic limbic seizures the attack is known to be accompanied by fear or anger, suggesting, as noted above, the excitation of a particular limbic locus correlated with these emotions; the 'lost feeling' that usually accompanies this type of attack can only manifest itself as a form of realization that one is 'cut off', isolated, in danger of dissolving and losing one's identity, implying that identity (self-assertion) is all-important to the patient. On other occasions, however, the patient may feel elation and tranquillity, 'together with a pantheistic experience of merging with the environment or the visual phenomena',[64] thus manifesting integrative tendencies and pointing to a different limbic locus as the brain correlate of this experience. Interestingly, in respect to animals, McLean has localized drives and self-preservation instincts in the lower half of the limbic system and those tendencies and instincts concerned with the 'preservation and welfare of the species' in the upper part. Needless to say that on the human level one must be careful not to be too literal in drawing parallels with the animal kingdom, as human emotions and cognitions have wider aspects than those of animals; bearing this qualification in mind, however, the dichotomy between self-assertive and integrative (self-transcending) tendencies may be maintained.

In many pathological cases resulting from anxiety and emotional stress, there may ensue a violent shift to the opposite (self-transcending) tendencies, i.e. one is *forced* to 'let go', causing in its turn a reaction towards the original mode activity, the final result being one of vacillation between the two extremes, first affirming and then negating a state of affairs. This kind of 'simultaneous' assertion-and-negation is also characteristic of many mystical experiences. In both cases the contradictions are resolved: in the latter case by 'seeing' that in a 'real' sense (real to the subject) all terms contain their opposites (indeed, *are* their opposites), in the former case by creating what has been called a 'close system' in which nothing can be contradicted. This kind of logic, in which everything can be related to everything else, and ultimately everything is the same, is to be encountered in hypnagogia where its presence enables us, as already pointed out, to understand not only pathological and mystical mentation as analysed above but also the mental mechanics of creativity.

Thus, the mentality of the oldbrain, as it manifests itself in hypnagogia and adjacent states, traverses and intersects a number of FsR, drawing them together and relating them in paralogical ways, that is, it relates and assimilates images and concepts where 'logical' rules would not allow such activities. As we have seen (for instance in chapters 7 and 8), if the different sense modalities were thought of as different FsR, then synesthetic phenomena, as they occur in hypnagogia and related states, are clearly paralogical (non-cortical), and so are autosymbolic phenomena – thus also suggesting how the oldbrain can work independently of higher cortical centres. As argued, hypnagogia, and hypnagogic-like mentation in general, comprises innumerable imaginal and conceptual associations whose relevance is often a matter of our readiness and ability to fit them into a consistent FR. This is not always possible, which means that we may always have geniuses and lunatics in our midst, people who would not accept that their FsR are indeed irrelevant when these are not shown to be valid in *our* universe of discourse. This is not merely to say that the theoretical frameworks of such individuals are alien to, and outside, the possibilities of what can be structured according to rules of logic, but more importantly, that these are derived from paralogical experiences, experiences which carry with them their own logic and type of understanding.

As pointed out elsewhere in this discussion, to refer to hypnagogia as a strange state is simply to make a value judgment from a 'logically' operating waking state. But in the depths of hypnagogia itself no such judgment is relevant. It would appear that the hypnagogist, the mystic, the 'psychic', the 'mentally disturbed' person, and the creative individual enter into a state of mind that permits paralogical associations among a number of universes of discourse. These associations seem to them perfectly 'logical', and so far as they are concerned, it is the rest of the population who are unable to see them. Van Dusen, for instance, tells us that Swedenborg 'felt it was possible to deal with universal ideas, understanding at once all the implications of a thing' by means of the method of 'passive potency'.[65] Before him, Plotinus had practised a similar technique which he adapted from Plato's *Symposium*.[66] This method of inspiration, which appears to circumvent or cut through logical steps, cuts both ways: it may lead to great and empirically verifiable inspirational insights, or to irrelevant gibberishness (although it might still be argued that calling such statements 'unverifiable' may simply mean that we are only capable or willing to try and verify statements that render themselves verifiable according to *our* principles of verification).

Koestler suggests the concept of 'bisociation' as an explanatory notion of the conceptual activity wherein two disparate FsR ('matrices'), such as the phases of the moon and the tides, can be brought together. In fact, as already noted, in hypnagogia the subject is often faced with more than two intersecting matrices and may thus be said to be multisociating. In the above well-known example of Kepler's associating the phases of the moon with the tides, Galileo is said to have dismissed the idea as an 'occult fancy'. Similarly, in the case of hypnagogia we often talk of the irrelevancies of imaginal and conceptual associations which, not infrequently, have been labelled 'occult', partly because of their apparent autonomy but also because of their paralogical nature which, not surprisingly, may be found to relate, as in McLean's example above, such disparate objects as blood and flowers.

Hypnagogia also manifests, like the hypnotic and mystical states, the paradox of combining single-mindedness and self-transcendence. We might get closer to understanding the paradox if we keep constantly in mind the hypnagogist's sensorial and conceptual 'openness', that is, his all-round sensitivity and suggestibility. In this way we can see that hypnagogic associations are not 'irrelevant' because each one is fascinatedly attended to. Moreover, irrelevant data are such as cannot be 'logically' related to a FR, and in hypnagogia there is no single 'logically' constructed FR. In the depths of hypnagogia the subject is peculiarly single-minded since every image, concept, or association 'fascinates' his attention. This state of attention, we may remind ourselves, is similar to that reached by the meditator who sets out deliberately to concentrate on a particular object, image, or concept. The hypnagogist's fascination, which eliminates or prevents 'secondary consciousness', also dissolves his self-assertive tendencies. And here may be found an important clue to man's acquisition of self-consciousness: its genesis may lie in those instincts and needs generally related to the activities of the sympathetic-adrenal division and the emotions of hunger, fear, and anger.

Self-assertiveness vs. self-transcendence

As noted, McLean localized self-preservation and species-preservation instincts in the lower and higher parts of the limbic system of animals respectively, and, in humans, Koestler has elaborated the first group of instincts into the self-assertive tendencies and the second into the self-transcending or integrative tendencies. It will be noticed that there is a mutual implication between self-preservation and self-assertion: one asserts oneself in an effort to preserve oneself, and vice versa, he preserves himself in self-assertive efforts. The point to be made here is that the very notion of self-assertion (or self-preservation) implies the assumption that even at the primitive level of the oldbrain there is some form of instinctual self-awareness. Fear and anger may have arisen out of this need for self-preservation, and this is, perhaps, why in an epileptic fit loss of identity *and* fear sometimes manifest simultaneously – in this way also pointing, as already suggested, to a localization within the limbic system of a physical discharge which is strongly correlated with such cognitions and emotions.

Thus, through the need to *preserve* itself as a more or less self-contained unit, an organism *asserts* itself on its environment: but without some form of awareness of itself as a separate unit, self-assertion would be meaningless – and some support for this argument, in regard both to early mammals and humans, lies in the ability to feel fear and to be angry, which emotions, again, would be utterly meaningless and useless if they did not stem from some form of self-awareness. Obviously, it is not to be argued here that all animal life 'thinks' and 'emotes', at least not in an anthropomorphic sense, but that every time an animal attacks or withdraws from an attack *it asserts itself* at no matter what primitive level.[67] This leads me to the formulation of the hypothesis that the oldbrain does not merely provide the 'raw material' of awareness but also contains the correlate locus of the genesis of self-awareness. The 'schizophysiology' talked about by McLean and Koestler and argued as being the *'insufficient co-ordination* between archicortex and neocortex'[68] may in fact lie – in so far as there is such a state of affairs as schizophysiology – not so much in the lack of co-ordination between the two brains as between the self-assertive and self-transcending tendencies 'generated' in the oldbrain, and perhaps only emphasized and exaggerated by the neocortex.

The relevance of the above to the nature and function of hypnagogia lies in my describing the latter as a state characterized by integrative features and self-transcending tendencies, viz. LEBs, abandonment, lack of fear in general and in particular of identity loss, the implicit assumption that the environment is not inimical, the tendency to incorporate (internalize) and merge with the environment, loss of self-awareness (or, perhaps, willingness to relinquish self-awareness), and, therefore, absence of self-assertiveness. This might enable us, first, to tentatively correlate psychological aspects of hypnagogia with the activities of physiological loci in the oldbrain, and, second, to speculate as to the evolutionary genesis and significance of hypnagogia.

If self-awareness, in mammals, is closely related to the self-assertive instincts whose brain substrates – if McLean is correct – are localized in the lower limbic system, then we may speculate that self-awareness might also be correlated, at least in part, with the activities of the same or adjacent loci. Conversely, we would seek for the brain correlates of self-transcendence in the upper part of the limbic system, where McLean localized the species-preservation instincts, and in the thalamus. (This contains the assumption that a human being transcends itself in species-preservation activities which are in fact only one type of manifestation or ramification of a human's self-transcending tendencies.) The thalamus, which, among other things, as we have seen, acts as a relay station directing afferent (incoming) sensory signals to the cerebrum, can be separated into three nuclei one of which, the medial thalamic nucleus (intrinsic nuclei), is, in fact, that part of the brain that induces alpha, and other, slower rhythmic activities, in the cortex. In contrast to the lower region of the RAS which mediates arousal and alertness, the diffuse thalamic system is known to mediate depression of cortical excitability, and sleep.[69] It is thought that the raphé system in the upper brainstem inhibits the arousing action of the RAS and in this way allows the medial thalamus to exert its own inhibiting effects on the cortex.[70]

Thus, because of the close connection between cortical excitability and wakefulness, it is often argued that not only is awareness dependent on cortical activation but that consciousness *is* cortical activation, and that without the contribution of the old 'visceral' brain to provide us with internal bodily sensations 'the experience of our own reality would probably be absent'[61] – we should be, as McLean put it, 'disembodied spirits'.[71]

Now, I believe the arguments in the preceding paragraph to be wrong because of the criteria on which their premises are based. To begin with, they appear to view consciousness as a behaviourist 'thing' entirely dependent on the criteria of arousal, i.e. a person loses and gains consciousness depending on his EEG record and whether he opens his eyes or shows other signs of wakefulness or sleep, as the case may be. A considerable research has gone into demonstrating the existence of collateral afferents that branch off into the reticular formation from the main sensory pathways which carry signals, through relays, to the cortex. Attaching these findings to the above criteria of consciousness, the conclusion is drawn that 'when human consciousness is lost it is because of failure on the part of the reticular formation to send up a sufficiency of the non-specific or "activating" nerve impulses to the cortex'.[72] For instance, in animals that were given ether or the barbiturate drug thiopentone, electric shock to the leg resulted in a cortical evoked potential identical to that registered in the animals' normal state, whereas 'the evoked potential of the reticular formation of the anaesthetized animals was now very small.'[73] In this example the cortex is clearly responsive (awake?) to stimuli during the time the animal is drugged while the reticular formation's responsiveness is greatly diminished, and is thus surmised by the experimenters that the animal was not conscious of the stimuli. But surely, if signals reaching the cortex do not cause the animal to respond, this does not support the notion that consciousness 'resides' in the cortex; on the contrary, it rather suggests that the 'residence' of consciousness is to be sought for elsewhere (in the reticular formation?). In other experiments, where decorticate animals continued, as usual, to show variations of wakefulness, loss of learned habits was observed,[74] which demonstrates how habit learning is dependent on the cortex and, thus, how the cortex is responsible for the acquisition of relationships with the environment and, therefore, reversing McLean's argument that if the cortex were on its own it would yield 'disembodied spirits': it would seem that it is the cortex that supplies the 'reality anchorage' or reality testing principle so often invoked as a criterion for distinguishing between wakefulness and dreams or hallucinations.

A most important point to note is that decrease in cortical activity does not necessarily mean decrease in awareness. As noted earlier, the medial thalamus is capable of driving the cortex into synchronized slow rhythms some of which (alpha-theta) are, in fact, characteristic of meditation, some psi states (those we concerned ourselves with in this book), and certain stages of hypnagogia. Which implies that these states, when deliberately brought about, induce thalamic activity which in its turn 'damps down' the cortex. This, as we saw in Part Two, often has the effect of leading into sleep unless checked; conversely, hypnagogia is utilized as a general condition conducive to these states. In other words, whether spontaneous or induced these states, including hypnagogia, are characterized by the activation of the thalamus and other oldbrain structures which *cause* the cortex to 'idle'. It is an active organismic defunctionalization of the cortex, physiologically initiated by the oldbrain and causing a switch to oldbrain awareness.

It is of great relevance in this connection to note that, whereas cortical activity diminishes during REM (sleepdream) states, activity in the mesencephalic reticular formation is often higher in these periods than that recorded during wakefulness,[75] and that, similarly, yoga meditators are said to be concerned with merging themselves into 'the "indeterminate" awareness of the deep subcortical mechanism, the highest level of neural integration – the centrencephalon'.[76] It is also worth noting that meditators intensify their internal experiences by coupling their non-cortical centrencephalic concentration of attention with breathing exercises that create excessive carbon dioxide and a shortage of oxygen in the blood.[77] It is interesting in this latter respect that low blood oxygen is generally known to be one of the causes of hallucination,[78] and that some studies have found schizophrenics to be characterized by reduced oxygen consumption.[79] Moreover, alveolar carbon dioxide is also known to increase with relaxation, and most noticeably during sleep onset and the first two hours of sleep.[80] Now, we know that hypnagogia is characterized by relaxation and reduced respiration (and, therefore, by increase in carbon dioxide in the blood), by inwardly turned, diffuse-absorbed attention, and by dreamlike mentation which is linked to a diminution in cortical and, as noted above, to an increase in mesencephalic activity.

Such a state of affairs would explain the paralogical nature of hypnagogia and the 'strange' synesthetic and other phenomena encountered therein. Some of these, such as synesthesias and the vividness and lifelikeness of imagery, would be features indigenous to the oldbrain itself, whereas others, such as the *jamais vu* and some of the *déjà vu* experiences, might be due to the extrinsic association nuclei of the thalamus being prevented from, or hindered in, conveying concerted information to the relevant association areas of the cortex, and in particular to the memory areas. The feeling of loss of identity, too, might be of the latter nature in that if no information from the senses is conveyed through the thalamus to the cortex the person is deprived of his 'reality anchorage' and the preservation of his 'ego schema' which normally enables him to relate himself to his mental and physical environment: to reiterate a point made earlier, in order to retain – indeed, to acquire – ego schema and reality anchorage, information must be relayed to the cortex where the senses are represented in rich detail, thus indicating how the logic of 3D reality is 'localized' on this part of the brain.

It is tempting to distinguish between 'cortical consciousness' and 'oldbrain consciousness', as indeed both McLean and Koestler do. But when such a distinction is drawn the criteria on which it is based are of the utmost importance. My position is that the cortex is there to fill in the logical steps, so to speak, between the major premise and the conclusion which are provided by the oldbrain. As both Penfield and Thomson argued, the system essential to consciousness is not to be found in the cortex but in the subcortical structures, and in particular 'where the mesencephalon, sub-thalamus and thalamus meet'.[81] That is, consciousness as such does not 'reside' in the cortex but in the oldbrain: it is the specificity of consciousness that the cortex is concerned with – it provides sequential-temporal and spatial relationships, it particularizes and individualizes existence. Major premises, universal ideas, and generalizations, like beliefs, in a sense stand outside logic: they are assumptions supplied by the 'integrative' aspect of the oldbrain which also provides, in its 'self-assertive' aspect (separation, differentiation), the means for developing the specific logic of deduction and induction. It is possible that these tendencies of the oldbrain, as they are taken up and particularized by the cortex, become not only mentally but also physically polarized into the two cerebral hemispheres. If this be the case, it would be of great interest to seek for physiological relationships between areas of the oldbrain and areas of one or the other of the cerebral hemispheres that show strong and consistent correlations with self-transcending or integrative tendencies on the one hand and self-assertive tendencies on the other. A tentative hypothesis at this stage might argue for correlations (a) between the thalamus, upper limbic system, right cerebral hemisphere, and integrative tendencies, and (b) between the thalamus, lower limbic system, left cerebral hemisphere, and self-assertive tendencies.

The thalamus, the pineal, and the caduceus

Hitherto in this chapter I have referred to the brain structures below the cortex as if they constituted a unit. I did so mainly because I wanted to contrast the logic of the cortex with the paralogic of subcortical activities in general, the latter being related as a whole to hypnagogic phenomena. In fact, brain anatomists and neurophysiologists distinguish between three brains, viz. the central core (reptilian), the limbic system (paleomammalian), and the cerebral cortex (neomammalian). It is thought that at the reptilian level consciousness is concerned with sensorimotor experiences but does not differentiate between one's body and external space. At the limbic level (the 'archicortex', McLean's 'visceral brain'), consciousness deals with images which are basic to both perception and hallucination. At the cortical ('neocortical') level, objects become clearly recognizable as belonging to external space.[82]

One might conjecture from this that consciousness at one level would be well-nigh inaccessible to consciousness at another level, or, at least, it would appear very strange and foreign to it. What is conscious and 'logical' to one brain may be unconscious and/or paralogical to another.[83] This would explain the paralogical character of hypnagogic experiences, if, as I have argued, the latter transpire in a general state of oldbrain predominance. Interestingly enough, the thalamus, on which I placed some considerable emphasis as the centre of consciousness, is shared by both the reptilian brain and the limbic system, and has strong reciprocal links with the two cerebral hemispheres. Might this not explain the preconscious nature of hypnagogia which, standing on the verge of wakefulness and sleep, has access to experiences that emerge from different levels of consciousness, such as the lack of differentiation between the 'I' and the 'It' (reptilian level), the viewing of images both as internal, psychological entities and as objects 'out there', as 'actualities', hallucinations (limbic level), and the awareness that one is awake and observing dream activities in progress (cortical level)?

Moreover, the thalamic system contains that pea-size, conically shaped body (about 8 mm in length) which Descartes was held to have considered to

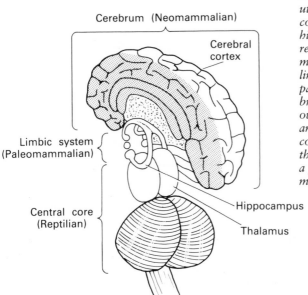

Cerebrum (Neomammalian)

Cerebral cortex

Limbic system (Paleomammalian)

Central core (Reptilian)

Hippocampus

Thalamus

Figure 10.4 *The three brains in mammalian evolution. These lie concentrically and hierarchically, with the reptilian at the lowest and most central position, the limbic system above and partly round the reptilian brain, and the cerebrum overlying the limbic system and part of the central core. Each of these areas of the 'triune brain' represents a fairly distinct type of mentation-cognition.*

be the 'seat' of the soul, namely the pineal. This is a strange little organ with a long and peculiar history both in the manner in which it has been viewed down the ages and in its phylogenetic and functional development. In the former respect, it was first pointed out by Herophilos (325–280 BC) and Erasistratos (310–250 BC) of the University of Alexandria, both of whom ascribed to it psychic and intellectual functions and considered it to be the substrate for the development of knowledge. In the second century AD, Galenos of Pergamon stripped it of its purported psychic functions and viewed it merely as a lymph gland. In the following centuries, other authors occupied themselves with its study, or speculated concerning its psychic and biological importance, culminating with Descartes's theory which did not so much speak of the seat of the soul as of the organ that distilled the 'spirit' from the blood and distributed it, through the ventricles, to the periphery of the body. After Steno's criticism of Descartes's theory in the seventeenth century, interest dwindled, but since the realization of the existence of endocrine glands researchers turned their attention once more to it, and in recent years it has become a focus of attention.

From a phylogenetic point of view, the pineal is extremely old, dating back to Devonian and Silurian tetrapods (as shown in fossil skulls), and much as its form and functions changed through the ages two of its main functions are still to be found in living vertebrates. The pineals of these animals are largely composed of photoreceptor elements that show both a photosensory and secretory function. In certain lower vertebrates, such as the reptile *Sphenodon*, the pineal, or rather, the epiphysis from which the mammalian pineal has developed, is made up of two distinct bodies, the *parietal organ*, which sits at the top of the head and constitutes a *parietal eye*, complete with cornea, lens and retina, and the *pineal organ*, which is glandular in character and secretes into the third ventricle. In mammals, including man, the parietal organ or eye appears quite clearly in early embryonic life but soon disappears while the pineal organ or gland remains. Like the parietal eye, the pineal gland is sensitive to light which it receives indirectly through the eyes and an accessory pathway but also by non-retinal pathways and without the involvement of the sympathetic nerves that connect with it, e.g. through the skull. Thus, the pineal has been called 'an indirectly photosensitive neuroendocrine organ',[84] or, more accurately, 'neuroendocrine transducer',[85] converting neural input to endocrine output.

Until about fifteen years ago the pineal was thought to be a body which, despite the fact that it lay within the cranium and was embryologically and topographically part of the brain to which it was connected by a stalk, in the adult mammal was not truly part of the brain but received its neuronal input from the peripheral autonomic nervous system.[84] More recently, however, various nerve fibres passing along its stalk from other areas of the brain have been clearly identified, and more are being found whose origins are as yet imprecise. Conversely, the pineal does not act directly on peripheral sense targets but on other glands and brain structures, and has been shown to be an endocrine gland of major regulatory importance thus gaining the title of 'regulator of regulators'.[86] Its effects are believed to be mainly inhibitory, and its hormones reach their targets through the cerebrospinal fluid and the circulatory system. It is also known to be the only organ that produces the aminoacid *melatonin* in mammals. Melatonin, which has been found to cause lightening of skin colour in some lower vertebrates, is the product of the neurotransmitter serotonin which, along with other transmitter substances, is present in large concentrations and has its largest circadian variations in this body. Various experiments have shown that melatonin affects the synthesis, release and levels of serotonin in the hypothalamus as well as the synthesis and levels of other neurotransmitters in other parts of the brain. It also affects the EEG, sleep, and behaviour.

The pineal shows very high basic activity, has an extraordinary blood supply (in this respect being second only to the kidney on a weight-for-weight basis), and when stimulated, e.g. by the presence of a tumour, produces high levels not only of melatonin and serotonin but also of other substances all of which are known to be of profound importance in maintaining body functions.[87] One effect of the excision of this gland is the disruption of the body's biological clock. Another is the elimination of the inhibitory influence which is exercised by the pineal melatonin on the gonadal system, with a resultant provocation of ovulation – a strong indication of the important part the pineal plays in the regulation of gonadal development: indeed, it is held by many researchers that this organ is possibly the mediator of the whole reproductive cycle. Disturbances in the pineal may result, for instance, in precocious puberty or delay in menarche.

Of special relevance to our present discussion is the observation that the mammalian pineal is extremely sensitive to environmental light, temperature variation, and stress – and other factors that generally affect the psychic and somatic equilibrium. Light, in particular, appears to inhibit the synthesis of melatonin and tends to produce results similar to those of pinealectomy – for instance it affects the oestrus and decreases the pineal weight, RNA, and protein. Conversely, darkness and a calming and relaxing environment, such as that necessary for the induction of hypnagogia, has the opposite effect of increasing the production of melatonin and pineal activity in general. Similarly, melatonim itself has a tranquillizing effect on the central nervous system, and is known to increase the sensitivity of the brain to barbiturates. Such observations may explain the absence of strong emotions during hypnagogia, and lend additional support to my general argument that, although cortical and strong sympathetic activities are not obviously present during hypnagogia, activities in and around the thalamus are on the increase. Another possible piece of evidence in this direction may lie in the suggestion that the pineal contains cholinergic nerve endings whose input might affect the enzyme HIOMT (hydroxyindole-O-methyltransferase) that catalyses the terminal step in melatonin biosynthesis. It is also very interesting that melatonin is believed to increase through meditation exercises[88] which include not only relaxation but, most importantly, visualization, the latter being very similar to, and often identical with, hypnagogic visual experiences. The stimulation of the pineal through meditation is, furthermore, thought to act on the hypothalamus in such a way as to inhibit strong affect, as is the case in hypnagogia, and loosen a person's tendency for attachment to things, people, places, etc., and, in effect, loosen one's ego boundaries. The same stimulation is also thought to reverse the 'earthing' of the sexual process, that is, to sublimate or re-invest sexuality into internal psychic processes such as those involving image formation in hypnagogia and related states.

The pineal gland appears to occupy the exact anatomical position of what in the Vedic literature is thought to be the 'organ' of spiritual vision, the 'third eye'. In the same tradition, it is believed that spiritual vision, which was originally readily available to man, is 'temporarily' (for some millions of years, that is) lost due to an evolutionary necessary descent into matter, to be regained in due course at a higher level. In the West, this latter level is often represented by the god Hermes's sceptre, the caduceus, depicting two snakes entwined around a central rod which culminates in a small sphere or cone flanked by two wings. Without going too deeply into the meaning of these symbols, it is worth noting that the snakes represent the two supposedly opposite sides of man, whereas the sphere or cone stands for the unity of consciousness. The two wings sprouting from the sphere are both higher representations of the two sides of man and the symbols of completion and of

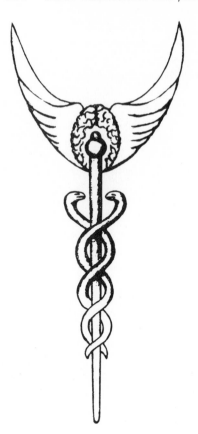

Figure 10.5 *The caduceus – the emblem of liberated consciousness. At its centre lies the 'cone' or pineal gland (conarium), the 'seat' of the soul.*

liberation of consciousness: they are the two cerebral hemispheres flanking, and practically encasing, the pineal gland. Could we not perhaps see in this scheme an evolution from primitive 'self-awareness' (at the 'egocentric' level where 'everything is in the self') to a more clearly defined notion of self which stands separate from its environment, and finally to a state of awareness in which 'the self is in everything' – the latter clearly being integrative and self-transcending? This would go some way to explaining mystical experiences in which a person 'returns' to an earlier stage of evolution but, as it were, on a spiral-fashion higher level. It might also explain some of the other states and experiences related to hypnagogia, and in particular how psychics and creative individuals appear to revert to an evolutionarily primitive mode of mentation.

It is also noteworthy that clinically defined death is generally referred to as 'brainstem death', thus again pointing a strong finger at the importance of this part of the brain in the function of consciousness. Paradoxically enough, even though death is thought of as the moment of ultimate and irreversible cessation of consciousness, there are numerous reports of 'death' and near-

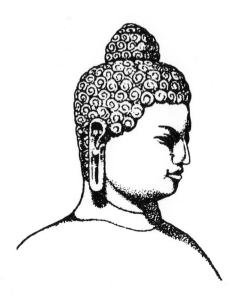

Figure 10.6   *Buddha with the conical 'crown', the symbol of illumination whose physiological correlate or substrate is thought to be the conically shaped pineal gland.*

death experiences in which consciousness appears to intensify rather than diminish or cease.[89] In such cases, as in some cases of hypnagogia and related states, the experients say that, during their 'death', they acquired incommunicable omniscience, were granted universal secrets which, however, were lost to them when they 'returned' to life. One wonders whether, in their 'liberated' state, these people did not function at a level of consciousness whose mode of cognition is so different from that of ordinary wakefulness that what is deemed knowledge in the former is utterly inexpressible in the latter, or simply 'forgotten' (see, for example, chapter 5 for similar cases in hypnagogia, meditation, and related states).

Finally, having argued fairly hard for the identification of the brain substrates of hypnagogic experiences, it becomes clear that the experiences themselves are subject to what I might call 'brainfields', that is, to 'fields of consciousness' that rise from, or give rise to, activities of *areas* of the brain. In other words, if, as I have argued, consciousness during hypnagogia is mainly concentrated around the thalamus, a given hypnagogic experience would be characterized by the degree to which this consciousness shifts, stretches, or relates to particular parts of the brain. Any such shift would create a 'field' whose features would condition the experience. Thus, a general shift to the reptilian level would be characterized by, for instance, a lessening of internal-external distinctions, whereas a shift to the cortical level would have the opposite effect (modified, of course, by the particular part of the cortex the 'field' relates to). Moreover, 'brainfields' need not be literally circumscribed by the anatomy and physiology of the brain but rather extend beyond them much in the fashion of electromagnetic fields which, although emanating from a definite source, are not spatially confined to it, nor is their mode of activity and influence restricted by the assumed three-dimensionality of their source.

11 · *The function and significance of hypnagogia*

The loosening of ego boundaries

Repeated reference has been made in earlier chapters to the paralogical and ontogenetically regressive character of hypnagogia, and in the last chapter this was tied in with a switch to predominating oldbrain activities which gave it a phylogenetic perspective. The frequent allusions to infantile and childhood psychological characteristics, which accord well with the general notion that 'ontogeny recapitulates phylogeny', are well justified both on physiological and psychological grounds. Physiologically, this can be seen in the pattern of gradual myelination of neural tracts in the fetus and neonate, and in the fact that the neuronal connections of an infant's cerebral cortex are lacking in the level of myelination and are immature in a variety of other respects[1] – observations which have led to the conclusion (noted in chapter 10) that infants are essentially precorticate. On the psychological level, depth psychologists and developmental theorists alike suggest that the perceptions and cognitions of human infants only gradually, and in tandem with their physiological growth, demonstrate differentiation and categorization of experience, and that neonates are characterized initially by a lack of ego boundaries. At a very early stage in the infant's life (and before it, in the life of the fetus) a fused, synesthetic mode may be naturally present and expressed in kinesthetic activity as the infant (or fetus) relates to an as yet undifferentiated universe.[2]

Similarly, we know that hypnagogia is strongly linked with the absence of directed, analytical (cortical) thinking and that the emergence, intensification and prolongation of hypnagogic imagery is connected with a passive-receptive attitude and a feeling of abandonment, of loosening of ego controls. The hypnagogist's general feeling of electrochemical field connection with his imagery, and his tendency to internalize and subjectify his environment, can also be seen as parallels to the infant's trophotropic attitude.

Thus, my relating hypnagogia both to oldbrain activities and to ontogenetically earlier mentation renders the presence of the phenomenon of LEBs in this state not merely plausible but necessary. Indeed, it appears to be a function of the state, and its presence not only would explain the occurrence of diverse phenomena in hypnagogia and related states but its nature is theoretically and experientially wide enough to encompass other concepts and theories formulated to account for the same and similar phenomena: Deikman's receptive mode, McKellar's autism, Oswald's dereism, Piaget's and Froeschels's egocentricism, Koestler's bisociationism, von Domarus's paralogical thinking, Freud's unconscious and preconscious mentation, Sidis's and Warcollier's subconscious and Prince's coconscious phenomena may all be fully, or to a very considerable extent, explained by the presence of the LEBs.

In order to understand the nature and conceptual breadth and potency of the LEBs we need to reflect on basic assumptions about the notions of mind and consciousness. To begin with, the idea that consciousness is equivalent to conscious awareness must be dismissed.. Ever since Descartes's assertion that 'the human soul is always conscious in any circumstances – even in the mother's womb',[3] implying that so long as there is mind this mind must exist in a variety of states of consciousness none of which could be thought of as constituting 'total unconsciousness', psychological research has strongly supported this claim. Sleep research and research in hypnosis have shown that the mind never really 'sleeps', that when it appears to be asleep or unconscious another part of it may be 'awake' and conscious, and that two or more levels of consciousness, layers or subsystems may exist concurrently and in seeming ignorance of one another.[4] Moreover, evidence afforded by reports of near-death experiences and the experiences of clinically 'dead' people argues that even at moments of behavioural and physiological 'total unconsciousness' mental activity may still carry on.

Now, in the process of maturing, along with the increase of cortical dominance there is a parallel development of ego sense. This is to be expected, since possibly the greatest achievement concomitant with cortical development is the acquisition of the ability to discriminate. But in order to discriminate barriers must be erected, restrictions imposed, and boundaries drawn. As discrimination becomes sharper and attention focal, and ego boundaries tighter and better defined, information processing changes from global and multidirectional to linear: 'filters' are formed to screen from focal attention 'unwanted' information. The formation of ego boundaries may be thought of as such a filter.

In filter theories, it is generally proposed that ordinary consciousness is characterized by small capacity, intolerance of ambiguity, and serial processing, typified by the operation of a 'dominant action system'. By contrast, preconsciousness has a much greater capacity, responds to multiple meanings of word stimuli and is a multichannel process.[5] In addition, it contains an enormous amount of material which normally remains on the borderline, checked by the dominant action system of ordinary waking consciousness. A great deal of this material often forms into 'semantic fields or systems' a number of which may exist in a person's unconscious and which, as noted, may be independent or even contrary to one another.[6] In preconscious hypnagogia, the LEBs effects a disengagement from, and a diffusion of, the dominant system, thus permitting the lifting of semantic inhibitions and the free and often simultaneous emergence of 'filtered-out' systems, complexes and mutli-aspected phenomena – a state of affairs that has been likened by McKellar to the listening to a number of radio programmes at once.

Two other important and related dimensions of the LEBs are vividness of imagery and sense of reality. Both of these markers feature prominently in psi, meditation, mystical, and schizophrenic experiences in all of which synesthetic and kinesthetic phenomena – which, too, are signs of the LEBs – are also to be found. Indeed, various workers have pointed out one or the other of these markers, either individually or as part of the wider complex of LEBs, as being responsible for the experience of hallucination.[7] In chapter 7 I invoked the notion of LEBs in order to explain not only hallucinations but many of the other phenomena of schizophrenia, and I offered similar explanations in regard to the creative process. What I consider basic, then, to hypnagogia and related states is this core phenomenon of the LEBs which appears in varying degrees and gives rise to a number of continua and thus to a variety of experiences.[8] Or, to put it in a way which extends my discussion of hypnagogia in Part Two, certain experiences which are variously ascribed to different 'states' are clearly seen to rise out of one core phenomenon whose occurrence in hypnagogia strips these experiences of their socially derived conceptual overstructures and points to their common basic aetiology.[9]

The LEBs ushers in a mental state whose functioning, as proposed in earlier chapters, seems to be governed by laws different from those operant in the ordinary waking state. In this connection, it is important to note, or rather remind ourselves, that hypnagogic phenomena, resulting as they do from the LEBs, tend to engage a person's cognitive processes in such a manner as to appear to him like episodes transpiring in a 'real' world. This is not to say that they are necessarily hallucinatory in the sense of the subject's believing that they are taking place in the physical world (although this, too, is not unusual in this state), but rather that they belong to a reality of their own which is just as valid and 'real' as the physical world but which answers to different criteria. As we shall see, the functioning in this reality, which one enters through the LEBs in hypnagogia, far from being 'merely imaginary' constitutes a most powerful organismic need. Indeed, it can be said that the LEBs in this state serves the important function of altering a person's structure of consciousness so as to enable him to satisfy this need.

But before embarking on the enterprise of justifying this claim, and for the sake of clarity, let us summarize the experiences that emerge from the root phenomenon of LEBs. This phenomenon, then, is characterized by regression to earlier modes of experience and cognition which is manifested in body schema alterations and dissolution, in the blurring of the distinction between ego and the external and internal environment, in synesthetic, kinesthetic and emphatic experiences, in intuitions, and in the primacy of reality sense over reality testing (and thus in vividness of imagery). It also endows the state of hypnagogia with the character of preconsciousness: that is, of sensitivity and openness both to external and internal stimuli that may lie beyond the normal reach of consciousness. It lifts the filters imposed on the mind by the consciousness and logic of the waking state. This permits the emergence of material and FsR from deeper layers of the mind, layers which are normally relegated to the unconscious domain. Not only is the person in this condition furnished with raw elements of experience that might otherwise not have reached a conscious level of mentation, but the emerging material and FsR may interact and fuse with one another to give rise to novel entities, concepts, and categories.[10]

The periodicity of hypnagogia

The function of hypnagogia, like that of everything else, is intimately related to its definition. Now, I began this book with a working definition of the state which was in fact the literal meaning of the term, and which confined the sense of hypnagogic experiences to a particular context, viz. that of leading into and coming out of sleep.[11] But the subsequent study of hypnagogic phenomena has shown that these do not always or necessarily lead to sleep. Maury himself, as we have seen, was the first to observe that attending to one's hypnagogic imagery might actually delay or prevent the onset of sleep. Other workers have noted that hypnagogic imagery may have nothing to do with sleep and drowsiness, and that it can take place while the subject is engaged in other mental activities.[12] Likewise, the phenomena of the hypnopompic end of the state occur mostly after the subject has awoken. We have also seen that visual imagery, as well as all the other phenomena of hypnagogia, are, not infrequently, experienced with open eyes. Indeed, as noted (chapter 9, 'Eidetic imagery'), in some cultures the hypnagogic period just prior to falling asleep is specifically used for voluntary recall and 'scanning' of the day's activities – an enterprise usually carried out in the darkness of a room with the imagery projected on to an imaginary screen.[13] Evidence and arguments along these lines have led to the broadening of the concept of hypnagogia and to its encompassing a number of other, qualitatively similar, states, processes and experiences. Moreover, a careful analysis of data has shown that the only necessary and sufficient conditions for the occurrence of this state are physical and psychological relaxation and an inward-turned passive-receptive attention. The satisfaction of these factors triggers off the LEBs whose features were summarized above.

Thus, the occurrence of hypnagogia does not seem to be integrally related to sleep, and their observed contiguity, although perhaps not entirely accidental, does not confine the former to the onset and end of sleep: what the latter does is to induce the type of psychophysical relaxation which promotes the occurrence of hypnagogia, and thus constitute a most obvious and strongly pronounced regular opportunity for experiencing hypnagogic episodes during the daily cycle. But there are indications suggesting that hypnagogia also occurs at other times during the day. As Tart, among others, observed, 'there are many times when we believe we are just "thinking deeply" or "concentrating" in which we momentarily slip into a hypnagogic state.'[14] Indeed, it can be argued that hypnagogia takes place periodically throughout the twenty-four-hour-day, and that it is linked to the fairly well established 'basic rest-activity cycle' (BRAC). This is 'a fundamental aspect of physiology, both functionally and in terms of the structural evolution of the CNS. The controlling mechanism has been localized to the brain stem, and in the absence of forebrain integration expresses its influence overtly as a periodic modulation of neuronal excitability.'[15] Measurements have shown that there is in fact a circadian 90- to 120-minute fluctuation in both physiological and mental activities which include stomach contractions, EEG rhythms, and dreaming or dreamlike occurrences.[16]

A basic misunderstanding about the BRAC, stemming from the confused definitions of its component terms, needs to be pointed out, however, before we continue with our discussion. The notion of the cycle originated in the now long-established alternation between REM and NREM sleep where the 'activity' component of the cycle is represented by REM sleep or dreaming (which is thought to be more active in certain respects than the waking state[17]). But in the diurnal manifestation of the cycle, daydreaming and dreamlike experiences, which are obvious parallels to nocturnal dreaming, are thought to represent the 'rest' component. It is clear that the confusion has arisen from comparing, on the one hand, REM with NREM sleep, and, on the other hand, daydreaming and fantasy with the more directed and controlled kind of wakeful mentation. In the event one is told that (REM)dreaming is 'active' and (day)dreaming 'restful'. The situation becomes interestingly problematic when we consider that full-blown dreams which are experientially indistinguishable from their REM counterparts are often experienced in the hypnagogic period prior to falling asleep, and are thus not only instances of 'restful' and invigorating dreaming but also examples of dreaming in the absence of sleep; and the same is, of course, true of the dream continuations on the hypnopompic side. This, in fact, makes hypnagogia a unique state indeed, a state which partakes both of the nature of the 'rest' periods of daily wakefulness and of the nature of the 'active' periods of nightly dreaming – while remaining primarily a 'restful' state.

Concerning the occurrence of dreaming in the absence of sleep, other workers have also proposed that dreaming as a whole has essentially nothing to do with sleep itself, but that it is merely during behavioural sleep that current techniques can measure its characteristic signs, such as EEG Stage 1, REMs, and decreased muscle activity.[18] Thus, it is argued that because of the ongoing state of wakefulness dream activity is difficult to detect although it might continue 'under conditions of reduced or impaired arousal which are ordinarily lumped within the waking category'.[19] The concept of 'arousal' and its behavioural criteria were, of course, questioned in chapters 4 and 10 where, in effect, it was argued that a dreaming person is not so much 'asleep' as imaginally involved and 'not interested' in responding directly to his physical environment[20] – although he *can* be 'awake' in his dreams. Conversely, it can be said that a wakeful person is prevented from paying full attention to his imagery by the distractions of the waking state. What all this amounts to is that, besides the strongly pronounced periods of diurnal wakefulness and nocturnal dreaming, there are also intervals of less pronounced dreaming or dreamlike experiences during wakefulness, and vice versa, and that these alternations follow the BRAC.

The REM sleep period is generally thought to be the time when most people dream, and there is strong evidence showing that when individuals are selectively deprived of it they experience what is known as 'REM rebound', that is, their successive REM periods increase, apparently in order to compensate for the loss.[21] People who do not show REM rebound seem to experience more dreams in the NREM period.[22] Also, schizophrenics who show no REM rebound are found to be actively hallucinating.[23] A similar kind of 'spillover' is found in persons under treatment with antidepressant drugs, such as imipramine. This drug, which is known to increase NREM while depriving the patient of REM sleep and the psychological phenomena associated with it, has been found to produce hypnagogic hallucinations.[24] As we have already seen (chapter 9), total sleep deprivation, which clearly prevents a person from having any sleepdreams at all, tends to produce hallucinations in what is behaviourally the waking state.

Now, in view of evidence supporting the notion that dreaming is an activity independent of sleep, and since the only kind of naturally occurring dream in the absence of sleep is the hypnagogic dream, it seems reasonable to propose that hypnagogic experiences may constitute that kind of human need and type of mentation which demonstrates itself as the REM dream during sleep and as a fantasy or hallucination during wakefulness. This view would accommodate arguments which propose that waking fantasies take the place of aborted dreams, as well as meet the suggestions of depth psychologists that sleepdreams may facilitate the gratification of wakeful fantasies: hypnagogia can, in fact, fulfil both of these functions without necessarily restricting itself to them.

The functions of hypnagogia

The view of hypnagogia as constituting the exemplification of a circadian organismic system gains more credence when seen as having a survival function. It has been suggested, for instance, that relaxation of the striate muscles and reduction of proprioceptive input, as we meet them in hypnagogia, cause a shift in the hypothalamic balance to the parasympathetic side. And it is instructive to note in this connection that such a shift is also thought to take place when small doses of tranquillizers are administered, 'resulting in calm and contentment, apparently similar to the state before falling asleep'.[25]

Relaxation, so typical of hypnagogia, has been shown to raise one's threshold of excitability and diminish the apparent unpleasantness of painful stimuli.[26] Also, the relaxation of skeletal muscles reduces the body's amount of blood lactate which is produced by the metabolism of these muscles and whose presence in high levels is thought to be instrumental in mediating anxiety.[27] Through the parasympathetic division, which as a whole has been related to the pleasurable emotions,[28] operates the trophotropic or energy-conserving system which functions as a protective mechanism against overstress, responding to attractive and peaceful stimuli and promoting the restorative processes.[29] In this regard, it will be recalled (chapter 3) that hypnagogia, and in particular the practice of observing hypnagogic imagery, is marked not only by conservation but by gaining of physical and psychical energy.[30] Other evidence concerning the function of hypnagogia comes from various studies on hypothalamic stimulation and physiological measurements which further show this process to be characterized by a general hypometabolic and parasympathetic shift marked by lowering of blood pressure and oxygen consumption, decrease in heart rate and respiration, facilitation of digestion and the disposal of body wastes, neutralization of excessive blood-sugar. Indeed, hypnagogia may constitute a protection from certain harmful effects of both wakefulness and REM sleep. In respect to the former, it is worth noting that beta EEG, which is characteristic of ordinary wakefulness, has also been associated with anxiety and various psychiatric disorders.[31] On the other hand, REM sleep has been found to exacerbate stomach ulcers and heart problems.[32]

It transpires, then, that hypnagogia has at least three functions. First, it has a hypometabolic function in that it acts as an anxiety-reducer, periodically drawing a person away from the tension-producing activities of the sympathetic system. Many reports emphasize the lack of affect and the sense of 'detached involvement' which is experienced by the hypnagogic subject. Second, it serves a trophotropic function by providing the individual with opportunities to conserve and maintain physical and psychic energy, and restore, regenerate and energize himself. Third, the psychological characteristics of hypnagogia are exactly those which might promote personal growth and development. It is obvious that an induced state of relaxation and detachment from the realities of the immediate environment would themselves have therapeutic consequences, as is appreciated by techniques for progressive relaxation and autogenic training.[33] But comparisons with creativity have shown that hypnagogia may additionally provide access to unconscious material and to novel conceptualizations. In other words, the loosening of the usual restrictions upon human cognition which is engendered by hypnagogia may enhance the solution of personal and abstract problems and promote physical and psychological health. In fact, it promotes exactly those attributes which are generally taken to be characteristic of the creative personality, namely, spontaneity, effortlessness, expressiveness, innocence, a lack of fear for the uncertain, ambiguous, or unknown, and an ability to tolerate bipolarity and to integrate opposites.

In evolutional perspective

Furthermore, seen in an evolutional perspective, hypnagogia indicates that it may have some other functions with farther-reaching implications. We saw earlier that there is considerable evidence arguing for the notion that human beings have a need to dream or engage in dreamlike or hypnagogic mentation on a periodic basis throughout the twenty-four-hour cycle. Counter-arguments have pointed out that this 'REM potential' theory is invalidated by evidence showing, first, that the REM rebound experienced by subjects deprived of REM sleep is much less than the amount of REM they were actually deprived of, and second, that those people in the normal population who were selectively deprived of REM sleep did not become obviously psychotic. However, what is ignored in these arguments is that REM-deprived subjects not only begin to have more dramatic dreams in the NREM period and hallucinations and 'microdreams' in behavioural wakefulness, but also that they experience changes of mood, and that the latter often produce or accompany subtle alterations in cognition signified by momentary diffusions of attention, 'drifting', misperceptions, and abstractions. Elsewhere, I have proposed that this 'need for dreaming' is better expressed not by saying that there are circadian REM potentials, as some workers have suggested, but rather that there are *potential periods of oneirosis* and that REM dreams form only one expression of this potential.[34] I have designated *oneirosis* as that psychological syndrome which includes dreams and dreamlike experiences such as hallucinations, quasihallucinations, psi and mystical experiences, is characterized by the person's LEBs, and, when spontaneous, is circadian following the BRAC.

Moreover, it is possible to argue that the phenomenon of oneirosis is evolutionally older than sleep and wakefulness. It has already been pointed out that hypnagogic experiences are correlated with oldbrain activities, that the mechanism which controls the BRAC has been localized to the brainstem, and that the trophotropic response is mediated by a hypothalamic nucleus through the parasympathetic nervous system. We have also seen that infants are spoken of as precorticate and that their experiences are thought to be characterized by a lack of ego boundaries. Other evidence shows that 'sleep does not exist in the newborn infant', nor in the newborn of many lower animals, and that the lives of these neonates merely alternate between dreaming and some form of wakefulness in which, as noted, there is practically no cortical participation.[35] If we accept the general idea that 'ontogeny recapitulates phylogeny', then this provides us with additional grounds for identifying oneirosis as an evolutionally old form of psychological mechanism. An important point to note here is that the term 'wakefulness' as applied to infants and precorticate animals does not carry the same sense as when used in reference to mature human beings. In this regard, an early form of wakefulness would be identified as a precorticate and phylogenetically 'primitive' kind of mentation, not dissimilar to oneirosis itself. Indeed, bearing in mind the arguments presented in the previous chapter in connection with the mentality of the oldbrain, it would be reasonable to infer that early forms of life must exist in a continuous state of oneirosis, perhaps alternating between deep oneirosis and hypnagogia. This would imply that, *inter alia*, the logic of wakefulness would be absent and that a different logic, that of empathy, fusion, a strong feeling of being inseparably part of a whole, lack of distinction between inside and outside, and lack of self-consciousness must be the qualities of such early life. Later, gradually, appears what we now call wakefulness. As noted above, this is indeed the case with human infants – their lives alternate between dreaming and waking. But, significantly, the quality of the early oneiric experiences also implies that there must be no feeling or need to fight for survival, the latter arriving on the scene with the appearance of the waking state and the direction of attention (which gradually acquires an 'active' component) to sensations, perceptions and, generally, to the external reality.[36] Thus emerge a dim self-consciousness and the need to survive as a separate entity. This is where, I believe, sleep as a separate state also makes its presence obvious: the emergence of the waking state does not obliterate the need to dream but merely overshadows it periodically; however, organismic life has begun to become individualized and the need to survive as an individual entity now utilizes the mechanism of sleep for the safe emergence of full oneiric activity. This line of argument suggests that one function of sleep must have been, and still is, to provide the conditions necessary for the occurrence of dreaming and at the same time secure the organism's safety during that most vulnerable period when its attention is withdrawn from the immediate physical surroundings. The organism's safety is secured by the induction of drowsiness which sends it looking for a safe place wherein to retire and give itself up to dream activity.

An interesting question might be raised at this juncture, namely that if physical survival were a prime concern of evolution, should we not by now have developed into non-sleeping beings adjusting the functions of sleep to some form of waking state, thus ensuring against our vulnerability during the regularly occurring abandonment in sleep? Also, if apart from providing conducive conditions for the emergence of oneiric activities, sleep has other physiological functions, e.g. physical recuperation and tissue repair, could these latter functions not be fulfilled without the person having always to abandon consciousness to the degree he does during sleep?

Now, a careful study of hypnagogia shows it to be the state most perfectly fulfilling both the functions of dreaming *and* sleep. Discussions throughout this book have shown hypnagogia to be, at times, indistinguishable physiologically and behaviourally from sleep. It has also been shown to be a dream state. Although it has often been stressed that the subject in hypnagogia is psychologically withdrawn and fascinatedly involved in imaginal activities, it has also been noted that many subjects can retain awareness of their external environment and hold conversations or have other thoughts unrelated to their concurrent hypnagogic imagery. It has been suggested that this is an ability that can be cultivated with appropriate training involving the manipulation of one's attentional state(s).[37]

Thus hypnagogia's conferring of double-consciousness on the subject, i.e. the ability to retain consciousness of one's surroundings while dreaming, is a definite evolutional advance over sleep dreaming: it enables a person to retain control over his external environment while investigating his internal terrain. An individual may, then, learn to oscillate in and out of hypnagogia to any desired degree. He may, for instance, return to the full waking state in order to attend to conditions requiring the employment of the waking mode, or move further into an oneiric state and become more deeply involved in internal imaginal activities. Of great importance here is the observation that in order to acquire double-consciousness in hypnagogia the subject must learn to relax physically, emotionally and intellectually. Significantly, these are precisely the conditions required for the induction of hypnagogia in the first place. In other words, learning to balance oneself in hypnagogia lies along evolutionally normal and natural directions. This is also borne out strongly by the advantages conferred on the subject through the very functions of hypnagogia.

But, since in hypnagogia there is the possibility of holding a 'dialogue with the unconscious' and dreaming without losing consciousness, the induction of this state should not be considered as a mere 'regression' to the evolutionally old oneiric state but perhaps more of a 'return' with the added advantages of an enriched consciousness. In this way, the oneirosis of hypnagogia, encompassing as it does numerous states of consciousness, may indeed be spoken of as a special state, and it is interesting to note in this respect that as far back as the tenth century AD a Tantric text advised the aspiring yogi that in order to acquire continuity of consciousness unaffected by sleep 'he must hold himself at the junction of all the states, i.e. in the half-sleep state, the link between waking and sleeping'.[38] Significantly, this state is designated by the exponents of the above tradition as the Fourth State, the other three being sleeping, dreaming and waking.

Indirect support for the above view comes from the fact that man needs less sleep than any other mammal which has been studied. If my theory concerning the nature of oneirosis is correct, then this could be explained by reference to man's acquisition of the ability to engage in oneiric activities during wakefulness, such as daydreaming, doing art, doing creative science, being creative in general, letting go without falling asleep (hypnagogizing). This could also explain why humans survive REM deprivation whereas animals, e.g. cats, become grossly aberrant and die.[39] The human ability, then, to relax and engage in oneiric activities may have as a result an overall reduction in the need to sleep and have sleepdreams. There is also evidence that some famous historical figures learned to take catnaps during the day, thus energizing themselves and reducing their need for nocturnal sleep considerably. Conversely, some yogis and occultists are said to be able to put their bodies to sleep for varying lengths of time while retaining consciousness and engaging in imaginal and other activities.[40] The same category of people also make use of particular times of the day and night for specific magical purposes. For example, a certain period in the afternoon is known for its 'psychic receptivity', the period after sunset is thought to be particularly conducive to invocations and 'conjuring', and so is the time around sunrise, whereas the period between 4 and 5 o'clock in the morning is believed to be very good for OBEs and lucid dreaming. It is interesting to note in this regard that many people have a tendency to doze for a while in the afternoon, and that various investigators have remarked on the relative ease with which they could conjure up imagery and recall past events, even 'unnoticed impressions' and material that 'struck the mind without its knowledge',[41] in hypnagogia as opposed to other times during the day when they were 'fully awake'. The time around 4 and 5 a.m. is generally known as the 'death hour' because of the high percentage of natural deaths occurring during this period. For the occultist, this is a time when the links between the physical body and the psyche are at their weakest, and it is therefore a naturally good time for 'astral projection'. This is also the period of the night when the great majority of people have their greatest amount of, and their most vivid, dreaming.

As the above arguments tend to suggest, there are signs indicating that conscious oneirosis, as experienced in hypnagogia during the relevant periods of the BRAC, is a likely future step in evolution. This has a number of implications which are made explicit by our existing knowledge of hypnagogia. For example, the ease with which hypnagogia is induced signifies the presence of a continuous undercurrent of oneiric activity which, as we have seen, can be contacted or brought to the fore by merely relaxing and turning one's passive-receptive attention inwards. Relaxation alone may satisfy all the physiological functions of sleep, but, coupled with a developed ability to have oneiric experiences while awake, a person would find himself in a position of not only enjoying experiences which emerge from strata governed by different logics but also of becoming capable of handling those of his mental processes which are generally thought to spring into consciousness only in sleepdreams, trances, 'paranormal' and abnormal states. This argues, in effect, that mind is not coextensive with consciousness, the latter, as already noted, often being wrongly identified with *self-consciousness*, and rational, logical, or 'cortical' thinking. But it has been shown in this book that forms of complex mentation exist outside focal consciousness and that they can be brought to the attention of the individual during hypnagogia, when, as Poincaré put it in respect to his hypnagogic-

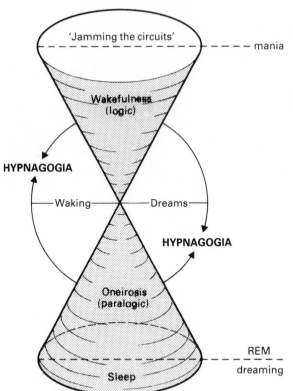

Figure 11.1 *The significance of hypnagogia. In this diagram we can see how hypnagogia can partake both of the logic of wakefulness and the paralogic of oneirosis, thus carrying into dreams and dreamlike phenomena a measure of wakefulness, and bringing to waking consciousness oneiric experiences, one important effect of such activities constituting waking dreams. (Sleep: bottom surface of lower cone. REM dreams: diameter of sleep area. Oneirosis: inside of lower cone. Wakefulness: inside of upper cone. 'Jamming the circuits': top surface of upper cone. Mania: diameter of 'jammed' area. Hypnagogia: conical surfaces.)*

creative experiences, 'one is present at his own unconscious work'.[42] The undercurrent of unconscious-nonrational mental activity which can be brought to the surface in hypnagogia reveals psychological dimensions which, as argued, need not, and perhaps should not, always be made to fit the evolutionally current mode of mentation encountered in the waking state, i.e. they should not always be interpreted according to cortical logic. As we have seen, these are more appropriately viewed from within their own frameworks without the assertive interference of the logic of ordinary wakefulness, a task ideally accomplished in hypnagogia which allows a person to be sufficiently 'awake' to register the experience while conferring on him the ability both to appreciate the phenomena in their own dimension and to see them, when applicable, as pertaining to solutions of problems or as references to his own state of mind and body. Thus, to reiterate an earlier point, this position would view hypnagogia not merely as a *regressive* state but rather as a *progressive* one in which the various aspects of consciousness and the bipolarity of rationality-nonrationality are brought to a synergetic relationship. This view I consider to be one of the main implications flowing from the evidence presented in this book, and one, moreover, which suggests a possible future line of evolution.

The multifariousness of oneiric experiences

As a prime example of oneirosis, hypnagogia reveals not only that there are many different types of dream but also that the latter are just one expression of the need to engage in oneiric experiences. As a dream state, it argues against some very important tenets of psychoanalysis. For instance, it shows, against Freud's contention,[43] that the function of dreams is not to protect sleep, but rather that the case is the other way round. Furthermore, the viewing of dreaming as an expression of oneirosis renders the Freudian 'censor' meaningless. That is, the presence of the censor implies the application of waking logic; the censor is logical – otherwise what would be the point of purportedly resorting to complex regressive mentation to evade it? The censor does not understand oneiric 'logic', it functions only in terms of waking logic. But, oneiric mentation is, as has been argued, both evolutionally older than waking cortical mentation and always present

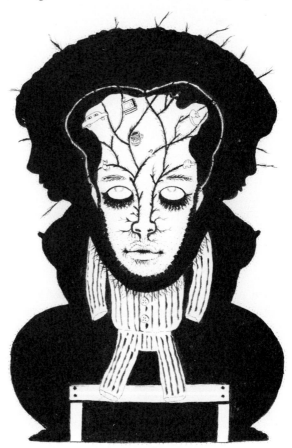

Figure 11.2 *A subject's general impression of hypnagogia. It is noteworthy that the eyes of the hypnagogist in this picture are depicted as being both shut and open, an attempt on the part of the subject to illustrate that hypnagogic phenomena are experienced in either condition and that in hypnagogia a person can 'dream' while awake or be awake while dreaming.*

unconsciously, becoming preconscious and reaching a conscious level of mentation when the original conditions of absence or diminution of cortical consciousness are fulfilled, viz. during states of oneirosis. These are natural organismic states whose type of mentation preceded the appearance of any logical censor, and whose functioning does not go anywhere near raising any question of 'evasion'.

This is not to deny, of course, that dream activity can ever be wish-fulfilling or that some dreams may constitute the mind's reaction in sleep to the experiences of the previous day, as Freudian psychoanalysis holds. However, wish-fulfilling dreams and those involved with the experiences of the previous day constitute only one or two species of the wider genus of oneirosis. As hypnagogia so clearly shows, oneiric imagery may refer to the present psychophysical state and mental preoccupations of a person (autosymbolic), contain solutions to problems, or point to future resolutions of present conflicts (anagogic).

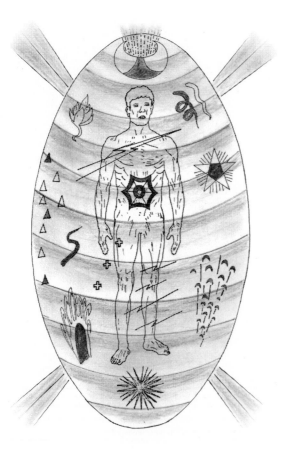

Figure 11.3 *Thought-forms (after Besant and Leadbeater 1975). According to psychic and occult traditions, thoughts, as well as emotions and sensations, are represented in a person's 'aura' by a variety of forms and colours, and can be seen by clairvoyants and people who enter a specific state of mind deliberately or accidentally. Such oneiric visions are comfortably encompassed within the experiential span of hypnagogia which, in its oneiric nature, displays a wealth of 'para' features.*

Moreover, oneiric experiences contain phenomena which are sometimes thought to arise from, or correlate with the functions and activities of, the various parts of one's body, and to carry their own very specific kind of mentation which, again, is incomprehensible to ordinary waking logic. Thus, Castaneda spoke of 'the awareness and memories and perceptions stored in our calves and thighs, in our back and shoulders and neck', and Ouspensky argued that our legs and arms and so on think, and that they 'think quite independently of and quite differently from the head'.[44] Other oneiric phenomena would include van Dusen's 'feeling-imagery' which is sometimes autosymbolic and on other occasions clearly telepathic or clairvoyant,[45] and the great variety of 'astral' thought-forms and other experiences ascribed by the mystical and occult traditions to the activities of paraphysical or extraphysical energo-cognitive centres or chakras which are 'localized' around a number of bodily areas.[46]

The multiplicity of realities

As pointed out in chapter 4 and subsequently, hypnagogia gives rise to the insight that there are many realities and that what we call wakefulness merely constitutes one of them. A further and very important realization is that the so-called waking state is hardly less a 'dream' state than the dream state experienced during sleep. In this insight, hypnagogia suggests the evolutionary possibility of a further expansion of consciousness, and poses a serious question concerning the nature of reality. The old philosophical polarization between 'real' and 'unreal' and the criteria proposed for distinguishing them are called into question, and referring to wakeful reality as a kind of 'dream' becomes no less meaningful than speaking of an oneiric experience as 'real'. The often invoked criteria for testing reality, namely, automatic reality testing, checking, and logical appraisal and learned counterweights,[47] are neither always sufficient to guarantee the 'reality' of an experience nor are they, as already noted, applicable to states of affairs beyond those pertaining to the physical world and to the state of consciousness loosely known as 'wakefulness'.

A polarized distinction is generally drawn between *reality sense* and *reality testing*. The former is nonrational, and the extent to which it is invested in external and internal phenomena is relative to the degree to which these phenomena enter the subject's ego boundaries and become 'egotized'[48] (cf. my argument for 'subjectification' of the object in chapter 3). It is intuitive, holistic, synthetic, complete in itself, has no need for confirmation, and its objects are absolute and unequivocal. By contrast, reality testing is intellectual, rational, dependent on common meanings, its objects are parts of a context whose relations must be determined, and its results are approximate and conditional.[49] Whereas the sense of reality has as its criterion the experience itself, reality testing is founded on the invariants of experience upon which the concept of reality rests. But, here's the rub: reality is far from being an absolute and invariant concept, it is elusive and variable. James, for one, replaced the notion of a single 'abstract' reality with that of many 'live' hypotheses.[50] It has been variously proposed that reality is dependent upon the conceptual correlation of systems of experience so that when we speak of something being real we are not so much referring to the object itself as stating our own logic and criteria in regard to an experience,[51] and that there are no absolute distinctions between real and unreal, thoughts and things, the world and the self.[52] It has also been pointed out that if the conceptual reference on which a current reality is based is changed, then features which were previously considered irrelevant become the 'invariants' of another type of reality; moreover, different modes of thinking contribute to the devleopment of different kinds of reality.[53]

It is peculiarly interesting that in our general scientific and philosophical thinking the physical 3D world still acts as a foundation and reference point for our viewing of other 'worlds' and 'realities'. The status we ascribe to imagery for instance, is closely related to, and dependent on, perception, and we describe images in a perceptual manner. And yet, imagery possesses characteristics which go well beyond those of physical objects and our perceptions of them. Moreover, without the ability to form and experience images we can hardly be in a position to perceive-conceive any world at all which we could consider relatively invariant and to whose features we could refer for reality testing.

An important question arising from the study of hypnagogia and related to the above discussion concerns the kind of space in which hypnagogic experiences take place. There is a general tendency to use the term 'mental space' in this connection and to refer to it as an 'analogue' (presumably of 'perceptual space'). But, as noted in the previous paragraph, images possess features which are not to be found in physical objects. On the other hand, imaginal objects, concepts, meanings, and relationships can be seen, constructed, manipulated; and consciousness can shift to any part of a person's body or move entirely outside it or become expanded to include, or merge with, other bodies and consciousness. Hypnagogic imagery can be shared, and it can be telepathic. At the same time, it does take place in some form of space, though clearly not in a space governed by the laws of the 3D physical world. Indications as to what sort of space this must be are afforded by the numerous reports cited throughout the book, and I have suggested a way of conceptualizing it by adopting the term 'electrochemical field' which I derived from the general feeling experienced in hypnagogia. It is interesting that other authors have used similar expressions in trying to explain the means of functioning in psi and related states.[54]

As noted earlier, the general impression gained in hypnagogia is that there are a number of realities; in our present discussion each of these realities would be characterized by its particular sense of space. In current scientific terms such space or spaces may be thought of as fields of energy of varying types and intensity whose concentration or diffusion, as the case may be, gives rise to a range of realities each of which constitutes a seemingly separate world populated by 'things', 'objects', etc., which are peculiar to its own level and type of energy concentration. In such a scheme, all worlds, all realities, would penetrate each other and exist in one Space, and their ultimate, as opposed to their 'emergent', nature, would be the same: sheer Energy. Of particular interest to the subject in hypnagogia is the feeling-cognition that this underlying energy is not so much physical as psychical, and that operating in any reality is a function of a person's adaptation and investment of that quantity of psychical energy which may happen to constitute at any given moment a schema, a structure, or an energy form, and which is identifiable as an 'I' or an 'individual'. This view would permit the experiencing of types of consciousness, such as encountered in hypnagogia and related states, in which the 'I' may be 'spread' or dissipated and the 'individual' may appear split, divided, or as a number of layers or psychical systems. Such experiences, as noted in chapter 7, have the unique mark of presenting a person simultaneously with phenomena of dissociation and fusion or integration, and as such they furnish the hypnagogist with a revealing and very intriguing psychical perspective of his own evolving nature.

Some practical and research implications

Before closing, it might be useful to indicate in brief certain practical and research implications arising from the present study of hypnagogia. These are clearly not exhaustive, and some have already been pointed out elsewhere in this book.

Hypnagogia may be put to therapeutic use in a variety of ways in the physical, psychosomatic, and purely psychological fields. Specifically, because of its triple dimension of relaxation (physical, emotional and intellectual) it may be used with particular stress on one or the other of these components. For instance, it may be employed to combat high blood pressure and excessive secretions in the stomach that might cause or exacerbate ulcers: people prone to such complaints may learn to take short hypnagogic 'naps' during the day. Psychosomatic illnesses, in general, may be treated in this way, and so can anxiety and neurotic and emotional disturbances. Such 'naps' can be effected either by combining hypnagogic relaxation with guided imagery and autogenic practices or by the use of the former on its own. That is, a person first learns to recognize the relaxed state of hypnagogia either by attending to it when it occurs naturally at sleep onset and on awaking or by producing it by means of biofeedback training. Then, he recalls and reproduces at will during the day the feelings of emotional calm (lack of affect), abandonment, tolerance, acceptance and lack of anxiety experienced during hypnagogia. The advantage this method has over similar ones already in clinical application is that one does not have to learn to do anything which one does not already know and practise: we all practise hypnagogia naturally and instinctively every day. All one needs to do is abstract hypnagogia from its 'traditional' presleep setting. Moreover, with some observation a person could discover his own natural BRAC and thus learn to take advantage of the 'rest' periods of this cycle by turning them into a series of deep, relaxing, and invigorating hypnagogic states. A further application of hypnagogia would be to make use of its autosuggestive element to bring about character changes and thus, again, effect somatic, psychosomatic and psychological healing.

On another level, it may be used to bring about intellectual disinhibition for purposes of creativity and psychological growth. In respect to creativity, a person may learn to 'hypnagogize' thus allowing the emergence of new FsR and their fusing into new combinations for the purpose of solving problems or arriving at inventions. On the other hand, hypnagogia opens up great vistas for internal exploration ranging from taking 'trips' for sheer enjoyment to exploring one's internal space and psychological structures in soul-searching quests. Such journeys of interior familiarization should inevitably bring about psychological integration and growth. A further psychological gain, or perhaps a corollary of the process, might be the achieving of insights into the nature of, and relationships between, the internal 'psychological' and the external 'physical' realms – these might be mystical, philosophical, or scientific insights, depending on the personality inclinations and training of a person. In regard to the close relationship between hypnagogia and psi states, a person can, again, learn to utilize the regular 'rest' periods of the BRAC, and in particular the strongly pronounced hypnagogia at either side of sleep, to test, practise, and extend the range of his own naturally occurring psi experiences. One other area in which hypnagogia might be put to practical use is that of education. Too much stress for too long has been placed on the converging 'blinkering' and 'filtering' kind of thinking. It would certainly be of psychological and intellectual benefit if school and college curricula included periods of guided hypnagogia for the express purpose of achieving the aims outlined in this paragraph, and for counteracting the restrictive effects of strictly rational, 'cortical' mentation.

Another kind of implication concerns future research directions. In this connection, all the practical applications of hypnagogia noted above could constitute experimental confirmation or disconfirmation of aspects of my arguments. For instance, hypnagogia could be experimentally tested for its conduciveness to the production of scientific and artistic insights and the facilitation of personal problem solving. In fact, this particular argument has already been partially confirmed in experimental settings.[55] A further area of research might be that of recovering long-forgotten data and remembering material that never entered the focal consciousness of the subject. Although this is an area in which hypnosis is already being applied, it would be of extra benefit to the subject if carried out in hypnagogia both because in the latter the subject need not lose consciousness of the situation and also because its practice would most likely increase his facility and access to similar material.

This closely relates to another area, namely, that of retaining consciousness and memory throughout hypnagogia and, in particular, in hypnagogic dreams. Extending the existing evidence, further research may direct itself to finding more individuals who can demonstrate that they can put themselves to sleep (physiologically, that is) but remain psychologically 'awake' while participating in a dream, i.e. be aware that they are dreaming and retain the capacity to respond to their environment. This would, then, be further strengthened by controlled experiments in which subjects are trained to enter hypnagogia and turn it into a dream state without relinquishing consciousness of the situation and awareness that they are dreaming. Important observations to be made in these experiments would be in their effects on the subjects' sleeping and dreaming habits as a whole, and in particular whether the length of their customary sleep and dreams is shortened and whether their experimental training affects the nature of their spontaneous sleeping and dreaming, i.e. whether the latter turn into conscious experiences, and whether such effects are lasting.

Hypnagogia could also be further tested for its psi-conduciveness. This can be carried out in two different ways. First, subjects can be tested for psi performance in laboratories at their normal bedtime, and second, at any time during the day or night when they feel spontaneously the 'oneiric need', e.g. when they feel like 'drowsing', 'drifting', 'daydreaming' or needing a 'rest'. In addition, inquiries could be made to ascertain the length and type of sleep and sleepdreams of 'practising' mystics, occultists, and psychics, who in a sense could be said to be actively 'hallucinating'.

*   *   *

Finally, to encapsulate the study programme of this book, my task has been fourfold. First, to carry out an analysis of the subject's cognitive-experiential state during hypnagogia. Second, to provide a comprehensive conceptual framework for the varied phenomena of hypnagogia. Third, to carry out systematic analyses of the relationships between hypnagogia and other states, processes and experiences. Fourth, to investigate the function(s) of hypnagogia and gain understanding of its evolutionary significance. Without arrogantly asserting that I have completely fulfilled this task, I hope my efforts have gone some way to achieving it, and that the book as a whole has both contributed to human knowledge and has opened up avenues for further research.

Appendix I
Methods and procedures

Historically the methods employed for collecting data in the hypnagogic area are as follows: (1) Spontaneous self-observation and questionnaire-survey, (2) systematic self-observation, (3) experimental studies.[1]

The first group comprises observations made on oneself spontaneously by two categories of people: the first category is made up of authors who, having noted the experiences in themselves, set about publishing their findings. The second category includes those people who answered questionnaires regarding their hypnagogic experiences. The strength of this method lies in its spontaneity and purity of data. However, there are at least three major disadvantages with this approach. First, hypnagogic experiences are often not recorded immediately after they have taken place, thus allowing the possibility of elaboration or forgetting. Second, reported experiences are likely to be those most striking, thus not permitting, for instance, finer analysis of modality incidence. Third, in the case of questionnaire-surveys, people may be unwilling to admit to having these experiences for fear that to do so might indicate some pathology.

The second method involves (a) the systematic recording of hypnagogic experiences occurring spontaneously (i) to oneself, and (ii) to subjects who have been instructed to make such recordings over a period of time, and (b) the systematic observation of hypnagogic experiences wherein the subject, as in (i) and (ii) above, set deliberate watch for the recording of such experiences. Of these two approaches, the former clearly retains the spontaneity and purity of events, whereas the latter may suffer from some contamination due to deliberation.

The experimental method clearly has the advantage of controlling numerous physiological and psychological variables. Drawbacks of this method may lie (a) in the appropriateness or otherwise of hypnagogic interruptions which (i) may lead to the destruction of this delicate state, and (ii) require refined distinctions between states of consciousness at first interruptions during e.g. alpha REMs, SEMs, theta waves, etc., at subsequent interruptions with similar physiological and electroencephalographic parameters, and at subsequent interruptions *after* any of the above parameters, e.g. after an alpha REM period that occurred after a specific interruption;[2] (b) in the ultimate strength and utility of converging operations, i.e. the justification for generalizing from observed correlations since personality and constitutional variables may argue against such an enterprise; and (c) in the possible qualitative differences between spontaneously occurring hypnagogic phenomena and those taking place in a sleep laboratory either 'freely' or deliberately induced (e.g. biofeedback).

Induction of hypnagogia under controlled experimental conditions has been carried out by a number of workers, and in a variety of ways. Kubie and Margolin, for instance, devised an apparatus that fed back to the subject, via an amplifier and headphones, his own respiratory rhythm thus inducing a hypnagogic state through the employment of rhythm and monotony.[3] Kubie used this method mainly for psychotherapeutic purposes. One of his subjects had vivid images of himself as a child, and 'not only was such vivid recall quite absent from his usual associations, but he was able to add certain new items'.[4] Bertini *et al.* used a mild sensory deprivation technique wherein they covered their subjects' eyes with halved ping-pong balls, thus creating a ganzfeld, and had them speak continuously against a background of white noise. Some of their subject's experiences were images and feelings from childhood.[5] Gastaut deprived his subjects of sleep and then had them read a book until they fell asleep.[6]

To the above must be added a number of biofeedback studies in which the subjects are trained to attain and maintain a hypnagogic state by monitoring their own physiological arousal. Green and his co-workers, for example, have introduced a procedure involving a number of steps and culminating in a prolonged hypnagogic state.[7] First, their subjects learn to relax, then they undergo fifteen minutes of alpha-theta feedback which is followed by thirty minutes of theta feedback alone. When they have mastered this routine the subjects are asked to report their experiences during the thirty-minute theta feedback part of the session. The presence of theta and alpha is signalled by 400-Hz and 900-Hz tones respectively. These investigators have also introduced various devices that enable subjects to practise at prolonging their hypnagogic state on their own. One such device is a finger ring with a build-in mercury switch that closes a circuit when tilted more than twenty degrees in any direction, thus setting off a door chime which prevents the subject from falling asleep.

Unlike Green's *digital* auditory feedback procedure which simply tells the subjects whether they are in or out of, say, theta, Budzynski and Stoyva have been using an *analog* system which monitors physiological and EEG correlates continuously, thus informing the subjects how close they are to the desired state.[8] These workers use a 'biofeedback polygraph', developed by Budzynski himself, which records EEG (mainly alpha and theta), EMG from the frontalis muscles, and six other physiological parameters. The phenomena observed in these and similar studies are identical to those reported in the spontaneously occurring hypnagogia. Biofeedback-induced hypnagogia has found a number of applications, including clinical treatment, the encouragement of creativity, and sleep learning.[9]

Two other methods of inducing hypnagogia are deliberate increase of carbon dioxide in the blood by means of shallow breathing, and autohypnosis. The first of these is partly discussed in chapter 10, and in a similar context is also known to have been used by Swedenborg whose hypnagogia was closely connected with meditative practices.[10] Similarly, instructions for shallow breathing relating to the production of a normalized presleep state as a therapeutic procedure against insomnia yield, naturally, a hypnagogic state.[11] Again, autohypnosis, as with classical 'heterohypnosis' (see chapter 9), directed to aims other than the induction of hypnagogia, tends to produce hypnagogic phenomena, as in the case of the subject who experienced hypnagogic imagery when he resorted to self-hypnosis for the purpose of helping himself out of a breakdown.[12]

Other methods, outside experimental settings, and in the comfort of one's home, can also be used for the induction, prolongation and utilization of hypnagogia, and most of these are mentioned at various points in the book (e.g. chapters 3, 4, 6 and 8).

A fairly easy method, and one which inspired Green *et al.* to invent the mercury ring mentioned above, is given by Muldoon and Carrington who suggest that the subject should lie in bed, as in going to sleep, but keep his arm in a vertical position resting on the elbow; this would allow him to move into a hypnagogic state but prevent him from going to sleep because the decreased tonus in the muscles of the arm would cause the latter to fall and thus awaken him.[13] In chapter 8 we can see Edison and Dali employing a similar procedure to arrive at new ideas.

By far the easiest method of inducing hypnagogia outside a laboratory is simply by lying down or sitting in a chair comfortably, closing one's eyes, and employing progressive relaxation and psychological withdrawal; concentrating relaxedly on a mental image speeds up the process. Soon, images begin to rise spontaneously. I have employed this method in the past (see chapter 3 and Appendix III) with success and I am using it again in my current classes. New findings will hopefully appear in a later publication.

With the obvious exception of de Manacéine's early investigations, the only other authors who drew attention to the prolongation of the hypnopompic state are Ouspensky and various occultists.[14] Ouspensky (see chapter 4) used this state to achieve conscious dreaming while the occultists (see chapter 6) take advantage of the light paralysis experienced in it to 'project' out of their bodies. In all cases the person remains in, or re-enters, a dream or semidream state.

There are two main procedures of recording the occurrence of hypnagogic phenomena: (a) *after* the experiences have taken place and, (b) *during* the experiences. The first procedure is the most commonly employed and encompasses all three major methods of investigation outlined in this Appendix. The second has been employed mainly by McKellar who trained subjects to report their experiences as they occurred, and had them taperecorded in the process, by Elmer Green and his collaborators, and by myself as reported in chapter 3 and Appendix III. Although some biofeedback material appears to have been recorded by means of the second procedure this is not entirely clear of all the cases as most investigators using biofeedback speak of their subjects' *oscillating* in and out of hypnagogia. Nonetheless, many biofeedback verbal reports are clearly made while the subjects are still in hypnagogia although perhaps in a 'lighter' stage.

An important question that has been raised concerning induction procedures is that of the possible confounding of the criteria of antecedent conditions that may distinguish hypnagogia from adjacent states which share most or all of the hypnagogic features. Specifically, the hypnagogic induction procedures referred to above may be seen to be methods of inducing states other than hypnagogia. However, as I argue throughout this book, and in particular in Parts Two and Three, the presence of the same antecedent, and sometimes of the same consequent, conditions in both hypnagogia and other states and mental processes does not so much confound the former with any of the latter as much as point out strong relationships existing between hypnagogia and these other states, processes, phenomena or experiences.

Appendix II
Physiological correlates

The subjective experiences of hypnagogia have been related by various investigators to physiological and EEG activities. This is a specific application of the method of combining physiological measures and verbal reports to monitor psychological states; other areas that have received this attention more extensively include sleep, dreaming, meditation, and psi. Since hypnagogia is a state generally ascribed a position immediately preceding and following sleep (or even constituting part of sleep itself), I shall begin the examination of its physiological correlates with a brief introduction of the physiology and electroencephalography of sleep as a whole.

Following Berger's classic employment of non-polarizable electrodes to measure brain electric potentials, it has become a tradition in sleep research to use EEG recordings as indicators of the phases of sleep.[1] In their pioneering work Loomis et al. and Davis et al.[2] pointed out five successive stages of sleep which they designated with the letters A, B, C, D, E thus: A – alpha with interruptions; B – low voltage with alpha loss; C – appearance of 14 cps spindles and random delta; D – higher voltage of spindles and delta, with the latter becoming longer; E – increase of delta in voltage and wavelength with spindles becoming inconspicuous.

Dement and Kleitman[3] simplified the above categorization by suggesting four stages: *Stage 1* (descending), modified alpha moving to theta (7 cps), corresponding to late A and B in the Loomis et al. study; *Stage 2*, lower voltage activity (3-6 cps) with 14 cps spindles, as in C above; *Stage 3*, delta (4 cps) with spindling; *Stage 4*, slower delta without spindling, corresponding to D and E. This pattern runs for about 90 minutes. The re-emergence of a modified stage 1 (ascending) has been linked with dreaming activity (dreaming appears also in the other stages but there it is generally found to be less dramatic and more thought-like). This 90-minute cycle (it ranges from 70 to 110 minutes) is repeated throughout the night, but, whereas at the beginning stages 3 and 4 are predominant, as the night progresses more time is spent in ascending stage 1 (up to an hour) and the other stages are represented mainly by stage 2. K-complexes, a term coined by the Loomis et al. group to denote a short, sharp, diphasic change of potential (a negative wave followed by a positive one) which is superimposed on the background electrical activity of B and C (stages 2 and 3), often appear as a response to auditory stimuli or internal autonomic events such as gastrointestinal contractions.[4] Both, spindles and K-complexes, are linked with stages 2 and 3 of sleep.

Sleep is generally thought to consist of two types. The first, known variously as S (slow-wave), Q (quiet), or NREM (non-rapid eye movement) comprises stages 2, 3 and 4 (and, often, descending stage 1). The second, A (active) or D (deep, desynchronized, dreaming) is represented solely by re-emerging or ascending stage 1. The latter is characterized by two groups of features: (a) phasic features, e.g. REMs (rapid eye movements), twitches, PIP (phasic integrated potential), brief contractions of the middle ear, and other, major, movements of the body, and (b) tonic (longer-lasting) features such as muscle relaxation, penile erection or vaginal moistening. Usually the onset of D or REM sleep is heralded by a burst of theta waves whose intermittent presence throughout this stage, indeed, constitutes a main feature of the period. The theta waves of ascending stage 1 have a sawtooth appearance and frequently occur just before or during a REM.[5]

Several writers have pointed out a number of physiological differences between what have come to be called REM and NREM types of sleep.[6] These include the presence in REM sleep of hippocampal rhythmic theta activity, twitches and variability in blood pressure, heart rate and respiration. By contrast, in NREM sleep hippocampal electrical activity is variable, movements are few and gross, respiration is deep and regular, blood pressure is below waking-level, and heart rate slow and regular.

Davis *et al.* were the first to note correlations between hypnagogic phenomena and sleep onset EEG rhythms.[7] They extended the Loomis *et al.* study by concentrating on subdivisions between A and B stages. They pointed out five electrophysiological subdivisions, with the fifth possibly belonging to 'real sleep' (or C stage in the Loomis *et al.* classification). Davis *et al.* remarked that subjects losing the EEG alpha rhythm during sleep onset reported dreamlike visions, phantasies and feelings. Similar observations were made by Gastaut who divided the hypnagogic state into stage '1a1' (alpha rhythm), '1a2' (fragmented alpha), and '1b' (appearance of theta).[8] Dement and Kleitman's subjects, also, reported dreamlike reveries as they were interrupted in descending stage one sleep.

The physiological changes occurring during the passage from wakefulness to sleep can be summarized as follows: there is a fall in muscle tonus and a decrease in heart rate and respiration; the insensible perspiration, as measured by the rate of weight loss, increases paralleling a fall in rectal temperature; the electrical conductivity of the skin decreases; cortical activity shifts from low amplitude fast frequencies to high amplitude slow ones. There is a general shift to hypometabolic parasympathetic activity.[9]

In respect to respiration, Bülow found that in the hypnagogic state 'when the alpha activity in the EEG disappeared and theta waves developed, ventilation decreased'; similarly, the sporadic reappearance of alpha correlated with increased ventilation.[10] Timmons *et al.* reported that

> Respiratory movements of the abdomen and chest of human Ss were found to undergo progressive changes with loss of wakefulness. Abdominal-dominant breathing was associated with relaxed wakefulness, abdominal-thoracic equality with drowsiness, and thoracic-dominant breathing with sleep onset. During drowsiness, variations in amplitude of abdominal movements were closely related to vacillation between alpha and theta activity in the EEG.[11]

Drowsiness, being a condition preceding sleep, is characterized by slow eye movements (SEMs) which, as Liberson and Liberson point out, 'seem to be associated with a process preceding or initiating drowsiness and subsiding as soon as drowsiness reaches a certain level, 20 or more sec after its onset';[12] also irregularity of respiration during the first 20 sec of drowsiness is followed by recovery of this regularity. The state of drowsiness is here defined as 'the onset of occipital alpha-blocking'.

The Libersons noted that 'there is a delay of several seconds for most subjects in subjective recognition of initial drowsiness'. For instance, 'only about 40% have a subjective recognition of drowsiness 10 sec after and about 50% recognise it 20 sec after the onset of alpha-blocking reaction.' An earlier study had already pointed to the possibility that 'muscle tonus diminishes very soon after the alpha pattern is lost, but the level of consciousness is lowered more slowly'.[13] Drowsiness, the Libersons noted, is a progressive affair, the subject slipping in and out of this state, staying in it for no more than 10 sec, and gradually remaining in it for increasingly longer periods as drowsiness becomes 'deeper'. It has also been noted that 'the incidence of slow eye movements occurring a certain time before the onset of EEG drowsiness increases as the number of repeated drowsy periods increases', covering periods of interrupted EEG pattern of drowsiness thus suggesting 'the presence of a residual state of drowsiness even though the electroencephalogram shows an alert pattern'. Conversely, 'when drowsy patterns start to invade the resting electroencephalogram . . . the subject may continue to be subjectively alert.' This subjective component of alertness was graded by the Libersons on a four-category scale ranging from reports of 'here and now' characterized by the subject's concern about the experiment to reports of 'more vague types of thinking' such as 'I was floating, drifting, dreaming'. Reports on the 'here and now' show a high incidence (53 per cent) during alpha activity, declining rapidly during the first 10 sec after alpha-blocking and practically disappearing from the subjects' reports 15 sec after the onset of drowsiness.

Electroencephalographically the progression is from occipital alpha activity to alpha-blocking accompanied by a more anterior low amplitude (4-7 cps) theta activity that increases in amplitude leading to relatively high voltage vertex waves. As drowsiness deepens, theta rhythm and vertex waves predominate. The appearance of 'spindles' (12-14 cps) signals the onset of descending stage 2 of sleep. The subjective mental changes occurring through the appearance of these EEG patterns may, therefore, be related to them thus showing a progression from 'here and now' reports (alpha activity) to 'vague and general thinking' (theta rhythm and vertex waves), the latter reports correlating with continuous patterns of drowsiness lasting for periods longer than 10 sec which, as a rule, do not occur for such lengths of time at the early stages of drowsiness.[14]

The Libersons' electroencephalographic progression was a confirmation of the earlier results of Foulkes and Vogel who found an increase in drowsiness with successive EEG/EOG stages.[15] In their study Foulkes and Vogel took reports from nine young adult subjects from four categories of awakening 'reflecting characteristic sequential changes in EEG and EOG variables', namely, alpha EEG (continuous, with a few bursts of REM), alpha EEG (discontinuous, with SEMs), descending stage 1 EEG (mostly with SEMs), descending stage 2 EEG (usually with SEMs). The results showed a steady decline in their subjects volitional control and awareness of immediate environment and a steady rise in the frequency of hallucinatory experiences, the latter being defined by a 'loss of the sense that one's experience is purely mental rather than actually transpiring out in the "real" world'. This increase in hallucinatory experience was found to be concomitant with a decline of affect.

In regard to the hypnopompic state, an early investigation showed that the pulse during this state had 'an evident tendency to become lower' and irregular. Respiration, too, was found to be 'very irregular, showing acceleration and pauses'. The faces of half-awakened persons, it was further noted, 'had always a somewhat tumified look', especially around the eyelids.[16] Later studies showed a definite acceleration of heart rate as the subjects awake in the morning, and an increase in the magnitude of the muscle potentials, tonic, and respiratory activities.[17] As with the hypnagogic end, the hypnopompic is also characterized by the presence of 6-7 cps theta waves.[18] Subjects are generally found to perform worse in the hypnopompic than during the hypnagogic period.[19]

Appendix III
Some incidental observations on psi and meditation

This Appendix is essentially an explanatory note concerning certain incidental observations I made in respect of the nature of hypnagogia and its relationship to psi and meditation, while I was investigating and experimenting with techniques relating to changes of consciousness. The relevant observations to be reported below form part of three wider collections of data gathered by means of three different methods. The first collection comprises interviews with psychics, the second consists of observations made at 'psychic development circles', and the third is made up of observations of, and reports from, two groups of people I instructed in progressive relaxation and self-reporting of subjective phenomena. It must be clearly pointed out at the outset that in many of these cases it was not specifically my intention at the time of collecting the data to investigate their occurrence in relation to hypnagogic phenomenology. Indeed, a great deal of data had been gathered before I began my research into hypnagogia.

In respect to my interviews with psychics, these have been carried out over a period of several years: they range from informal talks to more formalized taperecorded interviews guided by a preset questionnaire, and include responses of established mediums as well as of budding psychics. My purpose at the time was to gather information on the *modus operandi* of individuals said to be functioning in paranormal states of consciousness. When, however, I came eventually to relate this information to the phenomenology of hypnagogia I found many striking similarities. These are very much the same as those discussed in chapter 6.

Invariably, the psychics I spoke to referred to their psi mental states as a 'switching off' of the analytic mind and a switching into a different channel or reality. As a rule they experience their physical surroundings as fading into the background, while the 'psychic' world becomes prominent. In the words of Ivy Northage:

> I switch off entirely. I forget 'me' entirely. I cease to exist. I'm not there, only as a point of relaying. Physically I, as me, cease to exist. Psychologically too, I am not concerned with myself. . . . I can see people in the audience whom I know quite well, and fail to recognise them. I sort of lose that [the physical] into this [the psychic], you see. They are not exactly invisible but they don't register. . . . Everything physical, you see, becomes secondary.[1]

The medium appears to be functioning primarily in a psychic reality wherein he/she tends to lose body-schema identification, but not sensation. As another medium, Joan McCleod, put it, 'You lose consciousness of your body but your senses become sharper.'[2] McCleod, like all the other psychics I spoke to, stressed the brightness of colours in her psi imagery and the sense of reality experienced in a psi state. Likewise, she pointed out that in such states she becomes highly absorbed and yet detached, she enters what I would call a state of *de-egotization* wherein the current psychic activity presents itself with a force of realness and engages her interest, but her interest, although deep, is clearly impersonal. In the case of trance this absorbed-yet-detached attitude is particularly pronounced. Northage likened the state of trance to 'having gas at the dentist's: "I don't think you are wholly conscious with gas. You know what's going on, but you are not taking any part in it at all."' Northage further reported that when having an OBE she experiences 'images' and 'convictions' which are related to herself, as opposed to those appearing during a demonstration, which are always related to other people. She recounted to me three hypnopompic experiences which she clearly considered paranormal, one of which seems to constitute a form of 'reversed' autosymbolism, that is, an experience containing a verbal explanation of its contents: 'I woke up feeling very refreshed and I was thinking to myself, "Oh, what a lovely night I've had", and was sort of slipping back into consciousness when a man's voice said: "Death is as simple as that" – as if he were answering and explaining the lovely state I was in.'

In regard to the phenomena reported in 'development circles', these are practically impossible to distinguish from the phenomena of hypnagogia. As in the case of my interviews with psychics, my attending numerous 'development circles' was connected with my interest in gaining information – and, in this case, first-hand experience – of the way one operates in a psi state. A psychic 'development circle' is made up of a group of people – ranging in number from half a dozen to two dozen – meeting regularly – usually once a week – under the leadership of a psychic, who instructs them on how to enter and function in a psi state. The instructions and exercises vary from one circle to another and from one leader to the next. Basically, however, the members of the group are asked to sit relaxedly in a darkened room and 'let go' or 'open up'. Although one is not asked specifically to close one's eyes, this is nearly always done as a means of aiding psychophysical withdrawal. Thus, in the early stages of psychic development, a person sits comfortably in a darkened room, lets go of his hold on the surrounding reality, turns inwards, and waits. In spiritualist 'development circles' the 'waiting' is specifically characterized as the period during which the developing psychic is gradually making contact with the 'spirit world', that is, by relaxing and 'letting go' (becoming passive-receptive) he places himself in a psychological state conducive to effecting communication with entities believed to inhabit a spiritual world. Thus phenomena experienced in this state are often interpreted as 'messages' from spirits.

Now, as clearly pointed out in the main body of the book, if a person sits comfortably in a darkened room, closes his eyes and lets go, the chances are he will fall asleep. This is particularly the case when he is instructed to 'blank' his mind, that is, to stop thinking, analyzing, worrying, or concerning himself with everyday 'claptrap'. In such circumstances all the known hypnagogic phenomena are abundantly demonstrated. My notes contain reports aplenty of body-schema alterations (shrinking, expanding, floating, numbness, facial distortion), total body-schema loss, sensations of cold and heat, the hearing of names, isolated words, apparently irrelevant sentences, intuitions, solutions to one's own or someone else's problems. The visions include the seeing of isolated symbolic figures and signs, seascapes, landscapes, faces, fragmented or complete scenes – indeed practically all the hypnagogic sensorimotor phenomena discussed in the main body of the book. However, given the psychological set of developing psychics and the setting in which such experiences transpire, the latter are invariably interpreted either as signs that the psychic is making progress in his development or as messages from spirit communicators. This is not to deny that meaningful and significant psi results are never obtained in these circumstances, but merely to note the occurrence of certain phenomena irrespective of set and setting.

In parallel with my research above I began holding my own two-hour weekly evening group meetings which were not spiritualistic in character and included meditation and visualization exercises. They were held at various Adult Education Institutes and Colleges in London and were designed to experiment with techniques of consciousness expansion and introspection. Although these classes ran for six academic years – with mostly different people every year – data have been collected methodically from only two thirty-week academic periods with two different groups of twenty persons each.

In these meetings all exercises and experiments were invariably preceded by psychophysical relaxation. This was carried out in semi-darkness with the members of the group sitting relaxedly on chairs or lying on the floor and listening to my instructions on relaxation delivered against a background of specially composed music. The relaxation period was then followed by either *opening-up* or *concentrative meditation*. Opening-up meditation consists basically of relaxing, letting go, and attending diffusedly to one's external or internal space. Concentrative meditation goes a step further than the previous kind in that attention is concentrated (in the diffused-absorbed manner discussed in this book) on a particular external object, sensation, or mental image. Traditionally, the opening-up meditation is employed either as a 'blanking' technique for its own sake, i.e. as a means of allowing one's inner, intuitive nature to come to the fore, or as a preparation to the exercise of concentrative meditation. In my classes these two forms of meditation were practised separately.

The instructions in respect to the opening-up meditation were to the effect of relaxing, letting go of one's concerns, ceasing to analyse, turning inwards, and becoming effortlessly aware of any subjective psychophysical occurrences, e.g. physical sensations, images, quality of thought, and intuitions. It can be readily seen that these instructions, if followed diligently, would lead into a state identical to that aimed at in 'development circles', the only characteristic distinguishing the two states being that of set and setting. Moreover, it can also be seen that psychophysical relaxation (muscular, emotional, and intellectual), letting go, turning inwards (psychologically withdrawing), are symptoms of spontaneously occurring hypnagogia – small wonder that I heard snoring on occasion, both in my own classes and in 'development circles'! Subjective phenomena reported as occurring in this type of meditation fell well within the phenomenological span of hypnagogia and, allowing for the absence of a spiritualist setting, they were indistinguishable from those reported in 'development circles'.

In respect to concentrative meditation, this took the form of concentrating one's non-analytic attention either on a sensation (e.g. listening to the meditation music as if the latter were being played in the centre of one's head) or a mental image (visual, auditory, kinesthetic, tactile, or olfactory). Some relevant observations reported in this area include the following: on centring the hearing of music in one's head (internalizing, subjectifying), the sense of hearing became extremely – almost painfully – acute; the musical notes were felt somatically, as if the music were literally played in one's head or body. Concentrating on a mental image, e.g. an open red rose, often gave rise to visually related images, e.g. a rosebud, a withered rose, or a row of flowering plants on a windowsill. This did not seem to be the result of mental association but either grew out of the initial visualization, i.e. the open red rose, as though organically, or sprang forth directly and in vivid form from the very attempt to visualize an open red rose. Concentrative meditation facilitated introspection in two ways. First, it enhanced a person's familiarization with his internal space, and second, it enhanced his ability to control and manipulate not only his mental imagery but also his attentional state itself. These benefits reflected, within a few weeks of practice, in the reports of experiences during opening-up meditation. That is, opening-up meditation became richer in imagery (or, rather, one became aware of more imagery in this state), and one's ability at attaining and prolonging the state was enhanced.

Now, given the conditions and phenomenology of the opening-up meditation, the only criteria for distinguishing it from the spontaneously occurring hypnagogia are its deliberate induction and its prevention from leading to sleep – but these criteria, as argued in the main body of the book, cannot be invoked to distinguish the *experimentally induced hypnagogia* from a number of adjacent states, including meditation. Thus, in the exercises carried out in these classes, the opening-up meditation turned out to be a sustained hypnagogia in which a subject learned to balance himself between waking and sleeping and, in time, acquired the ability to report his experiences while the latter were in progress. This simultaneous reporting proved to have two advantages over the earlier routine of reporting *after* the experience had taken place, that is, at the conclusion of the exercise. First, it secured against forgetting the experiences themselves which was observed to be sometimes the case with the earlier routine, due mainly to the fascination and absorption experienced by subjects that prevented them from registering and remembering the experiences. Second, it secured against loss of awareness of surroundings and thus prevented a subject from falling asleep. Although this form of hypnagogic introspection initially led to a decrease in reported imagery frequency and vividness, as some subjects gradually became proficient in retaining double-consciousness (always remaining receptive and favouring the imaginal as opposed to the physical), their imaginal activities increased in amount, frequency and vividness, their relaxation deepened, and their ability to register hypnagogic phenomena was enhanced. Also noteworthy were the observations that the greater the amount and the more vivid the experiences one had, the more refreshed and invigorated one felt and the deeper one's relaxation. Thus, psychophysical relaxation was found to be not only a precondition for the occurrence of hypnagogia but also to be directly affected by the latter in a positive way, i.e. hypnagogic experiences deepened one's relaxation. These observations bear strongly on my arguments in respect to the hypometabolic or anabolic function of hypnagogia and the employment of this state as a means of immediate interpretation of 'dream' imagery while the subject retains awareness of his physical surroundings.

Finally, as with other reports cited in this book, some members of these groups had hypnagogic experiences which clearly constituted meaningful references to unknown, and unknowable by means of inference, aspects of the lives of other people. For instance, in the light of my experience with the phenomena of 'development circles' I asked my subjects in opening-up meditation to pose certain mental questions to themselves while experiencing hypnagogic imagery: they were to ask questions such as 'What does this image mean?', 'Who is it for?'. Conversely they were asked to concentrate diffusedly on one or other member of the group while drifting into hypnagogia. Some results were striking examples of clairvoyance and telepathy. This at least raises the question as to whether some seemingly 'irrelevant' hypnagogic images might not be meaningful phenomena belonging to another mind.

Notes and references

1 Introduction

1 Maury (1848; see also 1853, 1857, 1878).
2 Myers (1903).
3 Ellis (1897); McKellar (1979b) pointed out that if a distinction is to be made between them this must be made on the grounds that the former phenomena tend to 'form themselves' as one watches, while the latter variety, appearing as they do in the morning and being clear of perceptual experiences, are the sort one tends to 'come upon' already formed.
4 Aristotle (1931, 462a, 5-10).
5 Iamblichus (1895, pp. 115-17).
6 Leaning (1925a).
7 Hobbes (1651, part 1, ch. 2).
8 Cardano (1643, p. 160).
9 Ellis (1911, p. 30).
10 E.g. Swedenborg (1928-48, 1977); see also van Dusen (1972, 1975).
11 Poe (1949, p. 543).
12 Mitchell (1890).
13 Müller (1826, 1848).
14 Baillarger (1846).
15 Schacter (1976), Mavromatis and Richardson (1984).
16 McKellar and Simpson (1954).
17 Owens (1963).
18 Buck and Geers (1967).
19 McKellar (1972).
20 Richardson et al. (1981).
21 Richardson (1983).
22 McKellar (1972, p. 43).
23 Ibid.; see also Leroy (1933, pp. xiii-xiv) and earlier quotation from Aristotle.
24 Galton (1883), McKellar (1957), Oswald (1962), Holt (1964).
25 Foulkes (1971).
26 De Manacéine (1897).
27 Partridge (1898).
28 E.g. Leaning (1925a), Oswald (1962).
29 McKellar (1975).
30 See e.g. Burdach (1839), Herschel: cited by Leaning (1925a), Poe (1949), Collard (1953).
31 E.g. Baillarger (1846), Maury (1848, 1878), Hyslop (1908), Walsh (1920), Walter (1960), Oswald (1962); see also Leaning (1925a).
32 Walsh (1920), Critchley (1955), Oswald (1962).
33 Cited by Leaning (1925a).
34 Op.cit., p. 239.
35 See e.g. Foulkes and Vogel (1965), Foulkes et al. (1966), Vogel et al. (1969), Budzynski (1972, 1977), van Dusen (1972), Richardson (1984).
36 Op.cit., p. 123.
37 See e.g. Baillarger (1846), Maury (1848), Ellis (1897).
38 Op.cit., pp. 195-212.
39 Ouspensky (1978).
40 McKellar (1957).
41 E.g. Taine (1883), Titchener (1909), Hollingworth (1911); Leaning (1925a) also reported cases to the same effect.
42 Holt (1972).
43 Starker (1974).
44 Hypnagogic imagery per se has been relegated to various positions on imagery classification systems: see e.g. McKellar (1957), Richardson (1969), Horowitz (1978).
45 Vihvelin (1948).
46 Ibid.
47 Leroy (1933), Sartre (1978).

48 Arnold-Forster (1921).
49 Davis et al. (1938).
50 Liberson and Liberson (1966).
51 Gastaut (1969).
52 Stoyva (1973).
53 Vogel et al. (1969).
54 Oliver (1975, pp. 1-2); other workers who have pointed to the hypnagogic state as consisting of successive stages include Angyal (1927, 1930), Mayer-Gross (1929), Bizette (1931), Miyagi (1937), Critchley (1954, 1955), Linschoten (1956), Laird and Laird (1959).

2 Somatosensory phenomena

1 Collard (1953).
2 Gurney et al. (1886, p. 474).
3 See respectively: Saint-Denys (1982, p. 474), Gurney et al. (1886, pp. 390, 473), Letter-box of John O'London's Weekly (22 November 1930, p. 309).
4 See e.g. Müller (1826), Galton (1881, 1883), Greenwood (1882), Cane (1889), James (1890), Ladd (1892); one of the earliest reports is that of Vairo, Bishop of Pozzuolo (De Fascino, book 3, p. 112) in which he speaks of seeing a succession of colours, 'blue, green, red, white, etc. . . . ', while lying in bed and with the covers drawn over his head.
5 Galton (1881); see also Cane (1889).
6 'excitations of optic neurons arising from within the retina without benefit of light from the external world': Horowitz (1978, p. 25).
7 James (1890, p. 46).
8 McKellar (1957, p. 83); Holt (1972) found no correlation between awareness of entoptic phenomena and the occurrence of hypnagogic imagery, although this piece of evidence does not necessarily argue against the possibility that in most instances, as Galton (1883) and Ladd (1892) contended, hypnagogic images form themselves too quickly for the relaxing consciousness to be able to observe their formation.
9 Saint-Denys (1982, p. 136).
10 Greenwood (1882); see also Alexander (1909).
11 Leaning (1925a).
12 Light (24 February 1923, p. 117).
13 Gurney et al. (1886, p. 474, note 1).
14 'Faces in the dark', St. James's Gazette (15 February 1882, pp. 5-6).
15 Letter-box of John O'London's Weekly (6 December 1930, p. 427).
16 Letter-box of John O'London's Weekly (22 November 1930, p. 309).
17 This particular series of experiments was carried out at the end of lectures on hypnagogia, and the participants were mostly students. The extracts used here are from reports of student subjects at Bedford College (London) and Middlesex Polytechnic.
18 Ouspensky (1978, p. 282).
19 Maury, Le Sommeil et Les Rêves, Paris Didier et Cie (1861, pp. 133-4).
20 See e.g. Leroy (1933).
21 See also McKellar (1957, 1979a), McKellar and Simpson (1954), Lukianowicz (1959).
22 Dudley (1979, p. 86).
23 See e.g. Maury (1853, 1878), Gurney et al. (1886), Ladd (1892), McKellar (1975), Green and Green (1978).
24 J. of the Soc. for Psychical Research (hereafter J.SPR), (1899, vol.9, p. 121).
25 McKellar (1959).
26 McKellar (1979b, p. 101).
27 See James (1890) and Müller (1848) respectively.
28 McKellar (1972).
29 Taine (1883).
30 Leroy (1933, p. 86).
31 Ibid., p. 58.
32 Müller (1826, p. 20).
33 Ladd (1892).
34 Myers (1957).
35 J.SPR. (July 1898, pp. 269-70).
36 Oliver (1975, pp. 116-17).
37 Quoted by Leaning, op. cit.
38 Greenwood (1894).
39 Alexander (1909).
40 Ardis and McKellar (1956).
41 Freud (1953).
42 Quoted by Leaning, op. cit.
43 McKellar and Simpson (1954); see also Maury (1878), Hollingworth (1911).
44 Ardis and McKellar (1956); also Tournay (1941).
45 See e.g. Silberer (1965), Vihvelin (1948), Ardis and McKellar (1956).
46 Hollingworth (1911).
47 E.g. Maury (1878), Alexander (1909),

Leaning (1925a), Ardis and McKellar (1956), Oliver (1975).

48 See e.g. McNish (1830), Maury (1848, 1878), Alexander (1909), Rouquès (1946), Collard (1953), McKellar and Simpson (1954), Myers (1957), Green *et al.* (1970).

49 See e.g. Müller: cited by Leroy (1933); *St. James's Gazette* (15 February 1882, p. 5), Gurney *et al.* (1886, p. 474), Alexander (1909), Leaning (1925a), Leroy (1933), Rawcliffe (1952), Collard (1953), McKellar (1972), McKellar and Simpson (1954), Myers (1957).

50 Both reports are from McKeller (1979a, pp. 190-1).

51 Fox (1962, pp. 19-21).

52 Mitchell (1890), Critchley (1955).

53 See e.g. Maury (1848), McKellar (1957), Oswald (1962).

54 Kraepelin (1906), Froeschels (1946), Oswald (1962), van Dusen (1975) respectively.

55 See Note 19.

56 Hull (1962).

57 Alexander (1909), Schjelderup-Ebbe (1923), Archer (1935) respectively; Oswald (1962) mentions a collection of witty 'dream tags' that appeared in the *New Statesman* (1960, vol. 59, p. 930 and vol. 60, p. 42).

58 Archer (1935).

59 Maury (1878, p. 96).

60 Arnold-Forster (1921).

61 See e.g. Swedenborg (1977), van Dusen (1972), Hoche (1926), Oswald (1962).

62 Froeschels (1946).

63 Op. cit., p. 8.

64 McKellar (1975, 1979b).

65 Foulkes and Vogel (1965).

66 Maury (1878, p. 98), Leaning (1925a); see also Mitchell (1890).

67 See e.g. Galton (1883), Greenwood (1894), McKellar (1957), Dudley (1979).

68 Mitchell (1890).

69 Roger (1931).

70 Oswald (1962, p. 89).

71 Leaning (1925a), Critchley (1955), McKellar (1957), Lukianowicz (1959), Oswald (1962, p. 89), James (1975, p. 74).

72 McKellar (1979b), Sartre (1978), Isakower (1938).

73 Sartre (1978, pp. 45-6).

74 See e.g. McNish (1830), Roger (1931), McGlade (1942), Critchley (1955), Oswald (1959b, 1962).

75 Oswald (1962); see also de Lizi (1932), Pintus and Falqui (1934).

76 Oswald (1962, p. 90).

77 Harriman (1939), Oswald (1962).

78 Harriman (1939), McKellar (1957).

79 McKellar (1979b, p. 104). On the other hand, Foulkes and Vogel (1965) encountered only 1 per cent of falling experiences in their subjects' reports and an extremely low incidence of other bodily distortion experiences. These writers argue that the high incidence reported by other investigators is probably due to the fact that these experiences are startling and tend to arouse the subject 'whereas other, more frequent hypnagogic experiences go unnoticed because they are less unusual'. However, the Foulkes and Vogel study may suffer from at least two methodological inadequacies. First, there was unequal sex representation (eight males, one female) in the sampling. In fact, the one and only female in the sample contributed some of the most exceptional material (see also Vogel *et al.* 1966); it is possible, for instance, that females are more susceptible to falling experiences than males, and this was prevented from being demonstrated because of the unequal representation. Second, it is not known yet how hypnagogic interruptions affect subsequent hypnagogic experiences, that is, it is possible that interruptions are not at all conducive to the appearance of falling or to any of the other phenomena mentioned in this section.

In respect to the aetiology of these phenomena, Oswald (1962, p. 95) proposed what I consider to be an unsupported hypothesis. He argues that

the sudden sensory and motor phenomena could be thought to be due to an abrupt increase of cortical facilitation accompanying arousal. Many people may experience the 'fall' or the jerk as causing arousal rather than *vice versa*, but I do not think one can rely on this subjective impression of the sleeper . . . the belief that a fall, a bang or a jerk was responsible for awakening is a simple rationalization.

This argument of 'sudden arousal response' is unsound on both logical and evidential grounds. First, it is a peculiar assertion to say that a person wakes and *then* feels a jerk, a bang, sees a flash of light or feels as if falling, because such an argument necessarily ignores the fact that *something* caused the subject to wake in the first place. Now, Oswald wants to argue that that something is arousal itself, that is, the subject wakes suddenly and the very suddenness of 'cortical facilitation' in arousal is experienced as jerks, bangs, flashes of light or falling. The argument, however, is not only counterintuitive but also does not answer those occasions where husbands and wives are shaken by their partners in the midst of their myoclonic jerks, while falling asleep, to catch themselves kicking or twitching, or, in the case of being awakened at the end of a series of jerks, to deny actually having had them. In fact, Oswald himself provides evidence and arguments in support of the latter case, thus appearing to posit that *sometimes* the jerks take place during light sleep (and the hypnagogic state) and may on some occasions go unnoticed by the subject.

Moreover, there is an obvious absence of reports of bangs, jerks, etc., by subjects awakened from light sleep in sleep laboratories: if these phenomena were due to a 'sudden arousal response' then subjects shaken out of their sleep and questioned about their immediate experiences should have furnished us with a wealth of such reports. On the other hand, most of these experiences appear to take place at sleep onset, that is, during a process of diminishing cortical activity, and the phenomena are nearly always reported as causing the subject to return to wakefulness. In such cases, the subject is clearly 'brought back' either while in the middle of the event or afterwards, or in the middle of a psychological incorporation and transformation of the event into a dream experience such as hearing a pistol shot or falling off a cliff. In the latter, for instance, it is clearly the case that one 'dreams' of falling, or at least *feels* as if falling, and *then* wakes up: there have been no cases where the

falling experience was reported as taking place *after* the person had woken up. To say that one cannot rely on the subjective impression of the person who is in fact having the experience is to cast doubt on the very method of collecting reports in the whole area of sleep.

Oswald draws attention to the argument that even a wakeful person's judgment of the time relations of two nearly simultaneous events may be unreliable and that this, too, may be determined by the subjective significance he attaches to the events (see also Titchener 1908 on this). My criticism is not to support any argument to the effect that a sleeping or half-sleeping person's judgment of serial happenings is always to be taken on its face value but rather to point out that (a) such reports as there are must be taken together with other converging data, such as laboratory records, and (b) evidence cannot be dismissed merely on theoretical grounds, especially if this evidence appears to support an already existing hypothesis whose formulation is the end product of accumulated reports.

It is possible, and this point is developed in the later chapters, that cortical arousal or wakefulness plays a secondary role in the experiencing, and possibly no role at all in the causation, of the majority of hypnagogic events. This, of course, is not to deny that a certain degree of arousal during the occurrence of a hypnagogic event is necessary for the registering of the experience. Indeed, in some cases the process of awakening itself may be a requirement for both the occurrence and the registering of the event.

80 Gurney, *et al.* (1886, p. 391, note 2).
81 Myers (1903, p. 125); see also Aristotle (1931, 462a).
82 Quoted by Leaning (1925a, pp 353-4) from Pollock (1912).
83 Gurney *et al.* (1886, pp. 390-91).
84 De Manacéine (1897, pp. 280-1).
85 McKellar (1975, p. 23).
86 See e.g. de Manacéine (1897, pp. 278-81) and Leaning (1925a) for a number of examples.
87 E.g. Alexander (1909), Leaning (1925a), Archer (1935, p. 82), Prince (1952, p. 204), Green and McCreery (1975, p. 70),

James (1975, pp. 76-7).
88 McNish (1830, p. 82).
89 Kanner (1957).
90 *Proc. of the Soc. for Psychical Research*, vol. 10, p. 82.
91 Dudley (1979, p. 87).
92 Leaning (1925a); see also Iamblichus (1895, pp. 115-17).
93 De Becker (1968, pp. 97-9).
94 Fiss *et al.* (1966), Lavie and Giora (1973), Lavie (1974).
95 See e.g. Ellis (1911), Lukianowicz (1959), McKellar (1975).
96 Mintz (1948).
97 Maury (1857); see also Oswald (1962).
98 Cited by Vihvelin (1948).
99 Schultz (1930).
100 Vihvelin (1948).
101 McKellar (1957).
102 Myers (1957).
103 Richardson (1969).
104 By Schneider: cited by Vihvelin (1948).
105 See Ward (1883), Myers (1892), Titchener (1916), Hanawalt (1954), Warren (1921), McKellar (1957); also Oswald (1962).
106 See also Mayer-Gross (1929), Leroy (1933), Silberer (1965), van Dusen (1972).
107 Aristotle (1931, 462a) was the first to mention this kind of vision about which he noted, 'some very young persons, if it is dark, though looking with wide open eyes, see multitudes of phantom figures moving before them, so that they often cover up their heads in terror.'
108 McKellar (1979b, p. 95).
109 Op. cit., p. 28.
110 Titchener (1916, p. 75).
111 Quoted by Hanawalt (1954).
112 Ibid.
113 Jaensch (1930).
114 Richardson (1969, pp. 22-3).
115 Maury (1878, p. 87).
116 This is not to say that we cannot possibly 'see' inside our retinas but rather that whatever we see, we see it in front of us. It is of course entirely possible that, under certain circumstances, we could see an image as if it were from within it, or rather from within it and outside it simultaneously (see Collard's example above); but in such case reference to retina is irrelevant.
117 op. cit., p. 23.
118 See also Leaning (1925a), Lhermitte and Sigwald (1941).
119 McKellar (1957, p. 43).
120 See also Oliver (1975, p. 116) and earlier examples in this chapter.

3 Cognitive and affective characteristics

1 See e.g. Hollingworth (1911), Varendonck (1921).
2 Op. cit.
3 Arnold-Forster (1921, p. 161 *et seq.*).
4 Davis *et al.* (1939b).
5 Williams *et al.* (1962), Weitzman and Kremen (1965), Ornitz *et al.* (1967), Fruhstorfer and Bergström (1969), Fruhstorfer *et al.* (1971).
6 Op. cit.
7 De Lizi (1932), Oswald (1959b).
8 Op. cit., p. 157; Jastrow and McDowell are quoted in the same source, pp. 157 and 159.
9 E.g. Taine (1857, p. 42), Trömner (1911), Leaning (1925a), Leroy (1933, p. 1), Rosett (1939), Critchley (1955), Barber (1957), Sartre (1978).
10 Op. cit., pp. 46-7.
11 Alexander (1909).
12 Leaning (1925a).
13 Leroy (1933, pp. 18 and 45).
14 Budzynski (1977). Budzynski also makes reference in this respect to Lozanov's 'suggestopedic' method which entails relaxing and listening to classical music while ignoring verbal information conveyed by an instructor who modulates her voice according to the tempo of the music. It is claimed by Lozanov that suggestopedic learning is more intuitive and holistic and that information is retained longer than when received under alert conditions.
15 E.g. Simon and Emmons (1955, 1956), Rubin (1968).
16 In all fairness, however, it must be said that 'sleep learning' is still a highly controversial area riddled with much contradictory evidence.
17 De Manacéine (1897).
18 Vihvelin (1948).
19 Silberer (1965: original 1909); see also Alexander (1909).

20 Foulkes and Vogel (1965), who specifically pointed out the absence of this phenomenon in the reports of their subjects, conceded that they 'did not obtain the second of the two conditions which Silberer felt necessary for its occurrence', that is, 'an effort to think'.

21 Slight (1924).

22 Op. cit., pp. 44-7.

23 Rapaport (1967a).

24 Maury (1878, p. 451).

25 Jung (1953-79, vol. 9, part i, p. 132).

26 Van Dusen (1972): material quoted in this section is taken from pp. 97-105 of this work.

27 Greenwood (1882).

28 See e.g. Galton (1883), Alexander (1909), Leroy (1933), Vihvelin (1948), Sartre (1978).

29 Green and Green (1978, pp. 131-2).

30 See e.g. Hollingworth (1911), Leaning (1925a), McKellar (1979a).

31 See Werner (1948), Werner and Kaplan (1967).

32 Freud (1900).

33 McKellar (1957, p. 45).

34 Bergson (1901, 1902).

35 Jung (1944).

36 Quoted by Jung (1944, p.11).

37 A term introduced by Bleuler (1950).

38 Oswald (1962): this is another term introduced by Bleuler (1924); other workers who specifically noted the change in quality of thought in hypnagogia include Maury (1878), Archer (1935), Mintz (1948), Vihvelin (1948), Mayer-Gross (cited by Vihvelin), Critchley (1955), Foulkes and Vogel (1965), van Dusen (1972), Vogel *et al.* (1972), Stoyva (1973).

39 Piaget (1951).

40 Rapaport (1967a).

41 Singer (1966, p. 41).

42 Quoted by Critchley (1955, pp. 102-3).

43 Forbes (1949).

44 Froeschels (1949).

45 Op. cit., pp. 42-3.

46 See Drever (1964, p. 244).

47 Tappeiner (1977).

48 Deikman (1971).

49 For positive correlations between the experiencing of hypnagogic phenomena and the ability to become absorbed see e.g. Richardson (1983, 1984).

50 See Tellegen and Atkinson (1974).

51 See e.g. Maslow (1968) on 'fascination' and 'complete absorption', and Schachtel (1959) on the 'allocentric' perceptual mode.

52 House (1967, pp. 118-19).

53 Op. cit.: material quoted in this chapter is taken from pp. 48-51 of this work.

54 Ellis (1911, pp. 25-26).

55 Poe (1949, p. 544).

56 *J. of the Soc. for Psychical Research* (July 1898, p. 269).

57 Cited by de Manacéine (1897, p. 239); see also Fox (1962, p. 19) on the use of a similar method.

58 Myers (1957).

59 Cited by Galton (1883, p. 115).

60 Mitchell (1896).

61 Ladd (1892); see also Binet (1894).

62 Op. cit., pp. 115-18.

63 See Delage (1903).

64 Op. cit., p. 93.

65 Cited by Leaning (1925a).

66 Oliver (1975, p. 116).

67 McKellar (1957, p. 41; 1979a, p. 193).

68 Warren (1921).

69 Ardis and McKellar (1956).

70 Op. cit., p. 59.

71 Edmunds (1968, p. 248).

72 Sherwood (1965, p. 87).

73 Op. cit., p. 543.

74 Op. cit., p. 250.

75 McKellar (1979a, p. 193).

76 See e.g. Alexander (1909), Leroy (1933), Myers (1957).

77 Foulkes *et al.* (1966).

78 See e.g. Wallace and Benson (1973, pp. 363-4).

79 Oliver (1975, p. 12).

80 Ibid., p. 117.

81 Rouquès (1946).

82 See Buber (1958).

83 Bertini *et al.* (1969); see also Oliver (1975).

84 Oliver (1975) and McKellar (1979b) have also used this method with good results; see also Gurney *et al.* (1886, p. 474, note 1).

85 In fact, relaxation alone is often sufficient not only to induce hypnagogia but also to lead straight into sleep: see e.g. Coriat (1912), Kleitman (1923), Lovell and Morgan (1942).

86 Archer (1935, p. 45); see also de Manacéine (1897), Slight (1924),

Ouspensky (1978).

87 West (1962), Stoyva (1973).

88 See also Leroy (1933, p. 125) and Isakower (1938) on the 'reality' of hypnagogic experiences.

89 See Tart (1975) on 'discrete' states of consciousness and Ouspensky (1949) on Gurdjieff's multiplicity of 'I's.

90 Davis *et al.* (1937); see also Stoyva (1973, p. 394) and Oliver (1975, pp. 1-2).

91 Horowitz (1978, pp. 13-14).

92 Op. cit., pp. 28, 41, 44.

4   *Dreams*

1 Myers (1957).

2 Collard (1953).

3 Maury (1878, pp. 68, 100).

4 Leroy (1901).

5 Arnold-Forster (1921, p. 148).

6 Archer (1935, pp. 26-7).

7 Gastaut (1969, p. 41).

8 See Davis *et al.* (1938).

9 See e.g. Maury (1848, 1878), Leaning (1925a), Tournay (1941).

10 Leroy (1933): material quoted in this section is taken from pp. 97-118 of this work.

11 McKellar (1979a, p. 191).

12 McKellar (1957, p. 41).

13 Miller (1906).

14 Dudley (1979, p. 86).

15 Saint-Denys (1982): material quoted in this section is taken from pp. 43-6 of this work.

16 See Green and Green (1978, pp. 132-4).

17 McKellar (1979b, p. 89).

18 Foulkes and Vogel (1965); see also Foulkes *et al.* (1966), Singer (1976, pp. 47-8), Slap (1977).

19 On this see also Isakower (1938), McKellar (1957, 1979a), Budzynski (1972), Oliver (1975).

20 Foulkes and Vogel (1965).

21 See e.g. Kamiya (1961), Berger *et al.* (1962), Foulkes (1962), Rechtschaffen *et al.* (1963), Maron *et al.* (1964), Dement (1965), Berger (1967), Foulkes (1967), Niedermeyer and Lentz (1976), Singer (1976).

22 Vogel *et al.* (1969), basing their study on the Foulkes and Vogel data, found that

'there is a statistically significant tendency for each EEG stage (Alpha, stage 1 and stage 2) to be associated with a different combination of ego functioning'. This latter they called 'ego state'. They distinguished three ego states, viz. *I*, in which the ego remained intact or relatively intact, i.e. it either maintained both non-regressive content (secondary process mentation) and contact with reality or lost only one of them (this was observed mainly during alpha-EEG), *D*, in which the ego was relatively destructuralized, that is, both functions were impaired (usually during stage 1), and *R*, that is, relatively restructuralized, which was marked by a return to non-regressive mentation accompanied by complete loss of reality testing (usually during stage 2).

Although there were some exceptions to the observed correlations between each electroencephalographic stage and ego state, that is, I-D-R did not always correspond to Alpha EEG, stage 1, and stage 2 respectively, a closer analysis showed that the psychological I-D-R sequence was always present during sleep onset. Regarding the relationship of kinds of content (regressive/non-regressive) to loss of contact with reality, these investigators found that

some withdrawal precedes or accompanies the appearance of regressive content; that, following the appearance of regressive content, loss of reality testing (hallucination) precedes or accompanies a return to nonregressive content; and, finally, that withdrawal from the external environment (disorientation to time and place) precedes the appearance of hallucination.

Bearing the above in mind, Vogel, *et al.* offered a psychodynamic view of sleep onset according to which the desire for sleep produces a sequence of three de-cathexes (=withdrawal of energy investment, interest, or attention), namely, a decathexis of perceptual information, a decathexis of the perceptual apparatus, and a decathexis of the reality testing function. The second decathexis induces regressive changes in the ego which, although not necessary for sleep onset, appear to be the unavoidable side-effects of reduced sensory input, thus threatening the ego and producing the need for a defence. The consequent loss of reality testing which is followed by the re-appearance of non-regressive content is thought to constitute 'part of the needed defense which allows sleep to continue'. Individual differences (length, frequency, EEG stage) at sleep onset are seen as the way subjects are able to handle potential threats of regression (this is tied in with clinical impressions that the less anxious and rigid the subjects the earlier and richer their hypnagogic dreams).

The investigators' observation that in hypnagogic D dreams the instigator is the reduced sensory input or withdrawal which produces a regressed state indicates that Freud's (1900) contention that (a) dreams are instigated by unconscious wishes, and (b) dreams function to protect sleep, cannot be true of all dreams. Primarily, hypnagogic dreams are taken to represent regressed ego states rather than unconscious wishes, and the hypna-gogic D dream in particular is thought to represent 'a process which tends to disturb sleep' producing in turn the R dream, 'a defense against this potential disturbance'. Vogel *et al.* conclude that 'different kinds of dreams have different kinds of insti-gators, and . . . some dream instigators tend to disturb sleep and others to protect it'.

Two criticisms may be levelled against this study, one concerning the definition of 'regressive content' and the other the relationship and interpretation of the occurrence of D and R. In the first, content was rated as regressive only by the presence of one or more of six categories: (a) Single, isolated images, such as the number 2,081 hanging in mid air: . . . (b) An incomplete scene or bits and pieces of a scene, . . . (c) Bizarre, inappropriate, or distorted images, . . . (d) Bizarre sequence or superimposition of images, . . . (e) Dissociation of thought and image, e.g. one subject reported he was driving a car and simul-taneously thinking about a problem in linguistics. (f) Magical, omnipotent thinking.

Of the six categories, however, (a), (b) and (e) hardly warrant their inclusion in the definition. There is nothing regressive in the vision of an isolated image or an incomplete scene: they both can, and do, appear in normal memory and association. Category (e), too, displays nothing regres-sive. Besides the fact that there is nothing unusual in doing one thing and thinking about another in everyday life, (i) we may have memories of apparently unrelated events (e.g. about driving and linguistics) which deeper analysis might show to have been associated in a past experience, and (ii) since the investigators have not made an attempt to analyse the subject's imagery experience of driving a car in terms of symbolism, we are not in a position to deny the possibility that this experience is autosymbolic, that is, we do not know whether the subject did not have the hypnagogic experience of driving a car as a result-symbol of his thinking about a problem in linguistics. Naturally, if the latter were the case, we might still be dealing with regression in the sense that the scene of driving a car might be thought to be the resultant concrete symbol of an abstract linguistic problem. But, in that case, this particular kind of experience would not constitute a separate category but fall into category (a) or (b) and would come under the same criticism as those two categories. In addition, it should be noticed that 'isolated images' and 'incomplete scene' appear to deny the occurrence of hypnagogic images which are complete and set in a context and yet are not 'bizarre' (see Leaning's 1925a classification, in particular 'scenery' and 'scenes').

Second, in presenting a psychodynamic view of sleep onset, Vogel *et al.* contend that (a) the psychological sequence I-D-R is always present, and (b) loss of reality testing is necessary for the appearance of R. In the case of (a) the investigators' conclusions on the I-D-R- sequence do not appear to be applicable to the occurrence of, for instance, narcoleptic REM dreaming.

Their arguments with regard to (b) are simply not convincing enough. To begin with, it is not explained why reality testing should be lost as part of the defence against D if 'regressive changes are not in themselves necessary for sleep onset'. In other words, it is argued that a process-mentation of the importance of reality testing is sacrificed as part of a defence against a mere 'side effect' (D). This does not make very good sense in terms of evolution and survival. On the other hand, the appearance of R, which is defined as non-regressive mentation, i.e. 'plausible, realistic, coherent and undistorted', could hardly warrant the loss of reality testing: what is the point (necessity) of losing the reality testing ability if the resultant mentation is 'realistic'? It seems that either the definition of non-regressive mentation is wrong (or wrongly interpreted in individual cases) or that reality testing is lost for other reasons than those offered by Vogel *et al.* If the first is true, then the concept of non-regressive (as well as that of regressive, in addition to earlier arguments against the latter), is illdefined, in which case it may point to the second possibility and lend support to a more plausible hypothesis, namely that the loss of reality testing follows or accompanies a deepening D state, and that the emergence of the R state that follows is merely an indication of the ego's 'acceptance' of the new reality and its ability to 'structuralize' it, i.e. make sense of it, once the reality-unreality barrierthreat has been overcome. This would explain the experiences of subject 9 in the study under discussion whose D reports were all in alpha REM with R taking up almost all of stages 1 and 2, that is, the early destructuralization (implying physical and mental relaxation and lack of fear of regression) allowed for an early and long R state. It might also explain (and this point will be developed more fully later) why psychics – whose state of functioning appears to have many similarities with hypnagogia – experience, maintain, and develop lengthy periods of 'regressive' mentation accompanied by a nonregressive and 'coherent' commentary.

23 See Appendix II for stages of sleep.
24 Van Eeden (1969: original 1913).
25 See e.g. Evans-Wentz (1978, p. 216) and chapter 6.
26 Aristotle (1931, 462a, 5-10).
27 Quoted by de Becker (1968, p. 99) from Baillet's *La Vie de Monsieur Descartes*, Paris, 1901; see also Descartes (1934, p. 212).
28 See e.g. Arnold-Forster (1921), Green (1968a), Faraday (1972), Garfield (1976), Sparrow (1976), Watkins (1976), Corriere and Hart (1977), Hearne (1978, 1981, 1982), La Berge (1981), Fenwick *et al.* (1984).
29 See e.g. La Berge (1981).
30 McKellar (1968, p. 106).
31 McKellar (1979b, pp. 87-8).
32 Op. cit., 1933, pp. 115-18.
33 Tart (1967); see also Hearne (1981).
34 Oliver (1975, pp. 2-3).
35 Critchley (1955); see also Ellis (1897) and Hyslop (1908).
36 Kant (1900: original 1766).
37 Swedenborg (1928, para. 7387: original 1746).
38 Ouspensky (1978): material quoted in this section is taken from chapter 7 of this work.
39 See e.g. Steiner (1979, pp. 34-5).
40 Malcolm (1967): quotations are from pp. 50-9, 65-6, 109, 112 of this work.
41 Sullivan (1953, pp. 331-2).
42 Op. cit., p. 109.
43 This shows, incidentally, how blundering armchair philosophers can be, and how easily they tend to forget that 'logic' is merely a specific mental tool whose correct employment is utterly dependent on the antecedent establishment of, not logically but experientially, true premises.
44 See e.g. La Berge (1980, 1981), Hearne (1981), Fenwick *et al.* (1984).
45 Hearne (1981).
46 Green *et al.* (1971a).
47 Fox (1962).
48 See e.g. Muldoon and Carrington (1965, p. 126).
49 A subject once told me, for instance, how he used it to gain relief from pressing sexual needs. During a period of his life when he was lonely, depressed, and in great need of female sexual companionship, he discovered that at sleep onset, and as the hypnagogic pictures began to appear, he could easily visualize scenes in which he fully participated, and in which he would have sexual relationships with

women that left him as fully satisfied as any normal sexual act during wakefulness. In these experiences he was fully aware that he was dreaming, but this awareness did not detract one bit from the realness of the situation over which he appeared to have full control. This is a report from a normal individual, but in the clinical literature one comes across cases where at sleep onset a person is visited by a 'demon' who engages in sexual activities with the patient as a result of which the latter is relieved from headaches and other physical pains and psychological stresses (see e.g. Medlicott 1958).

50 Tart (1969).
51 Kamiya (1961).

5   Meditation

1 See e.g. Vivekananda (1955), Mishra (1967).
2 Honorton (1977).
3 See e.g. Wallace (1970), Wallace *et al.* (1971), Wallace and Benson (1973).
4 See Anand *et al.* (1961), Kasamatsu and Hirai (1963, 1966).
5 Gastaut (1969).
6 See e.g. Wada and Hamm (1973), Younger *et al.* (1975), Pagano *et al.* (1976).
7 Bagchi and Wenger (1959).
8 Regardie (1979, p. 102).
9 Ibid., pp. 101-5.
10 Van Dusen (1975, pp. 19-20).
11 Swedenborg (1950).
12 Op. cit., pp. 23-4.
13 Ibid., p.25.
14 Deikman (1969a).
15 Deikman (1969b).
16 Deikman (1971).
17 Gill and Brenman (1959, p. 178).
18 Werner (1948).
19 Quotations in respect to these features are from Deikman (1969b).
20 Silberer (1965).
21 Leary (1964).
22 Koestler (1974, p. 58).
23 This is reminiscent of the well-known phenomenon in physics in which the more accurately the location of an electron is determined the more uncertain its velocity becomes, and when its velocity is determined the electron becomes a blur.

24 Leaning (1925b).
25 See e.g. Baker (1980).
26 See also Trömner (1911) on this.
27 See e.g. Werner (1948), von Senden (1960), and Shapiro (1960) on the developmental organization of perception and cognition.
28 See also Suraci (1964) on this.
29 Schachtel (1959, p. 284).
30 Quoted by Deikman (1969b, p. 41).
31 Ehrenzweig (1964).
32 Van Dusen (1972, p. 104).
33 Poe (1949, p. 543).
34 Sherwood (1965, p. 90).
35 Wambach (1979, pp. 16-17).
36 Myers (1903), Ouspensky (1978), and Leroy (1933) respectively.
37 Suzuki (1969).
38 James (1975).
39 See Buck and Geers (1967).
40 Ellis (1897).
41 Stace (1960, p. 10).
42 Stace (1973, p. 232).
43 Organ (1975, p. 174).
44 Translated by Wolters (1977, ch. 43).
45 Castaneda (1976, pp. 186-7 and 197).
46 Koestler (1954).
47 Aurobindo (1949).
48 Staal (1975, p. 42).
49 Ibid., p. 43.
50 See also Bunge (1962) on this.
51 Op. cit., p. 79.
52 Underhill (1955).
53 Op. cit., pp. 543-4.
54 Mylonas (1974, p. 262).
55 Ayer (1977, p. 5).
56 Crichton-Browne (1895).
57 On this point see also Isakower's (1938) comments in respect to hypnagogia.
58 Van Dusen (1975, p. 25).

6   Psi

1 See e.g. Krippner (1970), Panati (1975).
2 See e.g. Green and Green (1978).
3 Carrington (1975).
4 Leaning (1925a), Edmunds (1968).
5 Myers (1957).
6 See e.g. Honorton and Harper (1974), Braud *et al.* (1975).
7 Leaning (1925a).
8 Sinclair (1930, pp. 181-2).
9 Butler (1968, pp.46-8).
10 Roberts (1964, p. 28).

11 Edwards (undated, p. 9); see also Carrington (1966, p. 31).
12 Bennett (1973).
13 Huson (1977, p. 64).
14 See Schmoll (1887), Barrett (1882, 1883, 1924), Rhine (1934, 1937), Tyrrell (1936), Dessoir (1886), Garrett (1941, 1950, p. 230), Carlson (cited by White 1964), Heywood (1964, p. 201), Le Shan (1973, p. 38).
15 White (1964).
16 Honorton (1974, 1977).
17 Braud and Braud (1975).
18 Honorton (1977).
19 See Stanford (1977); also chapter 10 for my arguments in reference to oldbrain predominance in the production of hypnagogic and related phenomena.
20 See e.g. Morris (1976), Stanford (1977).
21 See e.g. Braud and Braud (1973) on the relaxation component, and Stanford (1971) and Stanford and Lovin (1970) on alphoid EEG correlations.
22 For instance, Sinclair (1930, pp. 186-7) writes, 'After you have practised the exercise of concentrating on a flower. . . . Hold your mind a blank.' See also Carlson (cited by White 1964). On the other hand, Rush (1949) notes, 'In receiving, J.H.R.'s practice was to clear his mind as nearly as possible of sensory distraction, frequently sitting in darkness, and then to stop the usual stream of rational "daydream" imagery, thus creating a subjective blank screen upon which incoherent, unanticipated forms might take shape.' See also Barrett (1882), Lodge (1884), Dessoir (1886), Schmoll (1887), Schmoll and Mabire (1888), Rawson (1895), Thomas (1905), Usher and Burt (1909), Warcollier (1938, p. 20).
23 Rhine (1934).
24 Warcollier (1938, p. 51; 1948, p. 28).
25 Murphy and Dale (1943).
26 Gibson (1937).
27 Tyrrell (1938).
28 Murphy (1944).
29 Op. cit., pp. 184-5.
30 Warcollier (1938, p. 20 and pp. 222-3).
31 Op. cit., p. 186.
32 Leaning (1925a), McKellar (1979a), van Dusen (1972), Delage (1903), Ardis and McKellar (1956), Green *et al.* (1970).

33 See Trömner (1911) on this in respect to hypnagogia.
34 See e.g. Richet (1889).
35 Op. cit., pp. 10 and 16.
36 Garrett (1941, pp. 52-3).
37 Arnold-Forster (1921), Ornitz *et al.* (1967).
38 Op. cit., pp. 4 and 17.
39 Northage (1973, p. 49).
40 Op. cit., p. 18.
41 Ibid., p. 21.
42 Garrett (1941, p. 175).
43 Op. cit., pp. 200-1; see also Dessoir (1886), Schmoll (1887), Schmoll and Mabire (1888), Turvey (1911, pp. 41 and 56), Sidgwick (1924).
44 See e.g. Edwards (undated, pp. 26-8). Also Northage (personal communication, March 1981).
45 See Collard (1953) and Leroy (1933, p. 86) respectively.
46 Op. cit., pp. 64-5.
47 Op. cit., pp. 51-4.
48 Butler (1969, p. 62).
49 Butler (1973, p. 10).
50 Archer (1935, pp. 28, 33, 42-3); see also Miller (1906) for a more detailed case involving Red Indians.
51 Leroy (1933, p. 23, obs. xi).
52 Garrett (1941, pp. 131-2).
53 Slight (1924, pp. 278-9); see also Schneck (1968) for a similar case.
54 Op. cit., p. 23.
55 Edwards (undated, p. 23).
56 See also Kubie (1943) on the use of induced hypnagogic reverie for the recovery of repressed amnesic data.
57 Garrett (1941, p. 178). Sinclair (1930, p. 200), for instance, says, 'When the true visions came there usually came with them a "something" which I called a "hunch".' Johnson (Tyrrell 1936) states that a true psychic experience 'has the settled feeling of finality about it. It impels you and simply does not let you doubt it.'
58 Butler (1973, pp. 42 and 45). Likewise, White (1964) notes, 'Sometimes this impression [of an image] appears spontaneously; at these moments the percipients almost universally report a strong feeling of conviction that the impression is the correct one. But very often, on the other hand, the impressions

are neither so "single nor as singular".'

59 Garrett (1941, pp. 10 and 11).

60 Le Shan (1973, 1974, 1976).

61 Stanford (1977).

62 Green (1968b, p. 51): the immediately following quotations are from pp. 51, 84, 50, 54, 57-9 of this work.

63 Monroe (1974, p. 200).

64 Muldoon and Carrington (1965, p. 232).

65 Ibid., pp. 124-5.

66 E.g. Fox (1962, p. 138), Monroe (1974, pp. 200-2), Carrington (1978), Frost and Frost (1982, pp. 54-5). See also Blackmore's (1983) comprehensive review.

67 Fox (1962, p. 20) believes that this 'vibrating curtain of circular cells . . . is always present at the back of things, if one concentrates upon it, though it will often remain unnoticed because of the more arresting nature of other phenomena'.

68 Green (1968b, pp. 69-80).

69 See e.g. Walsh (quoted by Muldoon and Carrington, 1965, p. 69), Leroy (1933), Sartre (1978).

70 Fox (1962, p. 126); it must be said, however, that Fox's advocating 'a substantial repast' before undertaking an experiment in ecsomatosis is not supported by other psychics and occultists who generally advise against it on the ground that it makes one too sleepy.

71 Green (1968b, pp. 98 and 94).

72 Ibid., pp. 94-5.

73 Ibid., pp. 82 and 102.

74 E.g. Leroy (1933, pp. 18-19), Critchley (1939), McKellar (1979a, pp. 190-1, 1979b, p. 96).

75 Green (1968b, p. 119).

76 See e.g. Hollingworth (1911) and van Dusen (1972, 1975).

77 For reports of near-death experiences accompanied by a feeling of omniscience see Moody (1978, pp. 9-14).

78 Op. cit.

79 Green and McCreery (1975, pp. 75-9); see also Heisenberg (1971, ch. 11), who retails the occurrence of a hypnopompic dream which he felt was premonitory in character.

80 Gurney *et al.* (1886, pp. 399-456).

81 Collard (1953).

82 See letter-box of *John O'London's Weekly*

(6 December 1930, p. 427).

83 Garrett (1941).

84 Leaning (1925a) found that her correspondents fell into four groups according to the significance they attached to their hypnagogic visions, viz. those who believed that their visions were : (a) scenes from previous lives, (b) premonitions, (c) scenes of events taking place somewhere at the present time, (d) symbols of moral value.

85 Forman (cited by Ellis 1911), Iamblichus (1895), Poe (1949); see also Swedenborg (1928-48, 1977).

86 E.g. Roheim (1952), McKellar and Simpson (1954), Liddon (1967).

87 Maury (1878).

88 Tappeiner (1977).

89 Tappeiner's 'hypnagogic' interpretation of religious 'revelatory' phenomena found unexpected support when, after a lecture on hypnagogia at Bedford College's Psychological Society, I was approached by a student who told me that such experiences were very common in the religious group she belonged to. Since then I have found that such phenomena are fairly common in many religious groups.

90 Cited by Warcollier (1938, p. 219).

91 See Evans-Wentz (1978).

92 Garrett (1941, pp. 36-7 and 143-4).

93 For comparison, see a purported telepathic example containing neologisms, comparable to those occurring in hypnagogia, in Sinclair (1930, p. 37) where Mrs Sinclair 'received' and wrote down a string of German and near-German words.

94 Garrett (1941, p. 43).

95 Garrett (1949, p. 182).

96 Galton (1883).

97 Warcollier (1938, p. 111).

98 Alexander (1909).

99 Warcollier (1948, p. 55).

100 Muldoon and Carrington, op. cit., p. 50.

101 Le Shan (1973, p. 94).

102 Heywood (1964, p. 201).

103 Van Dusen (1972), Le Shan (1973).

104 Alexander (1909); see also Maury (1848), Budzynski (1972), Huson (1977).

105 Monroe (1974, pp. 200-1); see also van Dusen (1975) on Swedenborg's hypnagogic practices.

106 See e.g. Maury (1848), Alexander (1909),

Rouquès (1946), Collard (1953), McKellar and Simpson (1954), Myers (1957).

107 It is of interest that even great psychics, who are thought to be born with their psychic abilities, appear to undergo some form of 'psychic development' which typically begins with trances or trance-like states.

7 Schizophrenia

1 McKellar and Simpson (1954).
2 For an excellent account of dissenting arguments on the concept of schizophrenia see Clare (1976).
3 Mayer-Gross *et al.* (1969, pp. 277-8).
4 Cited by Mayer-Gross *et al.* (1969).
5 Bleuler (1950).
6 Jung (1909).
7 Berze (1914).
8 Op. cit., p. 265.
9 Cited by Mayer-Gross *et al.* (1969, pp. 265-6).
10 Payne (1962).
11 McReynolds (1960).
12 Op. cit., pp. 266-7.
13 Ibid., p. 267 and transcript of Plate VIII.
14 Jaspers (1959, p. 209).
15 Green (1973).
16 Despert (quoted by Froeschels, 1946), Benjamin (1964), and Cameron (1964) respectively.
17 McKellar (1957, p. 47).
18 Schjelderup-Ebbe (1923).
19 Trömner (1911).
20 Archer (1935, p. 35).
21 Froeschels (1946). This writer compares aspects of hypnagogic thinking to that encountered in schizophrenia and epilepsy and in the speech of small children, dysarthrics, dyslalics, dysphasics, para-noiacs, the feeble-minded, and aphasics.
22 McKellar (1957), van Dusen (1972), Oswald (1976).
23 Alexander (1909).
24 Schultz (1930).
25 Mintz (1948).
26 Froeschels (1949).
27 Poincaré (1978).
28 And perhaps, conversely, a valid logical transaction is not always accompanied by a feeling of certainty. Prime examples to illustrate this argument would be the philosophers Locke (1964) and Hume (1962): the former consistently refused to draw conclusions from valid arguments when such conclusions appeared to go against 'common sense', and the latter commented on the 'coldness' of his most important and validly drawn conclusions and drew attention to the non-logical grounds of knowledge.
29 Isakower (1938).
30 Federn (1952); see also Trömner (1911) on word-salad in respect to hypnagogia.
31 See e.g. Schultz (1930), and chapter 5.
32 See e.g. Weckowicz and Blewett (1959).
33 Op. cit., p. 275; see e.g. Leroy (1933) for identical remarks concerning hypnagogic hallucinations.
34 Schneider: cited by Mayer-Gross *et al.* (1969, p. 274).
35 Fish (1961).
36 Kubie (1943), Maury (1857).
37 Maury (1848).
38 Maury (1857). Quotations and references in the following section are from this work.
39 Berze (1914) and Bleuler (1950) respect-ively.
40 Op. cit., p. 270.
41 Ibid., p. 271.
42 Oswald (1962, p. 186).
43 McKellar (1979b, p. 96).
44 Singer (1976, p. 47).
45 Cited by Oswald (1962, p. 114).
46 Kasanin (1964).
47 Angyal (1964).
48 Von Domarus (1964).
49 See also Hyman (1953) and Arieti (1955) on the tendency of schizophrenics to conceptualize on the basis of 'partial' similarities.
50 Storch (1922).
51 See e.g. Frazer (1976), Eliade (1976).
52 Cameron (1939), Chapman and Taylor (1957), McGaughran and Moran (1956) respectively.
53 Peters (1952).
54 Lecky (1945), Rogers (1951), Festinger (1957), Peak (1955), Kelly (1955) re-spectively.
55 Hyman (1953), Arieti (1955).
56 West (1962).
57 Baillarger (1846); see also Mitchell (1890) regarding this view.
58 De Manacéine (1897).

59 Vogel *et al.* (1972).
60 Mitchell (1890).
61 See e.g. Gurney *et al.* (1886, p. 391, note 2).

8   Creativity

1 See Greenwood (1894), Myers (1903), Maury (1857, p. 164), Gurney *et al.* (1886, p. 493) respectively.
2 See Sartre (1978, p. 47), Crichton-Browne (1895), Novalis (quoted by Béguin 1939, p. 210) respectively.
3 For poems, see e.g. Miller (1906), Prince (1952), Bécquer (Lewin 1969), Moss (1970) and Koestler (1981); for stories and novels see Stearn (1973) on Caldwell and Panati (1975) on Leader. In general, according to one study (Marsh 1906), artistic and literary creative people appear to be at their best in the early morning and late evening.
4 E.g. M. Twain, E.A. Poe, R.L. Stevenson (Hollingworth 1911), Ernst (1952), Oster (1966), Wagner, Bradbury, C. Lamb, T. de Quincey (McKellar 1957, 1979b), Tolstoy (Panati 1975). In his *Moby Dick*, Melville describes a tactile hypnagogic experience as occurring to Ishmael, one of the characters in the novel (see Schneck 1977 for discussion). E. Brontë also describes hypnagogic imagery in *Wuthering Heights*, and in *Villette* C. Brontë describes what she calls an opium vision which she personally experienced not as a result of taking opium – she denied ever having taken any – but as the outcome of having thought about it on numerous occasions before sleep: 'The vision itself', McKellar (1963, p. 141) reports, 'emerged on one occasion after waking up in the morning.'
5 See Abell (1964) on Brahms, Gowan (1976) on Puccini and Wagner, and Watson (1974, p. 229) on Goethe.
6 Kekulé (Japp 1898), Arnold-Forster (1921), Varendonck (1921), Hadamard (1949), W. Scott, J. Brindley (Beveridge 1950), Stanford (1977), Edison (Bernd 1978), Poincaré (1978), Einstein (Koestler 1981).
7 Bernd (1978, pp. 28-9).

8 See e.g. Green *et al.* (1970), Cade and Coxhead (1979).
9 Hallman (1967).
10 See Bruner (1962), McKellar (1957), Kubie (1958), Murray (1959), Ghiselin (1952) respectively.
11 Galton (1883), Katz (1948).
12 Hudson (1968).
13 See e.g. Leroy (1933) and Rapaport (1967a) on this.
14 Miller (1906).
15 Koestler (1981, p. 167).
16 Coleridge (1952).
17 Prince (1952).
18 Hadamard (1949, p. 8).
19 Quoted by Newbold (1897, p. 12).
20 Cocteau (1952).
21 Leader: quoted by Panati (1975, p. 135).
22 Poincaré (1978).
23 Quoted by Japp (1898).
24 McKellar (1963, p. 134).
25 Ibid., p. 144.
26 Aristotle (1969: 1459a).
27 Nietzsche (1952).
28 Kretschmer: quoted by Koestler 1981, pp. 325 and 322).
29 Einstein (1952), Bartlett (1932, p. 226), Richardson (1969, p. 12), Paivio (1971, 1974), McClelland (1964), Schaefer (1975).
30 Green *et al.* (1970).
31 Wallas (1978).
32 Walkup (1965).
33 Bugelski (1970); see also Arnheim (1969) and Richardson (1969, p. 124) on this. Aristotle is probably the first known author to argue that all cognition involves imagery.
34 See e.g. Titchener (1909), Koffka (1912), Binet (1921), Arnheim (1969) on this.
35 Poincaré (1978), Mednick (1962), Cropley (1978) respectively.
36 Jones: cited by Milner (1981, pp. 161-2).
37 E.g. Ryle (1976) and the school of philosophical behaviourism.
38 Barron (1963, p. 249), Popper (1977, p. 32), Koestler (1981, p. 178), Hallman (1967), Nietzsche (quoted by Jung 1957, p. 104), Jung (1957, p. 105).
39 Quoted by Koestler (1981, p. 117).
40 Pinard (1957).
41 Gowan (1975, pp. 313 and 124).
42 Op. cit., p. 317.
43 Scott and Brindley are cited by Beveridge

(1950, pp. 73-4); see also McKellar
(1957) and Stoney (1974) on E. Blyton's
process of writing her stories.

44 See Kubie (1958), Rogers (1959, 1961),
Murray (1959), Gerard (1961), Taylor
(1959), Ghiselin (1952) respectively.

45 McKellar (1957) and Wilson *et al.* (1953)
respectively.

46 McKellar's (1977) comparison.

47 Koestler (1981, p. 201).

48 Brèton (1924).

49 Schmeller (1960, pp. 10 and 14).

50 Ernst (1952).

51 Dali (1976, pp. 436-7).

52 Dali: quoted by Wilson (1980, p. 18).

53 Quoted by Wilson (1980, p. 18).

54 Ibid.

55 McKellar (1963, p. 142 and 1979b, p.
101).

56 Guilford (1967).

57 Op. cit., pp. 170-1.

58 Quoted by Koestler (1981, pp. 125-6).

59 Housman (1952).

60 Plato (*Phaedrus*, 245 A): quoted by
Housman, ibid.

61 Cited by Koestler (1981, p. 339).

62 See Mednick (1962).

63 Williams (1922).

64 Op. cit., p. 211.

65 Hutchinson (1939).

66 Berne (1949).

67 Kris (1939).

68 Rogers (1961, p. 353).

69 Guilford (1950).

70 McKellar (1963, pp. 131-2).

71 Hudson (1975).

72 See Maslow (1956).

73 E.g. Vogel *et al.* (1969), Green *et al.*
(1971b), Budzynski (1972, 1977),
van Dusen (1972), Stoyva (1973).

74 E.g. Crichton-Browne (1895), Tauber
and Green (1959), Green *et al.* (1971b).

75 Greeley (1974).

76 Maslow (1968).

77 See e.g. Silberer (1965), Leaning (1925a),
Vihvelin (1948), Oswald (1962),
van Dusen (1972). Germane to this aspect
of hypnagogia are also Head's (1901)
findings concerning the mental changes
and images that accompany visceral
diseases. In the same vein, Leaning
(1925a) notes that attacks of headache
may be accompanied by visions of 'the
battlements of a fortress'.

78 See e.g. Silberer (1965), Slight (1924),
Kubie (1943), McKellar (1957),
Ouspensky (1960), Foulkes and Vogel
(1965), Vogel *et al.* (1966), Schneck
(1968), van Dusen (1972), Oliver (1976),
Budzynski (1977).

79 Silberer (1965, 1971).

80 Foulkes *et al.* (1966).

81 Green and Green (1978, p. 149).

82 See Budzynski (1972, 1977).

9 Other relevant areas of experience

1 James (1890), de Manacéine (1897),
Arnold-Forster (1921).

2 Hilgard (1968, p. 26).

3 Gill and Brenman (1959, pp. 57-8); see
also Sheehan (1979).

4 Orne (1959).

5 Hilgard (1968, p. 22). There are, of
course, various other means of inducing
hypnosis, e.g. by spinning or whirling and
rocking, and through shock or 'paralysing'
fear, but these are not directly relevant to
the subject in hand.

6 Kubie and Margolin (1944b).

7 It is a well supported fact that many
schizophrenics have schizoid parents who
continually frustrate them with broken
promises and unjustified and inexplicable
changes of attitude towards them. Some
workers consider this family atmosphere
to be the cause, or one of the main
causes, of schizophrenia.

8 See e.g. Erickson (1964) on the origination
and uses of the technique.

9 Zeig (1980, p. 17; and pp. 6-26).

10 Tart (1975).

11 See also Erickson *et al.* (1976, p. 300).

12 Ibid., p. 306.

13 See e.g. Braid (1843) and White (Sarbin
1950) on monoideism; Tellegen and
Atkinson (1974) on absorption; Hilgard
(1968) on dissociation.

14 See e.g. Hilgard (1973).

15 See e.g. Sherman (1971).

16 See e.g. Lilly (1977), Freedman and
Greenblatt (1960), Freedman *et al.* (1962).

17 See e.g. Leiderman (1964), Bexton *et al.*
(1954), Zuckerman and Cohen (1964).

18 They have been variously called 'visual'
and 'auditory' images (Bexton *et al.* 1954),
'hallucinations' (Vernon *et al.* 1958;

Vernon 1966), a kind of 'hypnagogic imagery' (Freedman *et al.* 1962), 'reported visual senations' (Myers and Murphy 1962), 'non-object-bound sensory phenomena' (Scheibel and Scheibel 1962).

19 See Brownfield (1965) for a more detailed discussion.

20 Sidis (1909, p. 54); see also Bolton (1894), Jacobson (1929), Kleitman (1967), Lovell and Morgan (1942), Kubie and Margolin (1944b).

21 Schacter (1976); see also Goldberger and Holt (1958), Holt and Goldberger (1961), Zuckerman *et al.* (1962), Zuckerman and Cohen (1964), Zuckerman and Hopkins (1966).

22 Leiderman (1964).

23 See e.g. Hebb (1954), Myers and Murphy (1962), Zuckerman (1964).

24 See Zuckerman (1964).

25 E.g. Freedman *et al.* (1962); Holt's (1972) correlations, however, were insignificant.

26 See Holt and Goldberger (1959, 1961).

27 Foulkes *et al.* (1966).

28 See Holt (1964) and Schacter (1976) respectively.

29 See respectively: Costa (1953), Smythies (1960), Freedman and Marks (1965), Horowitz (1967); Knoll and Kugler (1959, 1964), Knoll *et al.* (1962); Penfield and Rasmussen (1950), Penfield (1958), Ishibashi *et al.* (1964), Horowitz *et al.* (1968), Horowitz (1978).

30 See Holt and Goldberger (1959), Goldberger and Holt (1961), Foulkes *et al.* (1966), Richardson (1969).

31 See Freedman and Marks (1965), Richardson (1969).

32 Mahl *et al.* (1964); see also Horowitz (1978).

33 See e.g. de Boismont (1859), Galton (1883), Kleitman (1967).

34 Bliss and Clark (1962); see also Bjerner (1949), Oswald (1962).

35 Bliss and Clark (1962).

36 See e.g. Tyler (1955), Bliss *et al.* (1959), Brauchi and West (1959), Cappon and Banks (1960), Morris *et al.* (1960), Oswald (1962).

37 Bliss *et al.* (1959).

38 Horowitz (1978, p. 16); see also Horowitz *et al.* (1967).

39 Saul (1965).

40 Forbes (1949).

41 Horowitz (1978, p. 17); see also Horowitz (1966).

42 Mitchell (1896).

43 E.g. Hollingworth (1911), Klüver (1928b, 1942), Rawcliffe (1952), McKellar and Simpson (1954), Ardis and McKellar (1956), Caldwell (1968).

44 Klüver (1928b).

45 See also Leuner (1963) on this.

46 Klüver (1942).

47 Ardis and McKellar (1956).

48 See e.g. Tart (1971).

49 Richardson (1969).

50 Holt (1972).

51 See e.g. Galton (1880), Allport (1924, 1928), Klüver (1926, 1928a, 1930, 1932), Gengerilli (1930), Jaensch (1930), Teasdale (1934), Purdy (1936), Meenes and Morton (1936), Doob (1964, 1965, 1966), Haber and Haber (1964), Sheehan (1968), Haber (1969, 1979), Hatakeyama (1975).

52 Ahsen (1977).

53 Marks and McKellar (1982).

54 Doob (1964).

55 McKellar (1979b, p. 101).

56 Oswald (1962, p. 96).

57 Crichton-Browne (1895); see also Griffiths and Fox (1938), Oswald (1962).

58 See e.g. Jackson (1958), Mitchell (1890), Crichton-Browne (1895), Sedman (1964, 1966).

59 Beck and Guthrie (1956).

60 Sedman (1964).

61 Penfield and Perot (1963).

62 Sedman (1964), McLean (1964).

63 Slater and Beard (1963).

64 Sedman (1966).

65 McLean (1964), Koestler (1978).

66 See e.g. Mitchell (1890), Oswald (1962).

67 Buck and Geers (1967).

68 Ellis (1897).

69 Isakower (1938).

10 *The old versus the new brain*

1 E.g. Iamblichus (1895), Swedenborg (cited by van Dusen 1975), Forman (cited by Ellis 1911), Tappeiner (1977).

2 Alexander (1909), Leaning (1925a), Edmunds (1968).

3 See e.g. Isakower (1938), Vogel *et al.* (1969).

4 See e.g. Herschels (cited by Leaning, 1925a), Alexander (1909), Froeschels (1946, 1949), van Dusen (1972).

5 See e.g. Ladd (1892), Ellis (1911).

6 See e.g. Hollingworth (1911), Leroy (1933), Archer (1935), Hanawalt (1954), Oswald (1962), Ouspensky (1978); see also Vihvelin's (1948) 'synesthetic visions', Silberer's (1965) 'somatic phenomena', and reproductive and perserverative hypnagogic phenomena as reported by e.g. Titchener (1916), Warren (1921), Slight (1924), Leaning (1925a), Aristotle (1931); Monroe (1974, p. 201) has also proposed that some visual hypnagogic phenomena 'may merely be forms of neural discharge', and some schools of occultism call them *vrittis* and refer to them as 'thought-forms which constitute part of the relaxed brain's excretory mechanism' (Baker 1980).

7 See respectively: Cane (1889); de Manacéine (1887), Ellis (1897), Lhermitte and Sigwald (1941); Maury (1848, 1878), Guyon (1903); Kelly (1962), van Dusen (1975).

8 See e.g. Gruithuisen (1812), Müller (1826), Maury (1848, 1878), Radestock (1879), Ladd (1892), Binet (1894), de Manacéine (1897), Ellis (1911), Warren (1921), Hicks (1924), Griffitts (1927), Archer (1935), McKellar and Simpson (1954). Of interest in this respect is the list of entoptic phenomena compounded by Hyslop (cited by de Manacéine, 1897, p. 238) in regard to visual hallucinations in general and which includes: shadows formed on the retina by opaque bodies, movements of the blood corpuscles in the retinal capillaries, the entoptical pulse, pressure phosphenes, electric phenomena, spectra arising from internal causes such as increased blood pressure through the retina; see also Klüver (1942), Jackson (1958), White and Levatin (1962), Horowitz (1978) on floaters in the eye (*muscae volitantes*) and their role in the origination of some hallucinations.

9 Alexander (1909); see also Leaning (1925a), Tournay (1941), Rouquès (1946), Saint-Denys (1982).

10 See e.g. Leroy (1933, pp. 64 and 70-1).

11 Janet (in Delage, 1903); see also Gellé (1903), Leroy (1933).

12 See e.g. Freud (1953), Jackson (1958), Evarts (1962b), Sheehan (1966), Hebb (1968), Zikmund (1972), Shepard and Podgorny (1978), Marks (1982).

13 Finke (1980).

14 Gruithuisen (1812, p. 256), Burdach (1839), Meyer, and Strümpel (cited by de Manacéine 1897, who also reported identical results in her own research), Alexander (1904).

15 Wundt (1863, p. 387), Féré (1885), Meyer (cited by James 1890, p. 67), Binet (1894, reporting on the work of Ladd), Klüver (1928a), Jaensch (1930), Weiskrantz (1950), Oswald (1957a, 1957b, 1959a).

16 See e.g. Binet and Féré (1890), Downey (1901), de Bechterev (1906), Erickson and Erickson (1938). Further support for a hypothesis of non-peripheral origin and formation of visual imagery comes from some old investigations carried out in regard to the dreams of the blind (e.g. Heermann 1838, Jastrow 1888, Hitschmann 1894: cited by de Manacéine 1897, pp. 302-8) which showed that when loss of eyesight occurred after the age of 7 the visual dreaming ability was often retained and when sight was only partially lost dream visions became distinctly more vivid than physically seen objects. In particular, Heermann noted that dream visions were still experienced after twenty years of blindness, by which time the patient's optic nerves must have atrophied. More recently, Walter and Yeager (1956) found some evidence suggestive of retention of visual imagery if sight is lost in later life.

17 See Penfield: in Penfield and Jasper (1954).

18 See e.g. Klüver (1941), ter Braak and van Vliet (1963), Weiskrantz (1963), Humphrey and Weiskrantz (1967), Brindley *et al.* (1969), Pasik *et al.* (1969), ter Braak *et al.* (1971), Schilder *et al.* (1972), Poeppel *et al.* (1973), Sanders *et al.* (1974). Such evidence has led to the postulation of the 'two visual systems' hypothesis according to which 'focal' vision is subserved by the visual cortex, and 'ambient' vision by the superior colliculus of the midbrain (see Trevarthen 1968, Perenin and Jeannerod 1975, Lewin 1975). It appears that in ambient vision

one's visual space is 'unconscious', as witnessed by the subjects' denial of 'seeing' a stimulus although they can locate it accurately. As Humphrey remarked in reference to Helen, a cortically blind rhesus monkey, 'in one sense she sees everything, and in another, nothing' (Lewin, 1975). Of particular psychological interest are the introspective reports of cortically blind patients regarding the way they 'see' the various stimuli. For instance, when Weiskrantz and Warrington asked their patient to describe how he determined differences in pattern discrimination tests – tests for discrimination between noughts and crosses – he said he could tell the difference by the '"feeling" of something jagged, or something smooth' (Lewin 1975).

19 See e.g. ter Braak (1971).

20 Schatzman (1982).

21 Golla (1948); other workers who have studied this problem in relation to sensory stimulation and states of attention include Jasper *et al.* (1935), Bagchi (1937), Williams (1939), Mundy-Castle (1951), Short (1953), Short and Walter (1954), Walter and Yeager (1956).

22 Romains (1924).

23 Ivanov (1964).

24 Novomeiskii (1965).

25 Schiller (1935).

26 Davis *et al.* (1938), Adie (1926), Walter (1948) respectively. See also Lhermitte and Tournay (1927), Walter and Dovey (1944).

27 See e.g. Gerebtzoff (cited by Walter 1948), Obrador (1943), Morris (1976).

28 See respectively: Le Gros Clark (quoted by Japser, in Penfield and Jasper 1954, p. 157); Walker (1938, p. 277); Dempsey and Morison (1942), Kennard and Nims (1942a, 1942b), Morison and Dempsey (1942), Kennard (1943), Adrian (1947), Jasper and Droogleever-Fortuyn (1947).

29 Jasper: in Penfield and Jasper (1954, pp. 222-3).

30 See Hunter and Jasper (1949).

31 Horowitz (1978, p. 267 *et seq.*); see also Horowitz *et al.* (1968).

32 E.g. Pribram and McLean (1953), Cuenod *et al.* (1965), McLean (1966).

33 Douglas (1967).

34 Pribram and McLean (1953).

35 For instance, Hoskins's (1933) findings in respect to the urine volume of schizophrenics suggest either 'disturbed function of the diencephalon or of the posterior lobe of the pituitary gland'. Hoskins also found that 'the patients as a group showed a characteristic hypometabolism' – low blood pressure, slow pulse, and reduced oxygen consumption – which led him to conclude that the metabolism of the resting but wakeful schizophrenic is strikingly similar to the normal person in sleep and that 'perhaps the characterization of the psychosis as a dream state is worthy of more literal acceptance than had previously been supposed'. Davison (1966) found 'an excess of diencephalic and brainstem lesion both absolutely and relatively to the hospital population' of fifty schizophrenic patients. He also noted that 'basal brain lesions induced a psychosis more quickly than hemisphere lesions'. Further, both Staehelin (cited by Mayer-Gross *et al.* 1969) and Labhardt (1963) propose that a disturbance of diencephalic and mesencephalic functions may be implicated in the onset of psychotic symptoms. Labhardt views the appearance of these symptoms as the result of extreme stress often threatening the continued existence of the personality. Similarly, Fish (1961), as we saw in chapter 7, associates severe anxiety with marked overactivity of the reticular system which latter he considers to be the cause of schizophrenia. Fish's claim seems to be supported by experimental evidence showing that amphetamine overdosage in normal subjects produces a psychosis which is clinically indistinguishable from paranoid schizophrenia (e.g. Connell 1958) and in which 'the subjective experience is nearly always felt to have a dream-like quality' (Mayer-Gross *et al.* 1969, p. 300). Significantly, and supporting my hypothesis that hypnagogic and related experiences are associated with subcortical activities, Bradley (1957) has produced evidence suggesting that in animals amphetamine stimulates activity in the reticular system below the midbrain level.

Lhermitte (1925, 1932) and van

Bogaert (1927) showed that lesions of the mesencephalic tegmentum produce hallucinatory phenomena, as do lesions or electrical stimulation of the upper brainstem core (e.g. Olds and Milner 1954, Roberts 1958). Lhermitte and Tournay (1927), van Bogaert (1927, 1968), Lhermitte (1938), Lhermitte and Sigwald (1941), Tournay (1941), Rouquès (1946), Ey (1957), and Reimer (1970) have related, and some of them identified, hypnagogic hallucinations with peduncular hallucinosis in brainstem perturbations. Lhermitte and Sigwald (1941) pointed out that hypnagogic experiences and peduncular hallucinosis are strongly related by dint of their connections with the sleep regulatory system located in the mesodiencephalic and peduncular region. They note that in mesencephalic disturbances 'the subject abandons real life and descends into a world wherein are unfurled the whims of an imagination free from all restraint or support.' They also relate hypnagogic hallucinations and cataplexy, as components of narcolepsy, to the loss of mesencephalic tonus. The latter may further be implicated in the production of hypnagogic phenomena in Huntington's chorea where these phenomena have been observed to wax and wane with the illness (Guyon 1903).

36 Scheibel and Scheibel (1962); see also Amassian and de Vito (1954), Scheibel et al. (1955), Brodal (1957), Eldred and Fujimori (1958), Scheibel and Scheibel (1958).

37 Fox (1962, pp. 126-7).

38 Muldoon and Carrington (1965, p. 51).

39 Ibid., p. 104; see also Green (1968b, p. 214).

40 See Huson (1977, p. 67) on Eusapia Palladino.

41 Garrett (1941, pp. 52-3).

42 Warcollier (1948, p. 61).

43 See e.g. Morris (1976, p. 241).

44 See e.g. Reik (1949). For a more detailed argument along these lines see J.R. Smythies (ed.) *Science and ESP* (1971), and in particular Hardy's article on 'Biology and ESP'.

45 See e.g. Walter and Dovey (1944), Cairns (1952), Nash (1970).

46 Luria and Vinogradova (1959).

47 Kretschmer: quoted by Koestler (1981, pp. 315-16).

48 Cairns (1952).

49 See e.g. Sperry (1968), Bogen (1969a, 1969b), Bogen and Bogen (1969), Sperry et al. (1969), Gazzaniga (1970), Galin and Ornstein (1972), Galin (1974).

50 Galin (1974).

51 Cairns (1952); see also Puech et al. (1947), Nielsen and Sedgwick (1949).

52 Jackson (cited by Bogen 1969b).

53 See Schlesinger (1962) on musical ability, and Goldenberg et al. (1985) and Kosslyn (1985) on mental imagery.

54 Aphasics suffering from injuries to the left hemisphere are often capable of using complex sentences, defects in language (including aphasias) can result from injuries to the right hemisphere (in left-handers the situation is more complicated), speech or utterances pertaining to a stroke are often correlated with an epileptogenic focus in the right temporal lobe, gross defect in speech comprehension usually results not from left hemisphere lesion alone but in conjunction with relevant deconnections in the right temporal lobe, an aphasiogenic left hemisphere lesion may give rise to the patient's composing poetry for the first time, and stimulation of the right hemisphere can result in vocalization as well as alteration of ongoing speech (summarized from Bogen 1969b). See also Russell (1982, pp. 65-77) for more arguments regarding the adaptability of the brain.

55 Hécaen et al. (cited by Bogen 1969b).

56 Fischer (1975).

57 Penfield and Jasper (1954, p. 156, footnote).

58 McLean (1964).

59 See e.g. Miller et al. (1960).

60 McLean (1960, p. 1737).

61 Koestler (1978, p. 289).

62 Ibid., pp. 286 and 283.

63 McLean: quoted by Koestler (1978, p. 287).

64 Sedman (1966).

65 Van Dusen (1975, p. 21).

66 See O'Brien (1975).

67 See Griffin (1976) for some interesting arguments ascribing conscious awareness and intentionality to phylogenetically very primitive animals.

68 Koestler (1978, p. 273).
69 See e.g. Magoun (1963).
70 See Jouvet (1967).
71 McLean (1958).
72 Oswald (1976, p. 37).
73 Ibid., p. 38.
74 See e.g. Kleitman (1967).
75 Huttenlocher (1961).
76 Bagchi and Wenger (1959, p. 136).
77 Also, in the East, meditators are known to withdraw to high altitudes on tall mountains both because of the rarefied atmosphere and for quietude; in addition, the vegetable diet of such people is known to be compensated for by a rise in the carbon dioxide in the blood – as opposed to a meat diet where blood acidity is compensated for by a lowering of the alveolar carbon dioxide pressure.
78 See e.g. Horowitz (1978, p. 248).
79 E.g. Hoskins (1933).
80 Haldane and Priestly (1935).
81 Penfield (1938, 1957), Thomson (1951); see also Thomson and Nielsen (1948).
82 See McLean (1970), Brown (1977); in fact, Brown proposes a fourth level which is to be found only in humans: this is the symbolic consciousness of the asymmetrical brain (left-right hemispheric asymmetrical specialization).
83 See Brown (1977). Some writers have, indeed, suggested that the different parts of our body have their own consciousness and memories (Castaneda 1976, p. 131; Ouspensky 1978, ch. 7) and even dream their own dreams which to our rational mind are utterly incomprehensible (Ouspensky, ibid.).
84 Kappers (1971).
85 Antón-Tay (1971).
86 It is, so far, known to modulate the activity of adenohypophysis, neurohypophysis, endocrine pancreas, parathyroids, adrenal cortex, adrenal medulla, and gonads (see De Vries and Kappers 1971, Relkin 1972, Kappers 1976, Reiter 1977, Klein 1978). For general reviews and some classical work on the pineal see also collections of articles in Kappers and Schadé (1965) and Wolstenholme and Knight (1971), and the book by Wurtman et al. (1968).
87 It causes, for instance, high level activities of norepinephrine, histamine, acetyl-choline, 5-methoxyindole and 5-hydroxyindole acetic acid, iodine 131 uptake, high aminoacid peptidase and succinic dehydrogenase (Baker 1979, p. 24).
88 Ibid., p. 27.
89 Moody (1978, pp. 9-14); see also Moody (1976), Kübler-Ross (1978), Ring (1984), Grey (1985).

11 The function and significance of hypnagogia

1 See Langworthy (1933), Conel (1939), Tanner (1961).
2 This activity is sometimes misconstrued as evidence of self-awareness (e.g. Verny and Kelly 1982), whereas it is merely empathic response to stimuli, suggestive of a diffuse-absorbed attentional state as in hypnagogia. Infants below the age of 5 months are purely kinesthetic: they even reach for the unseen source of a sound – this is done both by babies born blind and by sighted ones in the dark (Bower 1977). For the infant, everything must be touched, sucked and chewed – a clear indication that empathy and 'internalization' are the practising cognitive modes at this age. If, when reaching for an object, its hand comes into view, the baby forgets all about the object and stares at its hand – thus gradually coming to identify, inferentially at first, the existence of its own body, and learn that this body is, as it were, an object that can be externally located in relation to other objects. Before the age of 7 months a baby cannot differentiate between the self and the world, nor can it distinguish between 'same' and 'similar'.

The fetus is known to respond to the human voice, especially to that of its parents, and to react differently to different types of music and to other sounds. Human infants, even a few hours old, are found to mimic, and there have been many cases of adults who remembered, mostly under hypnosis, prenatal and early postnatal experiences. These well-documented data have been taken, again, by some workers to mean that the fetus or neonate is self-aware, and that, because of its ability to mimic, it has a 'well-developed (one could say adult) thinking, including the handling of abstract ideas' (Verny and Kelly 1982, p. 154). But these are doubtful inferences. To begin with, the responses of the fetus to sound are explicable solely on empathic principles. Its differential reactions to the human voice are partly instinctive (innate) and partly the result of conditioning. If my arguments concerning the nature of the LEBs are correct, the fetus and infant are open to all kinds of influence and conditioning. The observed mimicry is also explicable on the principles of empathy and lack of ego boundaries. The argument from the recall of early experiences is more complicated since the memories are taking place in the mind of an adult. This is not to deny the veridicality of such memories but to question the inference to self-awareness. I am not even denying that the fetus is endowed with a primitive (instinctive) form of self-awareness – in fact, I have defended a similar view in chapter 10. What I *am* saying is that infantile cognitive processes are functions of an extremely weak or entirely lacking ego schema, and that the fetus's and infant's interactions with the world are not to be interpreted on inferences which tacitly assume a clear awareness of a distinct self.

3 Descartes (1976, p. 266).
4 See e.g. Prince (1898, 1906, 1907, 1917, 1922, 1929), Sidis (1912), van Eeden (1969); see also McKellar (1979b) for a recent discussion on coconscious phenomena.
5 See e.g. Miller (1956), Broadbent (1958), Payne *et al.* (1959), Sperling (1960), Atkinson and Shiffrin (1971), Shallice (1972), Posner and Klein (1973), Erdelyi (1974), Shaffer (1975), Frith (1979).
6 Luria and Vinogradova (1959).
7 See e.g. Klüver (1942), Bleuler (1950), Schilder (1950), Fisher (1962), Goldstone (1962). See also Klopfer *et al.* (1954) on the link between vividness of projection and release of ego control in Rorschach research.
8 In some instances of schizophrenia one should perhaps speak not so much of 'loosening' as of 'rupturing' of the ego boundaries whereas, by contrast, most

cases of mystical ecstasy are the outcome of a gradual LEBs. However, such polarized categorization is often arbitrary and heavily dependent on current social and medical standards and definitions. In point of fact, many schools of mysticism and occultism explicitly forewarn the acolytes of the 'maddening' experiences they are to undergo, and usually forearm them with appropriate training – which is not to say that the aspirants are spared these experiences or that they always succeed in remaining 'sane'. Conversely, people classed as schizophrenic sometimes report mystical phenomena. For some vigorous attacks on the concept of madness see e.g. Laing (1976) and Szasz (1970).

9 There are, of course, other ways of inducing LEBs, and some of these were noted in chapter 9 ('Hypnosis'). But in hypnagogia this happens naturally and spontaneously and thus renders the state unique in explaining the occurrence of similar phenomena in other states.
10 It is interesting that a remarkably similar account of imaginal experience in general, purely from an information-processing perspective, has recently been given by Morris and Hampson (1983).
11 This restrictive view is held, for example, by Richardson (1969) who employs the criterion of 'antecedent conditions' to define hypnagogic imagery and relegate it to the status of a subcategory of 'imagination imagery'. For similar views see also McKellar (1957) and Horowitz (1978).
12 Rouquès (1946) in fact claimed that he could think of past events and make complicated calculations while the images unfolded, and that the only reason he had for considering them 'premonitory of sleep' was the mere fact of their regularly occurring prior to sleep.
13 See e.g. Doob (1964) on the Ibo of Nigeria. In fact, there have been reports in which subjects, who experienced visual hypnagogic imagery with open eyes, found that the images would become faint or disappear on closing their eyes (see Horowitz 1978, p. 134; Marks and McKellar 1982, p. 12).
14 Tart (1969, p. 74); see also Liberson and Liberson (1966).

15 Sterman (1972).

16 See e.g. Kleitman (1969), Kripke (1974).

17 See e.g. Snyder (1963, 1965).

18 Globus (1966); see also Snyder (1963), Ouspensky (1978, p. 295).

19 Snyder (1963).

20 In fact, there is ample evidence to support the view that a dreaming person can respond to external stimuli when sufficiently motivated; see e.g. Christake (1957), Rowland (1957), Toman et al. (1958), Oswald et al. (1960), Granda and Hammack (1961), Snyder (1963).

21 See e.g. Dement (1960).

22 See e.g. Cartwright et al. (1967).

23 Zarcone et al. (1968).

24 See Lehman et al. (1958), Klein (1965), Vogel (1975, 1977), Flemenbaum (1976), Huapaya (1976), Schlauch (1979), Hemmingsen and Rafaelsen (1980).

25 Gellhorn and Loofbourrow (1963).

26 Miller (1926).

27 Pitts and McLure (1967).

28 Allport, F.H. (1924).

29 Hess (1957), Gellhorn and Loofbourrow (1963).

30 It is noteworthy that Muldoon and Carrington (1965, pp. 122-5) have each explained the invigorating effects of the hypnagogic state by reference to what they have called the 'act of discoincidence' or a shift of the 'astral body' away from the physical which results in the person's being charged with 'cosmic energy'. What this amounts to is that the energizing a person feels in hypnagogia is not merely the result of physical relaxation but of a more complex, positive, and psychological process which is characterized by a shift and alteration in consciousness. In other words, it involves a change in 'mode'.

31 See Hill (in Hill and Parr 1950) and Finley (1944) respectively.

32 Meddis (1977, p. 137).

33 See Jacobson (1929), Schultz and Luthe (1959).

34 Mavromatis (1983).

35 Sterman (1972); see also Jouvet et al (1961), Kleitman (1969), Emde and Metcalf (1970).

36 It is interesting to note, in this respect, Collier's (1964) three-level theory of the evolution of consciousness. The first level is 'the simple, generalized contact-chemical-sense-feeling' which is 'seen as the phylogenetic basis for all later developments of consciousness'. The second level 'appears phylogenetically when sense modalities have become differentiated', and the third level is typified by 'the evolved capacity to become aware of the fact that one is aware or conscious', that is, by 'reflective consciousness'.

37 Similar states of consciousness appear to be aimed at by Desoille (1966) in his 'waking dream' practices in which he guides his subject-patients into an ever-deepening reverie. Desoille argues that not only is the psychological phenomenology of 'waking dreams' very similar to that present in nocturnal dreams but also the physiology of the former strongly resembles that of the latter: he found, for instance, that, as with nocturnal dreams, his subjects showed lowering of rectal temperature, slowing down of respiration, and lowering of respiratory metabolism.

38 Esnoul: quoted by de Becker (1968, p. 154).

39 See e.g. Rose (1976, p. 304).

40 See e.g. Green et al. (1971a) who reported that their yogi subject was accurately aware of the workers' activities in the EEG laboratory, in which he was being tested, while in deep sleep (his EEG rhythm was that of 4 cps).

41 Maury (1878, pp. 69, 96; 1857); see also Lhermitte and Sigwald (1941), Kubie (1943), Warcollier (1948), Muldoon and Carrington (1965), Budzynski (1977), Green and Green (1978).

42 Poincaré (1978).

43 Freud (1943, p. 118).

44 Castaneda (1976, p. 131), Ouspensky (1978, p. 281).

45 Van Dusen (1972).

46 See e.g. Leadbeater (1966), Besant and Leadbeater (1975).

47 See Horowitz (1978, pp. 132-9) for a discussion of these 'clinically discrete operations'.

48 Weiss (1950).

49 Weisman (1958). It is intriguing that both reality sense and reality testing appear to emerge from the same basic need, namely that of certainty. This need, like all other needs, is nonrational, and as such it can never be satisfied by reality testing. As

Popper (1977, p. 280) rightly remarked, 'the demand for scientific objectivity makes it inevitable that every scientific statement must remain *tentative for ever. . . .* Only in our subjective experiences of conviction, in our subjective faith, can we be "absolutely certain".' This is essentially a need to hold on to, or discover, something comprehensible in which the ego remains intact and whole, or regains its lost wholeness. That is perhaps why Hume liked to return to the warmth and reassurance of human companionship after his excursions into the 'cold' uncertainties of dissecting, differentiating, and analysing logic. And that is why both a schizophrenic and a subject in a 'confusion technique' experiment would clutch at anything that promises even a temporary respite from the torment of uncertainty. Significantly, in seemingly illogical mental exercises, as in asking a person to make sense of the question 'What is the sound of one hand clapping?', Zen Buddhism makes use of this need for certainty to loosen a person's grip on reality testing, thus eventually flooding him with a sense of reality and causing him to adopt a very different approach to reality testing.

50 James (1890).
51 Cassirer (1953).
52 Pepper (1948).
53 Weisman (1958).
54 For instance, Monroe (1974, p. 238) suggests that perception in an OBE 'is achieved by means of some force in the electromagnetic spectrum – by direct magnetic fields either received or induced, or through some force or field yet to be identified – rather than by counterparts of the physical mechanism'.
55 See e.g. Green *et al.* (1970, 1971a, 1971b, 1973, 1978), Budzynski (1972, 1977).

Archer (1935), Hanawalt (1954), Buck and Geers (1967), Hebb (1968), McKellar (1972), Richardson *et al.* (1981); (2): Maury (1848), Müller (1848), Ladd (1892), Silberer (1965), Hicks (1924), Leroy (1933), Froeschels (1946, 1949), Vihvelin (1948), Collard (1953), Rapaport (1967a, 1967b), Singer (1976), Sartre (1978); (3): de Manacéine (1897), Bertini *et al.* (1964), Green and Green (1978), Green *et al.* (1970, 1971a, 1971b, 1973), Foulkes and Vogel (1965), Dement (1965), Foulkes *et al.* (1966), Vogel *et al.* (1966), Liberson and Liberson (1966), Vogel *et al.* (1972), Budzynski (1972, 1977), Stoyva (1973), Schacter and Kelly (1975), Oliver (1975).

2 For more detailed arguments on this see Fiss *et al.* (1966), de Strooper and Broughton (1969), Lavie and Giora (1973), Lavie (1974), Schacter (1976).
3 Kubie and Margolin (1942, 1944a).
4 Kubie (1943); see also Slight (1924) and Cade and Coxhead (1979).
5 Bertini *et al.* (1969); see also Honorton and Harper (1974), Braud and Braud (1975).
6 Gastaut (1969).
7 Green *et al.* (1970), Green and Green (1978).
8 Budzynski and Stoyva (1969); see also Stoyva and Kamiya (1968), Budzynski (1969, 1972, 1977), Brown (1970), Stoyva (1973), Oliver (1975), Cade and Coxhead (1979).
9 See Budzynski (1977), Green *et al.* (1970), Budzynski (1972) respectively.
10 Swedenborg (1928, 1977).
11 Kelly (1962).
12 Woolley (1914).
13 Muldoon and Carrington (1965).
14 De Manacéine (1897), Ouspensky (1978), Fox (1962), Muldoon and Carrington (1965), Monroe (1974).

Appendix I   Methods and procedures

1 See respectively : (1): Müller (1848), Poe (1949), Ellis (1897), Alexander (1909), Hollingworth (1911), Arnold-Forster (1921), Varendonck (1921), Warren (1921), Slight (1924), Leaning (1925a),

Appendix II   Physiological correlates

1 Berger (1930).
2 Loomis *et al.* (1937), Davis *et al.* (1937, 1938).
3 Dement and Kleitman (1957).
4 See Davis *et al.* (1939a, 1939b), Roth

et al. (1956), Johnson and Karpan (1968).

5 Schwartz and Fishgold (1960), Berger *et al.* (1962).

6 E.g. Aserinsky and Kleitman (1955), Dement and Kleitman (1957), Berger (1961), Jacobson *et al.* (1964), Snyder *et al.* (1964), Broughton *et al.* (1965), Fisher *et al.* (1965), Williams and Cartwright (1969).

7 Davis *et al.* (1938).

8 Gastaut (1969).

9 Partly summarized from Kleitman (1967, p. 74).

10 Bülow (1963); see also Goldie and Green (1961).

11 Timmons *et al.* (1972).

12 Liberson and Liberson (1966).

13 Blake *et al.* (1939): cited by Kleitman (1967, p. 57).

14 The Libersons have noted, however, that this progression is not always observed as there are people 'who show an exaggerated amount of theta-activity preceding the onset of alpha-blocking', or have 'delta-waves of sleep suddenly replacing alpha-activity' and other types of unusual sleep onset such as 'occipital onset', 'micro-sleep', and narcoleptic REM dreaming. See also Vogel (1960), Rechtschaffen *et al.* (1963), Maron *et al.* (1964), Globus (1966), Liddon (1967).

15 Foulkes and Vogel (1965).

16 De Manacéine (1897, pp. 214-15).

17 Fleisch (1929), Grollman (1930), Boas and Goldschmidt (1932), de Lizi (1932), Max (1937).

18 Walter and Dovey (1944).

19 Omwake (1932).

Appendix III Some incidental observations on psi and meditation

1 Personal communication, March 1981.

2 Personal communication, May 1981.

Bibliography

Abell, A.M. *Talks with Great Composers*. Garmisch-Partenkirchen, Germany: G.E. Schroeder-Verlag, 1964.

Adie, W.J. Idiopathic narcolepsy. *Brain*, 1926, 49, 257-306.

Adrian, E.D. *The Physical Background of Perception*. Oxford: Clarendon Press, 1947.

Ahsen, A. Eidetics: An overview. *J. Mental Imagery*, 1977, 1, 5-38.

Alexander, H.B. Some observations on visual imagery. *Psychol. Review*, 1904, 11, 319-37.

Alexander, H.B. The subconscious in the light of dream imagery and imaginative expression: with introspective data. *Proc. Amer. SPR*, 1909, 3, 614-98.

Allport, F.H. *Social Psychology*. Boston: Houghton Mifflin, 1924.

Allport, G.W. Eidetic imagery. *Brit. J. Psychol.*, 1924, 15, 99-110.

Allport, G.W. The eidetic image and the after image. *Amer. J. Psychol.*, 1928, 40, 418-25.

Amassian, K. and de Vito, R. Unit activity in reticular formation and nearby structures. *J. Neurophysiol.*, 1954, 17, 575-603.

Anand, B.K., Chhina, G.S. and Singh, B. Some aspects of electroencephalographic studies. *Electroenceph. Clin. Neurophysiol.*, 1961, 13, 452-6.

Angyal, A. Der Schlummerzustand. *Z. Psychol.*, 1927, 103, 65-99.

Angyall, A. Sullo stato del dormiveglia. *Arch. Ital. Psicol.*, 1930, 8, 89-94.

Angyal, A. Disturbances of thinking in schizophrenia. In Kasanin, J.S. (ed.) *Language and Thought in Schizophrenia*. New York: Norton, 1964.

Antón-Tay, F. Pineal-brain relationships. In Wolstenholme, G. and Knight, J. (eds) *The Pineal Gland* (Ciba Foundation symposium). Edinburgh and London: Churchill Livingstone, 1971.

Archer, W. *On Dreams*. London: Methuen, 1935.

Ardis, J.A. and McKellar, P. Hypnagogic imagery and mescaline. *J. Ment. Science*, 1956, 102, 22-29.

Arieti, S. *Interpretation of Schizophrenia*. New York: Brunner, 1955.

Aristotle. De Somniis. Trans. by Beare, J. and Ross, G. In Ross, W. (ed.) *The Works of Aristotle* (vol. 3). London: Oxford University Press, 1931.

Aristotle. *Poetics*. Trans. by Warrington, J. London: Dent & Sons, 1969.

Arnheim, R. *Visual Thinking*. Berkeley: University of California Press, 1969.

Arnold-Forster, M. *Studies in Dreams*. London: Allen & Unwin, 1921.

Aserinsky, E. and Kleitman, N. Regularly occurring periods of eye motility, and concomitant phenomena, during sleep. *Science*, 1953, 118, 273-4.

Atkinson, R.C. and Shiffrin, R.M. The control of short-term memory. *Scient.*

American, 1971, 224, 82-90.

Aurobindo, S. *The Life Divine*. Calcutta: Arya Publishing House, 1949.

Ayer, A.J. *The Central Questions of Philosophy*. Harmondsworth: Penguin, 1977.

Bagchi, B.K. The adaptation and variability of response of the human brain rhythm. *J. Psychol.*, 1937, 3, 463-85.

Bagchi, B. and Wenger, M. Electrophysiological correlates of some Yogi exercises. In *First Int. Congr. Neurol. Sciences (Brussels 1957): Vol. 3: EEG, Clinical Neurophysiology and Epilepsy*. London: Pergamon Press, 1959.

Baillarger, M.J. De l'influence de l'état intermédiaire à la veille et au sommeil sur la production et la marche des hallucinations. *Mem. Acad.-Roy. Méd.*, 1846, 12, 476-516.

Baker, D.M. *Esoteric Anatomy*. Essendon, Herts: D. Baker, 1979.

Baker, D.M. *The Techniques of Astral Projection*. Essendon, Herts: D. Baker, 1980.

Barber, T.X. Experiments in hypnosis. *Scient. American*, 1957, 196, 54-61.

Barrett, W.F. First report on thought reading. *Proc. SPR*, 1882, I, 13-34.

Barrett, W.F. On some phenomena associated with abnormal conditions of mind. *Proc. SPR*, 1883, I, 238-44.

Barrett, W.F. Some reminiscences of fifty years' psychic research. *Proc. SPR*, 1924, 34, 275-97.

Barron, F. *Creativity and Psychological Health*. New York: Van Nostrand, 1963.

Bartlett, F. *Remembering*. Cambridge University Press, 1932.

Beck, A.T. and Guthrie, T. Psychological significance of visual auras. *Psychosom. Medicine*, 1956, 18, 133-42.

Béguin, A. *L'Âme romantique et le rêve: Essai sur le romantisme allemand et la poésie française*. Paris: Librarie J. Corti, 1939.

Benjamin, J.D. A method for distinguishing and evaluating formal thinking disorders in schizophrenia. In Kasanin, J.S. (ed.) *Language and Thought in Schizophrenia*. New York: Norton, 1964.

Bennett, C., *Practical Time-travel*. Wellingborough, Northants: Aquarian Press, 1973.

Berger, H. Ueber das Elektroenkephalogramm des Menschen. *J. Psychol. Neurol.*, 1930, 40, 160-79.

Berger, R.J. Tonus of extrinsic laryngeal muscles during sleep and dreaming. *Science*, 1961, 134, 840.

Berger, R.J. When is a dream is a dream is a dream? *Exp. Neurol. Suppl.*, 1967, 4, 15-28.

Berger, R.J., Olley, P. and Oswald, I. The EEG, eye-movements and dreams of the blind. *Quart. J. Exp. Psychol.*, 1962, 14, 183-6.

Bergson, H. Le rêve. *Rev. Scient.*, 1901, 15, 705-13.

Bergson, H. L'effort intellectuel. *Rev. philos.*, 1902, 53, 1-27.

Bernd, E. Jr. *Relax*. Orlando, Florida: Greun Madainn Foundation, 1978.

Berne, E. The nature of intuition. *Psychiat. Quart.*, 1949, 23, 203-16.

Bertini, M., Lewis, H.B. and Witkin, H.A. Some preliminary observations with an experimental procedure for the study of hypnagogic and related phenomena. In Tart, C. (ed.) *Altered States of Consciousness*. New York: John Wiley & Sons, 1969 (orig. 1964).

Berze, J. *Primary Insufficiency of Psychic Activity*. Vienna: Deuticke, 1914.

Besant, A. and Leadbeater, C.W. *Thought-forms*. Wheaton, Ill.: Theosophical Publishing House, 1975 (orig. 1901).

Beveridge, W.I. *The Art of Scientific Investigation*. London: Heinemann, 1950.

Bexton, W.H., Heron, W. and Scott, T.H. Effects of decreased variation in the sensory environment. *Canad. J. Psychol.*, 1954, 8, 70-6.

Binet, A. G.T. Ladd – Contrôle direct sur le champ de la rétine. *Année psychol.*, 1894, 1, 424-5.

Binet, A. *L'Étude experimentale de l'intelligence*. Paris: Costes, 1921.

Binet, A. and Féré, C. *Le Magnétisme animal*. Paris: F. Alcan, 1890.

Bizette, A. Remarques sur les phases du présommeil. *J. Psychol.* (Paris), 1931, 28, 647-51.

Bjerner, B. Alpha depression and lowered pulse rate during delayed actions in serial reaction tests: study in sleep deprivation. *Acta Physiol. Scand. Suppl.*, 1949, 19, Suppl. 65.

Blackmore, S. *Beyond the Body*. St Albans, Herts: Granada, 1983.

Blake, H., Gerard, R.W. and Kleitman, N. Factors influencing brain potentials during sleep. *J. Neurophysiol.*, 1939, 2, 48-60.

Bleuler, E. *Textbook of Psychiatry*. New York: Macmillan, 1924.

Bleuler, E. *Dementia Praecox or the Group of Schizophrenias*. New York: International Universities Press, 1950.

Bliss, E.L. and Clark, L.D. Visual hallucinations. In West L.J. (ed.) *Hallucinations*. New York: Grune & Stratton, 1962.

Bliss, E.L., Clark, L.D. and West, C.D. Studies of sleep deprivation: relationship to schizophrenia. *AMA Arch. Neurol. Psychiatry*, 1959, 81, 348-59.

Boas, E.P. and Goldschmidt, E.F. *The Heart Rate*. Springfield, Ill.: Thomas, 1932.

Bogen, J.E. The other side of the brain: I. Dysgraphia and dyscopia following cerebral commissurotomy. *Bull. Los Angeles Neurol. Soc.*, 1969, 34, 73-105. (a).

Bogen, J.E. The other side of the brain: II. An appositional mind. *Bull. Los Angeles Neurol. Soc.*, 1969, 34, 135-62. (b).

Bogen, J.E. and Bogen, G.M. The other side of the brain: III. The corpus callosum and creativity. *Bull. Los Angeles Neurol. Soc.*, 1969, 34, 191-220.

Bolton, T.L. Rhythm. *Amer. J. Psychol.*, 1894, 6, 145-239.

Bower, T. *The Perceptual World of the Child*. London: Fontana/Open Books, 1977.

Bradley, P.B. Recent observations on the action of some drugs in relation to the reticular formation of the brain. *EEG Clin. Neurophysiol.*, 1957, 9, 372-3.

Braid, J. *Neurypnology: Or the Rationale of Nervous Sleep Considered in Relation to Animal Magnetism*. London: Churchill, 1843.

Brauchi, J.T. and West, L.J. Sleep deprivation. *J. AMA*, 1959, 171, 11-14.

Braud, W.G. and Braud, L.W. Preliminary explorations of psi-conducive states: Progressive muscular relaxation. *J. Amer. SPR*, 1973, 67, 26-46.

Braud, W.G. and Braud, L.W. The psi-conducive syndrome: Free response GESP performance following evocation of 'left-hemispheric' vs. 'right-hemispheric' functioning. In Morris, J.D., Roll, W.G. and Morris, R.L. (eds) *Research in Parapsychology 1974*. Metuchen, New Jersey: Scarecrow Press, 1975.

Braud, W.G., Wood, R. and Braud, L.W. Free response GESP performance during an experimental hypnagogic state induced by visual and acoustic ganzfeld techniques: A replication and extension. *J. Amer. SPR*, 1975, 69, 105-14.

Brèton, A. *Manifeste du surréalisme*. Paris: Editions du Sagittaire, 1924.

Brindley, G., Gautier-Smith, P. and Lewin, W. Cortical blindness and the functions of the non-geniculate fibres of the optic tracts. *J. Neurol. Neurosurg. Psychiatry*, 1969, 32, 259-64.

Broadbent, D.F. *Perception and Communication*. London: Pergamon Press, 1958.

Brodal, A. *The Reticular Formation of the Brain Stem. Anatomical Aspects and Functional Correlations*. London: Oliver & Boyd, 1957.

Broughton, R.J., Poire, R. and Tassinari, C.A. The electrodermogram (Tarchanoff effect) during sleep. *Electroenceph. Clin. Neurophysiol.*, 1965, 18, 691-708.

Brown, B.B. Recognition of aspects of consciousness through association with EEG Alpha activity represented by a light signal. *Psychophysiology*, 1970, 6(4), 442-52.

Brown, J. *Mind, Brain, and Consciousness*. New York: Academic Press, 1977.

Brownfield, C.A. *Isolation: Clinical and Experimental Approaches*. New York: Alfred A. Knopf, 1965.

Bruner, J.S. *On Knowing*. Cambridge, Mass.: Belknap Press, 1962.

Buber, M. *I and Thou*. New York: Charles Scribner's Sons, 1958.

Buck, L.A. and Geers, M.B. Varieties of consciousness: Intercorrelations. *J. Clin. Psychol..*, 1967, 23, 151-2.

Budzynski, T.H. Feedback-induced muscle relaxation and activation level. Unpublished doctoral dissertation, University of Colorado, 1969.

Budzynski, T.H. Some applications of biofeedback-produced twilight states. *Fields Within Fields Within Fields*, 1972, 5, 105-14.

Budzynski, T.H. Tuning in on the twilight zone. *Psychology Today*, 1977, 11(3), 38-44.

Budzynski, T.H. and Stoyva, J.M. An instrument for producing deep muscle relaxation by means of analog information feedback. *J. Appl. Behav. Analysis*, 1969, 2(4), 231-7.

Bugelski, R.R. Words and things and images. *Amer. Psychologist*, 1970, 25, 1002-12.

Bülow, K. Respiration and wakefulness in man. *Acta Physiologica Scandinavica*, 1963, 59, Suppl. 209, 1-110.

Bunge, M. *Intuition and Science*. Englewood Cliffs, New Jersey: Prentice-Hall, 1962.

Burdach, K.F. *Die Physiologie als Erfahrungswissenschaft*. Leipzig: L. Vosz, 1839.

Butler, W.E. *How to Develop Clairvoyance*. London: Aquarian Press, 1968.

Butler, W.E. *The Magician: His Training and Work*. Hollywood, Cal.: Wilshire Book Co., 1969.

Butler, W.E. *How to Develop Psychometry*. Wellingborough, Northants: Aquarian Press, 1973.

Cade, C.M. and Coxhead, N. *The Awakened Mind*. London: Wildwood House, 1979.

Cairns, H. Disturbances of consciousness with lesions of the brain-stem and diencephalon. *Brain*, 1952, 75(2), 109-46.

Caldwell, W.V. *LSD Psychotherapy*. New York: Grove Press, 1968.

Cameron, N. Schizophrenic thinking in a problem-solving situation. *J. Ment. Science*, 1939, 85, 1012-35.

Cameron, N. Experimental analysis of schizophrenic thinking. In Kasanin, J.S. (ed.) *Language and Thought in Schizophrenia*. New York: Norton 1964.

Cane, F.E. The physiology of dreams. *The Lancet*, 1889, 2, 1330-1.

Cappon, D. and Banks, R. Preliminary study of endurance and perceptual change in sleep deprivation. *Perc. Mot. Skills*, 1960, 10, 99-104.

Cardano, H. *De Propria Vita Liber*. Paris: I. Villery, 1643.

Carrington, H. *Mental Telepathy*. Hollywood, Cal.: Wilshire Book Co., 1966.

Carrington, H. *Your Psychic Powers and How to Develop Them*. Newcastle Publishing Co., 1975.

Carrington, H. *Higher psychical development*. Wellingborough, Northants: Aquarian Press, 1978.

Cartwright, R.D., Monroe, L.J. and Palmer, C. Individual differences in response to REM deprivation. *Arch. Gen. Psychiatry*, 1967, 16, 297-303.

Cassirer, E. *Substance and Function*, New York: Dover, 1953.

Castaneda, C. *Tales of Power*. Harmondsworth: Penguin, 1976.

Chapman, L.J. and Taylor, J. Breadth of deviate concepts used by schizophrenics. *J. Abn. Social Psychol.*, 1957, 54, 118-23.

Christake, A. Conditioned emotional stimuli and arousal from sleep. *Amer. Psychologist*, 1957, 12, 405.

Clare, A. *Psychiatry in Dissent*. London: Tavistock Publications, 1976.

Cocteau, J. The process of inspiration. In Ghiselin, B. (ed.) *The Creative Process*. New York: New American Library, 1952.

Coleridge, S.M. Prefatory note to Kubla Khan. In Ghiselin, B. (ed.) *The Creative Process*. New York: New American Library, 1952.

Collard, P. Hypnagogic visions. *Light*, 1953, 73, 233-5.

Collier, R.M. Selected implications from a dynamic regulatory theory of consciousness. *Amer. Psychologist*, 1964, 19, 265-9.

Conel, J.L. *The Postnatal Development of the Human Cerebral Cortex. I. Cortex of the Newborn*. Cambridge, Mass.: Harvard University Press, 1939.

Connell, P.H. *Amphetamine Psychosis* (Maudsley Monograph no. 5). Institute of Psychiatry. London: Chapman, 1958.

Corriere, R. and Hart, J. *The Dream Makers*. New York: Funk & Wagnalls, 1977.

Costa, A.M. L'effetto geometrico-cromatico nella stimolazione intermittente della ochi chiuse. *Arch. Psicol. Neurol. Psic.*, 1953, 14, 632-5.

Crichton-Browne, J. Dreamy mental states. *The Lancet*, 1895, 2, 1-5 and 73-5.

Critchley, M. Neurological aspects of visual and auditory hallucinations. *Brit. Med. J.*, 1939, (23 September), 634-9.

Critchley, M. Sleep as a neurological problem. *Brit. Med. J.*, 1954, 2, 152-3.

Critchley, M. The pre-dormitum. *Rev. Neurologique*, 1955, 93, 101-6.

Cropley, A.J. S-R psychology and cognitive psychology. In Vernon, P.E. (ed.) *Creativity*. Harmondsworth: Penguin, 1978.

Cuenod, M., Casey, K. and McLean, P. Unit analysis of visual input to posterior limbic cortex. I. Photic stimulation. *J. Neurophysiol.*, 1965, 28, 1101-17.

Dali, S. Conquest of the irrational. In Dali, S. *The Secret Life of Salvador Dali*. London: Vision Press, 1976.

Davis, H., Davis, P.A., Loomis, A.L. Harvey, E.N. and Hobart, G. Changes in human brain potentials during the onset of sleep. *Science*, 1937, 86, 448-50.

Davis, H., Davis, P.A., Loomis, A.L., Harvey, E.N. and Hobart, G. Human brain potentials during the onset of sleep. *J. Neurophysiol.*, 1938, 1, 24-8.

Davis, H., Davis, P.A., Loomis, A.L., Harvey, E.N. and Hobart, G. Analysis of the electrical response of the human brain to auditory stimulation during sleep. *Amer. J. Physiol.*, 1939, 126, 474-5. (a).

Davis, H., Davis, P.A., Loomis, A.L., Harvey, E.N. and Hobart, G. Electrical reactions of human brain to auditory stimulation during sleep. *J. Neurophysiol.*, 1939, 2, 500-14. (b).

Davison, K. Schizophrenia-like psychoses associated with organic brain disease. Preliminary observations on fifty patients. *Newcastle Med. J.*, 1966, 30(3), 67-73.

De Bechterev, M.W. Des signes objectifs de la suggestion pendant le sommeil hypnotique. *Arch. de Psychol.*, 1906, 5, 103-7.

De Becker, R. *The Understanding of Dreams*. London: Allen & Unwin, 1968.

De Boismont, A.B. *On Hallucinations: A History and Explanation of Apparitions, Visions, Dreams, Ecstasy, Magnetism and Somnambulism*. Trans. by Hulme, R.T. London: H. Rehshaw, 1859.

Deikman, A. Experimental meditation. In Tart, C.T. (ed.) *Altered States of Consciousness*. New York: John Wiley & Sons, 1969. (a). (orig. 1963).

Deikman, A. De-automatization and the mystic experience. In Tart, C.T. (ed.) *Altered States of Consciousness*. New York: John Wiley, 1969. (b). (orig. 1966).

Deikman, A. Bimodal consciousness. *Arch. Gen. Psychiatry*, 1971, 25, 481-9.

Delage, Y. La nature des images hypnagogiques et le rôle des lueurs entoptiques dans le rêve. *Bull. Instit. Général Psychol.*, 1903 (August-September), 235-54.

De Lizi, L. Su di un fenomeno motorio costante del sonno normale: le mioclonie ipniche fisiologiche. *Riv. Pat. Nerv. Ment.*, 1932, 39, 481-96.

De Manacéine, M. *Sleep: Its Physiology, Pathology, Hygiene, and Psychology*. London: Scott, 1897.

Dement, W.C. The effect of dream deprivation. *Science*, 1960, 131, 1705-7.

Dement, W.C. Perception during sleep. In Hoch, P. and Zubin, J. (eds) *Psychopathology of Perception*. New York: Grune & Stratton, 1965.

Dement, W. and Kleitman, N. The relation of eye movements during sleep to dream activity: An objective method for the study of dreaming. *J. Exper. Psychol.*, 1957, 53(5), 339-46.

Dempsey, E. and Morison, R. The production of rhythmically recurrent cortical potentials after localized thalamic stimulations. *Amer. J. Physiol.*, 1942, 135, 293-300.

Descartes, R. *The Philosophical Works of Descartes*. 2 vols. Edited by Haldane, E. and Ross, G. Cambridge University Press, 1934.

Descartes, R. *Descartes: Philosophical Writings*. Trans. and edited by Anscombe, E. and Geach, P. Sunbury-on-Thames: Nelson, 1976.

Desoille, R. *The Directed Daydream*. New York: Psycho-synthesis Research Foundation, 1966.

Dessoir, M. Experiments in muscle-reading and thought-transference. *Proc. SPR*, 1886, 4, 111-26.

De Strooper, J. and Broughton, R. REM awakening latencies and a possible REM breakthrough phenomenon. *Psychophysiology*, 1969, 6, 216.

De Vries, R.A. and Kappers, J.A. Influence of the pineal gland on the neurosecretory activity of the supraoptic hypothalamic nucleus of the male rat. *Neuroendocrinology*, 1971, 8, 359-66.

Doob, L.W. Eidetic images among the Ibo. *Ethnology*, 1964, 3, 357-63.

Doob, L.W. Exploring eidetic imagery among the Kamba of central Kenya. *J. Soc. Psychol.*, 1965, 67, 3-22.

Doob, L.W. Eidetic imagery: a cross cultural will-o'-the wisp? *J. Psychol.*, 1966, 63, 13-34.

Douglas, R.J. The hippocampus and behaviour. *Psychol. Bull.*, 1967, 67, 416-42.

Downey, J.E. An experiment on getting an after-image from a mental image. *Psychol. Review*, 1901, 8, 42-55.

Drever, J. *A Dictionary of Psychology*. Harmondsworth: Penguin, 1964 (revised edn).

Dudley, G.A. *Dreams*. New York: Samuel Weiser, 1979.

Edmunds, H.T. *Psychism and the Unconscious Mind*. London: Theosophical Publishing House, 1968.

Edwards, H. *A Guide for the Development of Mediumship*. London: Spiritualist Association of Great Britain (1960s: undated).

Ehrenzweig, A. The undifferentiated matrix of artistic imagination. In Neusterberger, W. and Axelrad, S. (eds) *The Psychoanalytic Study of Society*. New York: International Universities Press, 1964.

Einstein, A. Letter to Jacques Hadamard. In Ghiselin, B. (ed.) *The Creative Process*. New York: New American Library, 1952.

Eldred, E. and Fujimori, B. Relations of the reticular formation to muscle spindle activity. In *The Reticular Formation of the Brain: International Symposium*. Boston: Little Brown, 1958.

Eliade, M. *Myths, Dreams, and Mysteries*. London: Collins, 1976.

Ellis, H. A note on hypnagogic paramnesia. *Mind*, 1897, 6 (ix-Notes), 283-7.

Ellis, H. *The World of Dreams*. London: Constable, 1911.

Emde, R. and Metcalf, D. An electroencephalographic study of behavioral rapid eye movement states in the human newborn. *J. Nerv. Ment. Dis.*, 1970, 150, 376-86.

Erdelyi, M.H. A new look at the new look: perceptual defence and vigilance. *Psychol. Review*, 1974, 81, 1-25.

Erickson, M.H. The confusion technique in hypnosis. *Amer. J. Clin. Hypnosis*, 1964, 6(3), 183-207.

Erickson, M.H. and Erickson, E.M. The hypnotic induction of hallucinatory colour vision followed by pseudo-negative after-images. *J. Exp. Psychol.*, 1938, 22, 581-8.

Erickson, M.H., Rossi, E.L. and Rossi, S.I. *Hypnotic Realities*. New York: Irvington, 1976.

Ernst, M. Inspiration to order. In Ghiselin, B. (ed.) *The Creative Process*. New York: New American Library, 1952.

Evans-Wentz, W.Y. (ed.) *Tibetan Yoga and Secret Doctrines*. New York: Oxford University Press, 1978.

Evarts, E.V. A neurophysiologic theory of hallucinations. In West, L.J. (ed.) *Hallucinations*. New York: Grune & Stratton, 1962.

Ey, H. Les hallucinoses. *L'Encephale*, 1957, 46, 564-73.

Faraday, A. *Dream Power*. London: Hodder & Stoughton, 1972.

Federn, P. *Ego Psychology and the Psychoses*. New York: Basic Books, 1952.

Fenwick, P., Schatzman, M., Worsley, A., Adams, J., Stone, S. and Baker, A. Lucid dreaming: Correspondence between dreamed and actual events in one subject during REM sleep. *Biol. Psychol.*, 1984, 18, 243-52.

Féré, C. Sensation et mouvement. *Rev. Phil.*, 1885, 20, 337-68.

Festinger, L. *A Theory of Cognitive Dissonance*. Evanston: Row, Peterson, 1957.

Finke, R.A. Levels of equivalence in imagery and perception. *Psychol. Review*, 1980, 87(2), 113-32.

Finley, K.H. On the occurrence of rapid frequency potential changes in the human electroencephalogram. *Amer. J. Psychiatry*, 1944, 101, 194-200.

Fischer, R. Transformations of consciousness. A cartography. I: The perception-hallucination continuum. *Conf. Psychiat.*, 1975, 18(4), 221-44.

Fischgold, H. and Safar, S. États de demi-sommeil et images hypnagogiques. In *Rêve et conscience*. Paris: Presses Universitaires de France, 1968.

Fish, F. A neurophysiological theory of schizophrenia. *J. Ment. Science*, 1961, 107, 828-38.

Fisher, S. Body image boundaries and hallucinations. In West, L.J. (ed.) *Hallucinations*. New York: Grune & Stratton, 1962.

Fiss, H., Klein, G.S. and Bokert, E. Waking fantasies following interruption of two types of sleep. *Arch. Gen. Psychiatry*, 1966, 14, 543-51.

Fleisch, A. Erregbarkeitsaenderung des Atmungszentrums durch Schlaf. *Pfluegers Arch.*, 1929, 221, 378-85

Flemenbaum, A. Pavor nocturnus: a complication of single daily tricyclics or neuroleptic dosage. *Amer. J. Psychiatry*, 1976, 133, 570-2.

Forbes, A. Dream scintillations. *Psychosom. Medicine*, 1949, 11, 160-2.

Foulkes, D. Dream reports from different stages of sleep. *J. Abn. Soc. Psychol.*, 1962, 65(1), 14-25.

Foulkes, D. Nonrapid eye movement mentation. In Clemente, C.D. (ed.) *Experimental Neurology Supplement 4: Physiological Correlates of Dreaming*, 1967.

Foulkes, D. Longitudinal studies of dreams in children. In Masserman J.H. (ed.) *Science and Psychoanalysis* (vol. 19). New York: Grune & Stratton, 1971.

Foulkes, D., Spear, P.S. and Symonds, J.D. Individual differences in mental activity at sleep onset. *J. Abn. Psychol.*, 1966, 71(4), 280-6.

Foulkes, D. and Vogel, G. Mental activity at sleep onset. *J. Abn. Psychol.*, 1965, 70, 231-43.

Fox, O. *Astral Projection*. New York: University Books, 1962 (new edn).

Frazer, J.G. *The Golden Bough: A Study in Magic and Religion*. London: Macmillan Press, 1976, (abr. edn).

Freedman, S.J. and Greenblatt, M. Studies in human isolation: II. Hallucinations and other cognitive findings. *US Armed Forces Med. J.*, 1960, 11, 1479-97.

Freedman, S.J., Grunebaum, H.V., Stare, F.A., and Greenblatt, M. Imagery in sensory deprivation. In West, L.J. (ed.) *Hallucinations*. New York: Grune & Stratton, 1962.

Freedman, S.J. and Marks, P.A. Visual imagery produced by rhythmic photic stimulation: personality correlates and phenomenology. *Brit. J. Psychol.*, 1965, 56(1), 95-112.

Freud, S. *A General Introduction to Psychoanalysis*. Garden City, New York: Doubleday, 1943.

Freud, S. The interpretation of dreams. In Strachey, J. (ed.) *Standard Edition of the Complete Psychological Works of Sigmund Freud*. London: Hogarth Press, 1953.

Frith, C.D. Consciousness, information processing and schizophrenia. *Brit. J. Psychiatry*, 1979, 134, 225-35.

Froeschels, E. A peculiar intermediary state between waking and sleep. *J. Clin. Psychopath. Psychotherapy*, 1946, 7(4), 825-33.

Froeschels, E. A peculiar intermediary state between waking and sleeping. *Amer. J. Psychotherapy*, 1949, 3, 19-25.

Frost, G. and Frost, Y. *Astral Travel*. St Albans, Herts: Granada, 1982.

Fruhstorfer, H. and Bergström, R.H. Human vigilance and auditory evoked responses. *Electroenceph. Clin. Neurophysiol.*, 1969, 27, 346-55.

Fruhstorfer, H., Partanen, J. and Lumio, J. Vertex sharp waves and heart action during the onset of sleep. *Electroenceph. Clin. Neurophysiol.*, 1971, 31, 614-17.

Galin, D. Implications for psychiatry of left and right cerebral specialization. *Arch. Gen. Psychiatry*, 1974, 31, 572-83.

Galin, D. and Ornstein, R. Lateral specialization of cognitive mode: An EEG study. *Psychophysiology*, 1972, 9, 412-18.

Galton, F. Statistics of mental imagery. *Mind*, 1880, 5, 300-18.

Galton, F. The visions of sane persons. *Fortnightly*, 1881, 35, 729-40.

Galton, F. *Inquiries into Human Faculty and its Development*. London: Macmillan, 1883.

Garfield, P. *Creative Dreaming*. London: Futura, 1976.

Garrett, E. *Telepathy: In Search of a Lost Faculty*. New York: Creative Age Press, 1941.

Garrett, E. *My Life as a Search for the Meaning of Mediumship*. London: Ryder, 1949.

Garrett, E. *The Sense and Nonsense of Prophesy*. New York: Creative Age Press, 1950.

Gastaut, H. Hypnosis and pre-sleep patterns. In Chertok, L. (ed.) *Psychophysiological Mechanisms of Hypnosis*. Berlin: Springer-Verlag, 1969.

Gazzaniga, M.S. *The Bisected Brain*. New York: Appleton-Century-Crofts, 1970.

Gellé, M. Communication submitted to the Société de Psychologie, 4 December 1903.

Gellhorn, E. and Loofbourrow, G. *Emotions and Emotional Disorders*. New York: Hoeber, 1963.

Gengerilli, J.A. Some quantitative experiments with eidetic imagery. *Amer. J. Psychol.*, 1930, 42, 399-404.

Gerard, R.W. What is imagination? In Harris, T. and Schawn, W. (eds) *Selected Readings on the Learning Process*. New York: Oxford University Press, 1961.

Ghiselin, B. (ed.) *The Creative Process: A Symposium*. New York: New American Library, 1952.

Gibson, E.P. A Study in comparative performance in several ESP procedures. *J. Parapsychol.*, 1937, I, 264-75.

Gill, M. and Brenman, M. *Hypnosis and Related States: Psychoanalytic Studies in Regression*. New York: International Universities Press, 1959.

Globus, G. Rapid eye movements in real time. *Arch. Gen. Psychiatry*, 1966, 15, 654-9.

Goldenberg, G., Podreka, I., Höll, K. and Steiner, M. Changes in cerebral blood flow pattern caused by visual imagery: an IMP-SPECT study. Paper presented at the 2nd International Imagery Conference, University College of Swansea, Wales, April 1985.

Goldberger, L. and Holt, R.R. Experimental interference with reality contact (perceptual isolation): method and group results. *J. Nerv. Ment. Dis.*, 1958, 127, 99-112.

Goldberger, L. and Holt, R.R. *A Comparison of Isolation Effects and their Personality Correlates in Two Divergent Samples*. ASD Tech. Rep. 61-417. Ohio: Wright-Patterson AFB, 1961.

Goldie, L. and Green, J.M. Changes in mode of respiration as an indication of level of awareness. *Nature*, 1961, 189, 581-2.

Goldstone, S. Psychophysics, reality and hallucinations. In West, L.J. (ed.) *Hallucinations*. New York: Grune & Stratton, 1962.

Golla, F. Electrophysiology in psychiatry. In Harris, N. (ed.) *Modern Trends in Psychological Medicine*. London: Butterworth, 1948.

Gowan, J.C. *Trance, Art and Creativity*. Buffalo: Creative Education Foundation, 1975.

Gowan, J.C. The view from myopia. *Gifted Child Quarterly*, 1976, 20, 378-87.

Granda, A. and Hammack, J. Operant behavior during sleep. *Science*, 1961, 133, 1485-6.

Greeley, A.M. *Ecstasy: A Way of Knowing*. Englewood Cliffs, New Jersey: Prentice Hall, 1974.

Green, C. *Lucid Dreams*. Oxford: Institute of Psychophysical research, 1968. (a).

Green, C. *Out of the Body Expreiences*. Oxford: Proc. Inst. Psychophys. Res., 1968, 2. (b).

Green, C. and McCreery, C. *Apparitions*. Oxford: Institute of Psychophysical Research, 1975.

Green, E. and Green, A. *Beyond Biofeedback*. London: Bell Press, 1978.

Green, E., Green, A. and Walters, D. Voluntary control of internal states: Psychological and physiological. *J. Transpers. Psychol.*, 1970, 1, 1-26.

Green, E., Green, A. and Walters, D. *Biofeedback for Mind-Body Self Regulation: Healing and Creativity* (mimeo). Topeka, Kansas: Menninger clinic, 1971. (a).

Green, E., Green, A. and Walters, D. *Psychophysiological training for creativity* (mimeo). Topeka, Kansas: Menninger Clinic, 1971. (b).

Green, H. Heat-craze my teeth in bitterest anger. Selection from *I Never Promised You a Rose Garden*. In Fadiman, J. and Kewman, D. (eds) *Exploring Madness: Experience, Theory, and Research*. Monterey, Cal.: Brooks/Cole, 1973.

Greenwood, F. Faces in the dark. *St James's Gazette*, 1882, 10 February.

Greenwood, F. *Imagination in Dreams and Their Study*. London: J. Lane, 1894.

Grey, M. *Return from Death*. London: Routledge & Kegan Paul, 1985.

Griffin, D.R. *The Question of Animal Awareness*. New York: Rockefeller University Press, 1976.

Griffiths, G.M. and Fox, J.T. Rhythm in epilepsy. *Lancet*, 1938, 235, 409-16.

Griffitts, C.H. Individual differences in imagery. *Psychol. Monogr.*, 1927, 37, whole no. 172.

Grollman, A. Physiological variations in the cardiac output of man. XI. Pulse rate, blood pressure, oxygen consumption, arterio-venous oxygen difference and cardiac output of man during normal nocturnal sleep. *Amer. J. Psysiol.*, 1930, 95, 274-84.

Gruithuisen, F.v.P. *Beyträge zur Physiognosie und Eautognosie. Für Freunde der Naturforschung auf dem Erfahrungswege*. Munich: I.J. Lentner, 1812.

Guilford, J.P. Creativity. *Amer. Psychologist*, 1950, 5, 444-54.

Guilford, J.P. Factors that aid and hinder creativity. In Gowan, J.C., Demos, G.D. and Torrance, E.P. (eds), *Creativity: Its Educational Implications*. New York: Wiley & Sons, 1967.

Gurney, E., Myers, F.W.H. and Podmore, F. *Phantasms of the Living*. London: Trubner, 1886.

Guyon, E. *Sur les Hallucinations hypnagogiques, en général et dans la chorée*. These fac. de méd. de Paris: Libr. Méd. et Scient. Jules Rousset, 1903.

Haber, R.N. Eidetic imagery – real or imagined? *Scient. American*, 1969, 220, 36-44.

Haber, R.N. Twenty years of haunting eidetic imagery: Where's the ghost? *Behav. Brain Sciences*, 1979, 2, 583-629.

Haber R.N. and Haber, R.B. Eidetic imagery I: Frequency. *Perc. Mot. Skills*, 1964, 19, 131-8.

Hadamard, J. *The Psychology of Invention in the Mathematical Field*. New Jersey: Princeton University Press, 1949.

Haldane, J. and Priestley, J. *Respiration*. Oxford: Clarendon Press, 1935.

Hallman, R.J. The necessary and sufficient conditions of creativity. In Gowan, J.C., Demos, G.D. and Torrance, E.P. (eds) *Creativity: Its Educational Implications*. New York: John Wiley & Sons, 1967.

Hanawalt, N.G. Recurrent images: New instances and a summary of the older ones. *Amer. J. Psychol.*, 1954, 67, 170-4.

Harriman, P.L. The dream of falling. *J. Gen. Psychol.*, 1939, 20, 229-33.

Hatakeyama, T. The constructive character of eidetic imagery. *Tohoku Psychologica Folia*, 1975, 34, 38-51.

Head, H. Certain mental changes that accompany visceral disease. *Brain*, 1901, 24(3), 345-429.

Hearne, K.M.T. Lucid dreams: an electrophysiological and psychological study. Unpublished PhD thesis, University of Liverpool, 1978.

Hearne, K.M.T. 'Lucid' dreams and ESP: An initial experiment using one subject. *J. of the SPR*, 1981, 51, 7-11.

Hearne, K.M.T. Effects of performing certain set tasks in the lucid-dream state. *Perc. Mot. Skills*, 1982, 54, 259-62.

Hebb, D.O. The problem of consciousness and introspection. In Delafresnaye, J.F. (ed.) *Brain Mechanisms and Consciousness*. Oxford: Blackwell, 1954.

Hebb, D.O. Concerning imagery. *Psychol. Review*, 1968, 75(6), 466-77.

Heisenberg, W. *Physics and Beyond*. London: Allen & Unwin, 1971.

Hemmingsen, R. and Rafaelsen, O. Hypnagogic and hypnopompic hallucinations during amitriptyline treatment. *Acta Psychiat. Scand.*, 1980, 62, 364-8.

Hess, W.R. *The Functional Organization of the Diencephalon*. New York: Grune & Stratton, 1957.

Heywood, R. *ESP: A Personal Memoir*. New York: Dutton, 1964.

Hicks, G.D. On the nature of images. *Brit. J. Psychol.*, 1924, 15, 121-48.

Hilgard, E.R. *The Experience of Hypnosis*. New York: Harcourt Brace Jovanovich, 1968.

Hilgard, E.R. A neodissociation interpretation of pain reduction in hypnosis. *Psychol. Review*, 1973, 80(5), 396-411.

Hill, D. and Parr, G. (eds) *Electroencephalography. A Symposium on its Various Aspects*. London: Macdonald, 1950.

Hobbes, T. *Leviathan*. London: A. Crooke, 1651.

Hoche, A. Der Traum. In Bethe, A., Bergmann, G.V., Embden, G. and Ellinger, A. (eds) *Handbuch der Normalen und Pathologischen Physiologie* (vol. 17), correlation III. Berlin: Julius Springer, 1926.

Hollingworth, H. The psychology of drowsiness. *Amer. J. Psychol.*, 1911, 22, 99-111.

Holt, R.R. Imagery: The return of the ostracized. *Amer. Psychologist*, 1964, 19, 254-64.

Holt. R.R. On the nature and generality of mental imagery. In Sheehan, P. (ed.) *The Function and Nature of Imagery*. New York: Academic Press, 1972.

Holt, R. and Goldberger, L. *Personological Correlates of Reactions to Perceptual Isolation*. W.A.D.C. Tech. Rep. 59-375. Ohio: Wright-Patterson AFB, 1959.

Holt, R. and Goldberger, L. Assessment of individual resistance to sensory alteration. In B. Flahery (ed.) *Psychophysiological Aspects of Space Flight*. New York: Columbia University Press, 1961.

Honorton, C. Psi-conducive states of awareness. In Mitchell, E.D. and White, J. (eds) *Psychic Exploration*. New York: Putnam's Sons, 1974.

Honorton, C. Psi and internal attention states. In Wolman, B.B. (ed.) *Handbook of Parapsychology*. New York: Van Nostrand Reinhold, 1977.

Honorton, C. and Harper, S. Psi-mediated imagery and ideation in an experimental procedure for regulating perceptual input. *J. Amer. SPR*, 1974, 68, 156-68.

Horowitz, M.J. Body image. *Arch. Gen. Psychiatry*, 1966, 14, 456-60.

Horowitz, M.J. Visual imagery and cognitive organization. *Amer. J. Psychiatry*, 1967, 123, 938-46.

Horowitz, M.J. *Image Formation and Cognition*. New York: Appleton-Century-Crofts, 1978.

Horowitz, M., Adams, J. and Rutkin, B. Dream scintillations. *Psychosom. Med.*, 1967, 29, 284-92.

Horowitz, M., Adams, J. and Rutkin, B. Visual imagery on brain stimulation. *Arch. Gen. Psychiatry*, 1968, 19, 469-86.

Hoskins, R.G. Schizophrenia from the physiological point of view. *Ann. Internat. Med.*, 1933, 7, 445-56.

House, H. *Aristotle's Poetics*. London: Rupert Hart-Davis, 1967.

Housman, A.E. The name and nature of poetry. In Ghiselin, B. (ed.) *The Creative Process*. New York: New American Library, 1952.

Huapaya, L. Somnambulism and bedtime medication. *Amer. J. Psychiatry*, 1976, 133, 1207.

Hudson, L. *Contrary Imaginations*. Harmondsworth: Penguin, 1968.

Hudson, L. *The Psychology of Human Experience*. Garden City, New York: Anchor Press/Doubleday, 1975.

Hull, C.L. Psychology of the scientist: IV. Passages from the 'Idea Books' of Clark L. Hull. *Perc. Mot. Skills*, 1962, 15, 807-82.

Hume, D. A treatise of human nature. Glasgow: Collins, 1975. (orig. 1739-40).

Humphrey, N. and Weiskrantz, L. Vision in monkeys after removal of the striate cortex. *Nature* (Lond.), 1967, 215, 595-7.

Hunter, J. and Jasper, H. Effects of thalamic stimulation in unanaesthetised animals. *Electroenceph. Clin. Neurophysiol.*, 1949, 1, 305-24.

Huson, P. *How to Test and Develop your ESP*. London: Sphere Books (Abacus), 1977.

Hutchinson, E.D. Varieties of insight in humans. *Psychiatry*, 1939, 2, 323-32.

Huttenlocher, P. Evoked and spontaneous activity in single units of medial brain stem during natural sleep and waking. *J. Neurophysiol.*, 1961, 24, 451-68.

Hyman, M. An investigation of cognitive process in schizophrenia. Unpublished doctoral dissertation. University of California, 1953.

Hyslop, J.H. Introduction to 'A further record of experiments'. *Proc. Amer. SPR*, 1908, 2(3), 378-453.

Iamblichus. The epistle of Porphyry to the Egyptian Anebo. In *Iamblichus on the Mysteries of the Egyptians, Chaldeans, and Assyrians*. Trans. by Taylor, T. London: B. Dobell, and Reeves & Turner, 1895.

Isakower, O. A contribution to the pathopsychology of phenomena associated with falling asleep. *Internat. J. Psychoanalysis*, 1938, 19, 331-45.

Ishibashi, T., Hori, H., Endo, K. and Sato, T. Hallucinations produced by electrical stimulation of the temporal lobes in schizophrenic patients. *Tohoku J. Exp. Medicine*, 1964, 82, 124-39.

Ivanov, A. Soviet experiments in 'eye-less vision'. *Internat. J. Parapsychology*, 1964, 6, 7-23.

Jackson, J.H. In Taylor, J. (ed.) *Selected Writings*, vol. 2. New York: Basic Books, 1958.

Jacobson, A., Kales, A., Lehmann, D. and Hoedemaker, F.S. Muscle tonus in human subjects during sleep and waking. *Exp. Neurol.*, 1964, 10, 418-24.

Jacobson, E. *Progressive Relaxation*. Chicago: University of Chicago Press, 1929.

Jádi, F. and Trixler, M. Hypnagogic hallucinations in art therapy. *Arts in Psychotherapy*, 1982, 67, 3-4.

Jaensch, E.R. *Eidetic Imagery*. London: Kegan Paul, 1930.

James, W. *Principles of Psychology*. London: Macmillan, 1890.

James, W. *The Varieties of Religious Experience*. London: Collins (Fontana), 1975.

Japp, F.R. Kekulé memorial lecture. *J. Chem. Society*, 1898, 73, 97-138.

Jasper, H., Cruikshank, R. and Howard, H. Action currents from the occipital region of the brain in man as affected by variables of attention and external stimulation. *Psychol. Bull.*, 1935, 32, 565.

Jasper, H. and Droogleever-Fortuyn, J. Experimental studies of the functional anatomy of petit mal epilepsy. *Res. Publ. Ass. Nerv. Ment. Dis.*, 1947, 26, 272-98.

Jaspers, K. *General Psychopathology*. Trans. (from 7th edn) by Hoenig, J. and Hamilton, M.W. Manchester: Manchester University Press, 1959. (orig. 1913).

Jéquier, M. Hallucinations hypnagogiques. *Rev. Med. Suisse Rom.*, 1940, 60, 530-9.

Johnson, L.C., and Karpan, W. Autonomic correlates of the spontaneous K-complex. *Psychophysiology*, 1968, 4, 444-52.

Jouvet, D., Valatx, J. and Jouvet, M. Étude polygraphique du sommeil du chaton. *C.R. Soc. Biol. (Par.)*, 1961, 155, 1660-4.

Jouvet, M. The stages of sleep. *Scient. Amer.*, 1967, 216, 62-72.

Jung, C.G. *The Psychology of Dementia Praecox*. Trans. by Peterson, F. and Brill, A. New York: Journal of Nervous and Mental Disease Publishing Co., 1909.

Jung, C.G. *Psychology of the Unconscious*. London: Kegan Paul, 1944. (orig. 1919).

Jung, C.G. *The Collected Works of C.G. Jung*. Ed. Read, H.J. Fordham, M. and Adler, G. London: Princeton University Press, 1953-9.

Kamiya, J. Behaviour, subjective, and physiological aspects of drowsiness and sleep. In Fiske, W. and Maddi, S. (eds) *Functions of Varied Experience*. Homewood, Ill.: Dorsey Press, 1961.

Kanner, L. *Child Psychiatry*. Springfield, Ill.: Charles C. Thomas, 1957, (3rd edn).

Kant, I. *Träume eines Geistersehers, erläutert durch Träume der Metaphysik*. Berlin: Georg Reimer, 1905. (orig. 1766).

Kappers, J.A. The pineal organ: an introduction. In Wolstenholme, G. and Knight, J. (eds) *The Pineal Gland* (Ciba Foundation symposium). Edinburgh and London: Churchill Livingstone, 1971.

Kappers, J.A. The mammalian pineal gland: a survey. *Acta Neurochir.*, 1976, 34, 109-49.

Kappers, J.A. and Schadé, J.P. (eds) Structure and functions of the epiphysis cerebri. *Prog. Brain Research*, 1965, 10.

Kasamatsu, A. and Hirai, T. Science of Zazen. *Psychologia*, 1963, 6, 86-91.

Kasamatsu, A. and Hirai, T. An electroencephalographic study of the Zen meditation (Zazen). *Folia Psychiat. Neurol. Jap.*, 1966, 20(4), 315-36.

Kasanin, J.S. Concluding remarks. In Kasanin, J.S. (ed.) *Language and Thought in Schizophrenia*. New York: Norton, 1964.

Katz, D. *Psychological Atlas*. New York: Philosophical Library, 1948.

Kelly, C.P. *The Natural Way to Healthful Sleep*. London: Darton, Longman & Todd, 1962.

Kelly, G. *The Psychology of Personal Constructs*. New York: Norton, 1955.

Kennard, M.A. Electroencephalogram of decorticate monkeys. *J. Neurophysiol.*, 1943, 6, 233-42.

Kennard, M. and Nims, L. Changes in normal electroencephalogram of Macaca mulatta with growth. *J. Neurophysiol.*, 1942, 5, 325-33. (a).

Kennard, M. and Nims, L. Effect on electroencephalogram of lesions of cerebral cortex and basal ganglia in Macaca Mulatta, *J. Neurophysiol.*, 1942, 5, 335-48. (b).

Klein, D.C. The Pineal gland: a model of neuroendocrine regulation. *Res. Publs Ass. Nerv. Ment. Dis.*, 1978, 56, 303-27.

Klein, D.F. Visual hallucinations with imipramine. *Amer. J. Psychiatry*, 1965, 121, 911-14.

Kleitman, N. *Sleep and Wakefulness*. Chicago: University of Chicago Press, 1967 (revised edn).

Kleitman, N. Basic rest activity cycle in relation to sleep and wakefulness. In Kales, A. (ed.) *Sleep: Physiology and Pathology*. Philadelphia: Lippincott, 1969.

Klopfer, B., Ainsworth, M., Klopfer, W. and Holt, R. *Developments in Rorschach Technique. I. Technique and Theory*. New York: World Book, 1954.

Klüver, H. An experimental study of the eidetic type. *Genet. Psychol. Monogr.*, 1926, i, 70-230.

Klüver, H. Studies on the eidetic type and on eidetic imagery. *Psychol. Bull.*, 1928, 25, 69-104. (a).

Klüver, H. *Mescal: The 'Divine' Plant and its Psychological Effects*. London: Kegan Paul, Trench, Trubner, 1928. (b).

Klüver, H. Fragmentary eidetic imagery. *Psychol. Review*, 1930, 37, 441-58.

Klüver, H. Eidetic phenomena. *Psychol. Bull.*, 1932, 29, 181-203.

Klüver, H. Visual functions after removal of the occipital lobes. *J. Psychol.*, 1941, 11, 23-45.

Klüver, H. Mechanisms of hallucinations. In McNemar, Q. and Merrill, M. (eds) *Studies in Personality: Contributed in Honour of Lewis M. Terman*. New York: McGraw-Hill, 1942.

Knoll, M. and Kugler, J. Subjective light pattern spectroscopy in the electroencephalographic frequency range. *Nature*, 1959, 184, 1823.

Knoll, M. and Kugler, J. *Pulse Current Analysis of Elementary Visual Hallucinations by Coincidence Circuits in the Brain*. Internat. Conf. Microwaves, Circuit Theory, Information Theory, part 2, Tokyo, 1964.

Knoll, M., Kugler, J., Eichmeier, J. and Höfer, O. Note on the spectroscopy of subjective light patterns. *J. Anal. Psychol.*, 1962, 7, 55-70.

Koestler, A. *The Invisible Writing*. New York: Macmillan, 1954.

Koestler, A. *The Roots of Coincidence*. London: Hutchinson, 1974.

Koestler, A. *The Ghost in the Machine*. London: Pan Books, 1978.

Koestler, A. *The Act of Creation*. London: Pan Books, 1981.

Koffka, K. *Zur Analyse der Vorstellungen und ihrer Gesetze*. Leipzig: Quelle & Meyer, 1912.

Kosslyn, S. Visual Imagery and cerebral lateralization: a computational approach. Paper presented at the 2nd International Imagery Conference, University College of Swansea, Wales, April 1985.

Kraepelin, E. *Über Sprachstorungen im Traume*. Leipzig: Engelman, 1906.

Kripke, D.F. Ultradian rhythms in sleep and wakefulness. In Weitzman, E.D. (ed.) *Advances in Sleep Research*, vol. 1. New York: Spectrum Publications, 1974.

Krippner, S. An Experiment in search of psi-favorable states of consciousness. Paper presented at Duke University, Durham, North Carolina, 10 October, 1970.

Kris, E. On inspiration. *Internat. J. Psychoanalysis*, 1939, 20, 377-89.

Kubie, L. The use of induced hypnagogic reveries in the recovery of repressed amnesic data. *Bull. Menninger Clinic*, 1943, 7, 172-82.

Kubie, L. *Neurotic Distortion in the Creative Process*. Kansas: University of Kansas Press, 1958.

Kubie, L. and Margolin, S. A physiological method for the induction of states of partial sleep, and securing free associations and early memories in such states. *Trans. Amer. Neurol. Assn.*, 1942, 68, 136-9.

Kubie, L. and Margolin, S. An apparatus for the use of breath sounds as a hypnagogic stimulus. *Amer. J. Psychiatry*, 1944, 100, 610. (a).

Kubie, L. and Margolin, S. The process of hypnotism and the nature of the hypnotic state. *Amer. J. Psychiatry*, 1944, 100, 611-22. (b).

Kübler-Ross, E. *Death: The Final Stages of Growth*. New Jersey: Prentice-Hall, 1978.

La Berge, S. Lucid dreaming: An exploratory study of consciousness during sleep. Unpublished doctoral dissertation. Stanford University, Cal., 1980.

La Berge, S. Lucid dreaming. *Psychology Today*, 1981 (January), 48-57.

Labhardt, F. *Die Schizophrenieähnlichen Emotionspsychosen*. Berlin: Springer, 1963.

Ladd, G.T. Contribution to the psychology of visual dreams. *Mind*, 1892, 1, 299-304.

Laing, R.D. *The Politics of Experience*. Harmondsworth: Penguin, 1976. (orig. 1967).

Laird, D. and Laird, E. *Sound Ways to Sound Sleep*. New York: McGraw-Hill, 1959.

Langworthy, O.R. Development of the behavior patterns and myelinization of the nervous system in the human fetus and infant. *Contributions to Embryology*, 1933, 24(139): Carnegie Institute Publication no. 443.

Lavie, P. Differential effects of REM and non-REM awakenings on the spiral after effect. *Physiol. Psychology*, 1974, 2, 107-8.

Lavie, P. and Giora, Z. Spiral aftereffect durations following awakening from REM sleep and non-REM sleep. *Perceptions and Psychophysics*, 1973, 14, 19-20.

Leadbeater, C.W. *The Chakras*. Adyar, Madras: Theosophical Publishing House, 1966, (orig. 1927).

Leaning, F.E. An introductory study of hypnagogic phenomena. *Proc. SPR*, 1925, 35, 289-409. (a).

Leaning, F.E. Hypnagogic phenomena. *Journal of the SPR*, 1925, 22, 146-54. (b).

Leary, T. The religious experience: Its production and interpretation. *Psychedelic Review*, 1964, 1, 324-46.

Lecky, P. *Self-consistency: A Theory of Personality*. New York: Island Press, 1945.

Lehman, H., Cahn, G. and De Verteuil, R. The treatment of depressive conditions with imipramine. *Canad. Psychol. Assn. J.*, 1958, 3, 155-64.

Leiderman, P.H. Imagery and sensory deprivation. *Proc. Third World Congress Psychiatry*, 1964, 227-31.

Leroy, E.B. *Les Visions du demi-sommeil*. Paris: Librarie Felix Alcan, 1933. (orig. 1926).

Leroy, E.B. and Tobolowska, J. Sur les relations qui existent entre certaines hallucinations du rêve et les images du langage intérieur. *Bull. Instit. Psychol. Internat.*, 1901, 5, 241-48.

Le Shan, L. *Toward a General Theory of the Paranormal: A Report of Work in Progress*. New York: Parapsychological Foundation, 1973.

Le Shan, L. *The Medium, the Mystic, and the Physicist*. New York: Viking Press, 1974.

Le Shan, L. *Alternate Realities*. London: Sheldon Press, 1976.

Leuner, H. The interpretation of visual hallucinations. In *Psychopathology and Pictorial Expression*. Sandoz, 1963.

Lewin, B.D. Remarks on creativity, imagery, and the dream. *J. Nerv. Ment. Dis.*, 1969, 149, 115-21.

Lewin, R. Blindsight. *Psychology Today*, 1975, 1(4), 53-61.

Lhermitte, J. *Le Sommeil*. Paris: Gautier-Villars, 1925.

Lhermitte, J. L'hallucinose pédonculaire. *L'Encéphale*, 1932, 27, 422-35.

Lhermitte, J. Désordre de la function hypnique et hallucinations. *Annales Med.-Psycholog.*, 1938, 15, 1-14.

Lhermitte, J. and Sigwald, J. Hypnagogisme, hallucinose et hallucinations. *Rev. Neurol.*, 1941, 73, 225-38.

Lhermitte, J. and Tournay, A. Le sommeil normal et pathologique. *Rev. Neurol.*, 1927, 1, 751-822 and 885-7.

Liberson, W.T. and Liberson, C.W. EEG records, reaction times, eye movements, respiration, and mental content during drowsiness. In Wortis, J. (ed.) *Recent Advances in Biological Psychiatry* (vol. 8). New York: Plenum Press, 1966.

Liddon, S.C. Sleep paralysis and hypnagogic hallucinations: Their relationship to the nightmare. *Arch. Gen. Psychiatry*, 1967, 17, 88-96.

Lilly, J.C. Mental effects of reduction of ordinary levels of physical stimuli on intact, healthy persons. In Lilly, J.C. *The Deep Self*. New York: Warner Books, 1977.

Linschoten, J. Ueber das Einschlafen. I. Einschlafen und Erleben. II. Einschlafen und Tun. *Psychol. Beitr.*, 1956, 2, 70-97 and 266-98.

Locke, J. *An Essay Concerning Human Understanding*. Glasgow: Collins, 1964. (orig. 1690).

Lodge, O. An account of some experiments in thought-transference. *Proc. SPR*, 1884, 2, 189-200.

Loomis, A.L., Harvey, E.N. and Hobart, G.A. Cerebral states during sleep, as studied by human brain potentials. *J. Exp. Psychol.*, 1937, 21, 127-44.

Lovell, G.D. and Morgan, J.J. Physiological and motor responses to a regularly recurring sound: a study in monotony. *J. Exp. Psychol.*, 1942, 30, 435-51.

Lukianowicz, N. Hallucinations à troix. *Arch. Gen. Psychiatry*, 1959, 1, 322-31.

Luria, A.R. and Vinogradova, O.S. An objective investigation of the dynamics of semantic systems. *Brit. J. Psychol.*, 1959, 50(2), 89-105.

McClelland, D.C. On the psychodynamics of creative physical scientists. In Gruber, H., Terrell, G. and Wertheimer, M. (eds) *Contemporary Approaches to Creative Thinking*. New York: Atheron Press, 1964.

McGaughran, L. and Moran, L. 'Conceptual level' vs. 'conceptual area' analysis of object-sorting behavior of schizophrenic and nonpsychiatric groups. *J. Abn. Social Psychol.*, 1956, 52, 43-50.

McGlade, H.B. This relationship between gastric motility, muscular twitching during sleep and dreaming. *Amer. J. Digest. Dis.*, 1942, 9, 137-40.

McKellar, P. *Imagination and Thinking*. London: Cohen & West, 1957. (Quotations are from the 3rd impression, 1967.)

McKellar, P. The mental images which precede sleep. *J. Amer. SPR*, 1959, 53, 23-27.

McKellar, P. Three aspects of the psychology of originality in human thinking. *Brit. J. Aesthetics*, 1963, 3, 129-47.

McKellar, P. *Experience and Behaviour*. Harmondsworth: Penguin, 1968.

McKellar, P. Imagery from the standpoint of introspection. In Sheehan, P. (ed.) *The Function and Nature of Imagery*. New York and London: Academic Press, 1972.

McKellar, P. Twixt waking and sleeping. *Psychology Today* (European edn), 1975, 4, 20-24.

McKellar, P. Autonomy, imagery, and dissociation. *J. Mental Imagery*, 1977, 1, 93-108.

McKellar, P. Between wakefulness and sleep: Hypnagogic fantasy. In Sheikh A.A. and Shaffer, J.T. (eds) *The Potential of Fantasy and Imagination*. New York: Brandon House, 1979. (a).

McKellar, P. *Mindsplit*. London: J.M. Dent, 1979. (b).

McKellar, P., and Simpson, L. Between wakefulness and sleep: Hypnagogic imagery. *Brit. J. Psychol.*, 1954, 45, 266-76.

McLean, P. Contrasting functions of limbic and neocortical systems of the brain and their relevance to psycho-physiological aspects of medicine. *Amer. J. Med.*, 1958, 25(4), 611-46.

McLean, P. Psychosomatics. In Field, J. *et al.* (eds) *Handbook of Physiology: Section 1. Neurophysiology* (vol. 3). Washington DC: Williams & Wilkins, 1960.

McLean, P. Man and his animal brains. *Modern Medicine*, 1964 (3 February), 95-106.

McLean, P. The limbic and visual cortex in phylogeny: Further insights from anatomic and microelectrode studies. In Hassler, R. and Stephen, H. (eds) *Evolution of the Forebrain*. Stuttgart: Thieme Verlag, 1966.

McLean, P. The triune brain, emotion, and scientific bias. In Schmitt, F. (ed.) *The Neurosciences: Second Study Program*. New York: Rockefeller University Press, 1970.

McNish, R. *The Philosophy of Sleep*. Glasgow: W.R. McPhun, 1830.

McReynolds, P. Anxiety, perception and schizophrenia. In Jackson, D. (ed.) *The Etiology of Schizophrenia*. New York: Basic Books, 1960.

Magoun, H.W. *The Waking Brain*. Springfield, Ill.: C. Thomas, 1963.

Mahl, G.F., Rothenberg, A., Delgado, J. and Hamlin, H. Psychological responses in the human to intracerebral electrical stimulation. *Psychosom. Medicine*, 1964, 26, 337-68.

Malcolm, N. *Dreaming*. London: Routledge & Kegan Paul, 1967.

Marks, D. Mental imagery and consciousness: A theoretical review. In Sheikh, A. (ed.) *Imagery: Current Theory, Research and Applications*. New York: Wiley, 1982.

Marks, D. and McKellar, P. The nature and function of eidetic imagery. *J. Mental Imagery*, 1982, 6(1), 1-124.

Maron, L., Rechtschaffen, A. and Wolpert, E. Sleep cycle during napping. *Arch. Gen. Psychiatry*, 1964, 11, 503-8.

Marsh, H.D. The diurnal course of efficiency. *Columbia University Contrib. Philos. Psychol.*, 1906, 14, 1-99.

Maslow, A.H. Personality problems and personality growth. In Moustakas, C.E. (ed.) *The Self*. New York: Harper & Row, 1956.

Maslow, A.H. *Toward a Psychology of Being*. Princeton, New Jersey: Van Nostrand, 1968, (2nd edn).

Maury, A. Des hallucinations hypnagogiques ou des erreurs des sens dans l'état intermédiaire entre la veille et le sommeil. *Ann. Medico-Psychol. Syst. Nerveux*, 1848, 11, 26-40.

Maury, A. Nouvelles observations sur les analogies des phénomènes du rêve et de l'aliénation mentale. *Ann. Med. Psychol.*, 1853, 5, 404-544.

Maury, A. De certains faits observés dans les rêves et dans l'état intermédiaire entre le sommeil et la veille. *Ann. Med. Psychol.*, 1857, 3, 157-76.

Maury, A. *Le Sommeil et les rêves*. Paris: Didier, 1878.

Mavromatis, A. Hypnagogia: The nature and function of the hypnagogic state. Unpublished doctoral dissertation, Brunel University, 1983.

Mavromatis, A. and Richardson, J.T.E. Hypnagogic imagery. *Internat. Review of Mental Imagery*, 1984, 1, 159-89.

Max, L.W. Action-current responses in the deaf during awakening, kinesthetic imagery and abstract-thinking. *J. Comp. Psychol.*, 1937, 24, 301-44.

Mayer-Gross, W. Zur Struktur des Einschlaferlebens. *Arch. Psychiat.*, 1929, 86, 313.

Mayer-Gross, W., Slater, E. and Roth, M. *Clinical Psychiatry*. London: Baillière, Tindall & Cassell, 1969 (3rd edn).

Meddis, R. *The Sleep Instinct*. London: Routledge & Kegan Paul, 1977.

Medlicott, R.W. An inquiry into the significance of hallucinations with special reference to their occurrence in the sane. *Internat. Record of Medicine*, 1958, 171, 664-77.

Mednick, S.A. The associative basis of the creative process. *Psychol. Review*, 1962, 69(3), 220-32.

Meenes, M. and Morton, M.A. Characteristics of the eidetic type. *J. Gen. Psychol.*, 1936, 14, 370-91.

Miller, F. Quelque faits d'imagination créatrice subconsciente. *Arch. Psychologie*, 1906, 5, 36-51.

Miller, G.A. The magical number seven plus or minus two: Some limits on our capacity for processing information. *Psychol. Review*, 1956, 63, 81-97.

Miller, G., Galanter, E. and Pribram, K. *Plans and the Structure of Behaviour*. New York: Holt, 1960.

Miller, M. Changes in the response to electric shock produced by varying muscular conditions. *J. Exp. Psychol.*, 1926, 9, 26-44.

Milner, M. *On Not Being Able to Paint*. London: Heinemann, 1981.

Mintz, A. Schizophrenic speech and sleepy speech. *J. Abn. Soc. Psychology*, 1948, 43, 548-9.

Mishra, R. *The Textbook of Yoga Psychology*. New York: Julian Press, 1967.

Mitchell, S.W. Some disorders of sleep. *Internat. J. Med. Sci.*, 1890, 100, 109-27.

Mitchell, S.W. Remarks on the effects of anhalonium lewinii (the mescal button). *Brit. Med. J.*, 1896, 2, 1625-8.

Miyagi, O. The hypnagogic neologisms. *Jap. J. Exp. Psychol.*, 1937, 4, 109-11.

Monroe, R.A. *Journeys Out of the Body*. London: Corgi Books, 1974.

Moody, R.A. Jr. *Life after Life*. New York: Corgi/Bantam Books, 1976.

Moody, R.A. Jr. *Reflections on 'Life after Life'*. New York: Bantam Books, 1978.

Morison, R. and Dempsey, E. A study of thalamo-cortical relations. *Amer. J. Physiol.*, 1942, 135, 281-92.

Morris, G.O., Williams, H.L. and Lubin, A. Misperception and disorientation during sleep deprivation. *Arch. Gen. Psychiatry*, 1960 2, 247-54.

Morris, P.E. and Hampson, P.J. *Imagery and Consciousness*. London: Academic Press, 1983.

Morris, R.L. The psychobiology of psi. In Mitchell, E.D. and White, J. (eds) *Psychic Explorations*. New York: Putnam's Sons, 1976.

Moss, T.S. Interview: Thelma S. Moss. *Psychic*, 1970 (July-August).

Muldoon, S. and Carrington, H. *The Projection of the Astral Body*. London: Rider, 1965.

Müller, J. *Ueber die phantastische Gesichtserscheinungen: Eine physiologische Untersuchung mit einer physiologischen Urkunde des Aristoteles über den Traum, den Philosophen, und Aerzten gewidmet.* Koblenz: J. Hölscher, 1826.

Müller, J. *The Physiology of the Senses, Voice, and Muscular Motion, with the Mental Faculties.* Trans. by Baly, W. London: Taylor, Walton & Maberly, 1848.

Mundy-Castle, A.F. Theta and beta rhythm in the electroencephalograms of normal adults. *Electroenceph. Clin. Neurophysiol.,* 1951, 3, 477-86.

Murphy, G. Removal of impediments to the paranormal. *J. Amer. SPR,* 1944, 38, 2-23.

Murphy, G. and Dale, L.A. Concentration versus relaxation. *J. Amer. SPR,* 1943, 37, 2-15.

Murray, H.A. Vicissitudes of creativity. In Anderson, H. (ed.) *Creativity and its Cultivation.* New York: Harper & Row, 1959.

Myers, F.W.H. Sensory automatism and induced hallucinations. *Proc. SPR,* 1892, 8, 436-536.

Myers, F.W.H. *Human Personality and its Survival of Bodily Death.* London: Longmans, Green & Co., 1903.

Myers, O.H. Images in the mind. *J. Amer. SPR,* 1957, 51, 62-73.

Myers, T.I. and Murphy, D.B. Reported visual sensations during brief exposure to reduced sensory input. In West, L.J. (ed.) *Hallucinations.* New York: Grune & Stratton, 1962.

Mylonas, G.E. *Eleusis and the Eleusinian Mysteries.* Princeton, New Jersey: Princeton University Press, 1974.

Nash, J. *Developmental Psychology: A Psychobiological Approach.* Englewood Cliffs, New Jersey: Prentice-Hall, 1970.

Newbold, W.R. Subconscious reasoning. *Proc. SPR,* 1897, 12, 11-20.

Niedermeyer, F. and Lentz, W. Dreaming in non-REM sleep: A preliminary study of brief diurnal sleep in the clinical EEG laboratory. *Waking & Sleeping,* 1976, 1, 49-51.

Nielsen, J. and Sedgwick, R. Instincts and emotions in an anencephalous monster. *J. Nerv. Ment. Dis.,* 1949, 110, 387-94.

Nietzsche, F. Composition of thus spake Zarathustra. In Ghiselin, B. (ed.) *The Creative Process.* New York: New American Library, 1952.

Northage, I. *The Mechanics of Mediumship.* London: Spiritualist Association of Great Britain, 1973.

Novomeiskii, A.S. The nature of the dermo-optic sense. *Internat. J. of Parapsychology,* 1965, 7(4), 341-67.

Obrador, S. Effect of hypothalamic lesions on electrical activity of cerebral cortex. *J. Neurophysiol.,* 1943, 6, 81-4.

O'Brien, E. *The Essential Plotinus.* Indianapolis: Hackett, 1975.

Olds, J. and Milner, P. Positive reinforcement produced by electrical stimulation of septal area and other regions of rat brain. *J. Comp. Physiol. Psychol.,* 1954, 47, 419-27.

Oliver, G.W. Symbolic aspects of hypnagogic imagery associated with theta feedback. Unpublished doctoral dissertation, California School of Professional Psychology, 1975.

Omwake, K.T. Effect on varying periods of sleep on nervous stability. *J. Appl. Psychol.,* 1932, 16, 623-32.

Organ, T.W. *Western Approaches to Eastern Philosophy.* Ohio University Press, 1975.

Orne, M.T. The nature of hypnosis: Artifact and essence. *J. Abn. Soc. Psychol.,* 1959, 58, 277-99.

Ornitz, E.M., Ritvo, E.R., Carr, E.M., La Franchi, S. and Walters, R.D. The effect of sleep onset on the auditory averaged evoked response. *Electroenceph. Clin. Neurophysiol.*, 1967, 23, 335-41.

Oster, G. Phosphenes. *Art Internat.*, 1966, 10, 34-46.

Oswald, I. After-images from retina and brain. *Quart. J. Exp. Psychology*, 1957, 9, 88-100. (a).

Oswald, I. The EEG, visual imagery and attention. *Quart. J. Exp Psychology*, 1957, 9, 113-18. (b).

Oswald, I. A case of fluctuation of awareness with the pulse. *Quart. J. Exp. Psychology*, 1959, 11, 45-48. (a).

Oswald, I. Sudden bodily jerks on falling asleep. *Brain*, 1959, 82, 92-103. (b).

Oswald, I. Falling asleep open-eyed during intense rhythmic stimulation. *Brit. Med. J.*, 1960, 1, 1450-5.

Oswald, I. *Sleeping and Waking*. Amsterdam: Elsevier, 1962.

Oswald, I. *Sleep*. Harmondsworth: Penguin, 1976.

Ouspensky, P. *In Search of the Miraculous*. New York: Harcourt, 1949.

Ouspensky, P. *A New Model of the Universe*. London: Routledge & Kegan Paul, 1978. (orig. 1931).

Owens, A.C. A study of imagination. Unpublished doctoral dissertation. University of Liverpool, 1963.

Pagano, R., Rose, R., Stivers, R. and Warrenburg, S. Sleep during transcendental meditation. *Science*, 1976, 191, 308-10.

Paivio, A. *Imagery and Verbal Processes*. New York: Holt, 1971.

Paivio, A. Neomentalism. *Canad. J. Psychol./Revised Canad. Psychology*, 1974, 29, 263-91.

Panati, C. *Super Senses*. London: Jonathan Cape, 1975.

Partridge, G.E. Reverie. *Pedagog. Seminary*, 1898, 5, 445-74.

Pasik, P., Pasik, T. and Schilder, P. Extrageniculostriate vision in the monkey: Discrimination of luminous flux-equated figures. *Exp. Neurol.*, 1969, 24, 421-37.

Payne, R.W. An object classification test as a measure of over-inclusive thinking in schizophrenic patients. *Brit. J. Soc. Clin. Psychol.*, 1962, 1(3), 213-21.

Payne, R., Matussek, P. and George, G. An experimental study of schizophrenic thought disorder. *J. Ment. Science*, 1959, 105, 627-52.

Peak, H. Attitude and motivation. In Jones, M. (ed.) *Nebraska Symposium on Motivation*. Lincoln: University of Nebraska Press, 1955.

Penfield, W. The cerebral cortex in man. I. The cerebral cortex and consciousness. *Arch. Neurol. Psychiatry*, 1938, 40, 417-42.

Penfield, W. Consciousness and the centrencephalic organization. (First Internat. Congr. Neurol. Sci., Seconde Journée Commune.) Brussels: *Acta Med. Belg.*, 1957, 7-18.

Penfield, W. Centrencephalic integrating system. *Brain*, 1958, 81, 231-4.

Penfield, W. and Jasper, H. *Epilepsy and the Functional Anatomy of the Human Brain*. London: Churchill, 1954.

Penfield, W. and Perot, P. The brain's record of auditory and visual experience. A final summary and discussion. *Brain*, 1963, 86, 595-696.

Penfield, W. and Rasmussen, T. *The Cerebral Cortex of Man*. New York: Macmillan, 1950.

Pepper, S. *World Hypotheses: A Study in Evidence*. Berkeley and Los Angeles: University of California Press, 1948.

Perenin, M. and Jeannerod, M. Residual vision in cortically blind hemifields. *Neuropsychologia*, 1975, 13, 1-7.

Peters, H. Supraordinality of associations and maladjustment. *J. Psychol.*, 1952, 33, 217-25.

Piaget, J. *Play, Dreams and Imitation*. London: Heinemann, 1951.

Pinard, W.J. Spontaneous imagery: Its nature, therapeutic value, and effect on personality structure. *Boston Univ. Grad. J.*, 1957, 5, 150-3.

Pintus, G. and Falqui, A. Sulla sede di origine delle 'mioclonie ipniche fisiologiche'. *Riv. Neurol.*, 1934, 7, 133-60.

Pitts, F. Jr. and McLure, J. Jr. Lactate metabolism in anxiety neurosis. *New England J. Med.*, 1967, 277, 1329-36.

Poe, E.A. Marginalia. In Slater, M. (ed.) *The Centenary Poe*. London: Bodley Head, 1949. (orig. in *Graham's American Monthly Magazine*, 1846, vol. 28, part 3).

Poeppel, E., Held, R. and Frost, D. Residual visual function after brain wounds involving the central visual pathways in man. *Nature* (Lond.), 1973, 243, 295-6.

Poincaré, H. Mathematical creation. In Vernon, P.E. (ed.) *Creativity*. Harmondsworth: Penguin, 1978. (orig. 1913).

Popper, K.R. *The Logic of Scientific Discovery*. London: Hutchinson, 1977. (orig. 1959).

Posner, M.I. and Klein, R.M. On the functions of consciousness. In Kornblum, S. (ed.) *Attention and Performance IV*. London: Academic Press, 1973.

Pribram, K. and McLean, P. Neuronographic analysis of medial and basal cerebral cortex. II: Monkey. *J. Neurophysiol.*, 1953, 16, 324-40.

Prince, M. An experimental study of visions. *Brain*, 1898, 84, 528-46.

Prince, M. *The Dissociation of a Personality*. London: Longmans, 1906.

Prince, M. A symposium on the subconscious. *J. Abn. Psychol.*, 1907, 2, 67-80.

Prince, M. Coconscious images. *J. Abn. Psychol.*, 1917, 12(5), 289-316.

Prince, M. An experimental study of the mechanism of hallucinations. *Brit. J. Psychol. (Med. Section)*, 1922, 2(3), 165-208.

Prince, M. *The Unconscious*. New York: Macmillan, 1929.

Prince, M. Subconscious intelligence underlying dreams. In Ghiselin B. (ed.) *The Creative Process*. New York: New American Library, 1952.

Puech, P., Guilly, P., Fischgold, H. and Bunes, G. Un cas d'anencéphalie hydrocephalique. Etude électroencéphalographique. *Rev. Neurol.*, 1947, 79, 116-24.

Purdy, D.M. Eidetic imagery and plasticity of perception. *J. Gen. Psychol.*, 1936, 15, 437-54.

Radestock, P. *Schlaf und Traum: Eine physiologisch-psychologische Untersuchung*. Leipzig: Breitkopf & Haertel, 1879.

Rapaport, D. Cognitive structures. In Gill M.M. (ed.) *The Collected Papers of David Rapaport*. New York: Basic Books, 1967. (a).

Rapaport, D. States of consciousness: A psychopathological and psychodynamic view. In Gill M.M. (ed.) *The Collected Papers of David Rapaport*. New York: Basic Books, 1967. (b).

Rawcliffe, D.H. *The Psychology of the Occult*. London: Ridgeway, 1952.

Rawson, H.G. Experiments in thought-transference. *Proc. SPR*, 1895, 11, 2-17.

Rechtschaffen, A., Wolpert, E.A., Dement, W.C., Mitchell, S.A. and Fisher, C. Nocturnal sleep of narcoleptics. *Electroenceph. Clin. Neurophysiol.*, 1963, 15, 599-609.

Regardie, I. *Foundations of Practical Magic.* Wellingborough, Northants: Aquarian Press, 1979.

Reik, T. *Listening with the Third Ear.* New York: Farrar, Straus, 1949.

Reimer, F. *Der Syndrom der optischen Halluzinose.* Stuttgart: Thieme Verlag, 1970.

Reiter, R.J. *The Pineal – 1977* (Annual research reviews). Montreal: Eden Press, 1977.

Relkin, R. Effect of pinealectomy on adrenal secretion of testosterone in castrate cats. *Acta Endocrinol. Panam.*, 1972, 3, 129-33.

Rhine, J.B. *Extra-sensory Perception.* Boston: Bruce Humphries, 1934.

Rhine, J.B. *New Frontiers of the Mind.* New York: Farrar & Rinehart, 1937.

Richardson, A. *Mental Imagery.* London: Routledge & Kegan Paul, 1969.

Richardson, A. Imagery: Definition and types. In Sheikh, A. (ed.) *Imagery: Current Theory, Research, and Application.* New York: Wiley, 1983.

Richardson, A. *The Experiential Dimension of Psychology.* St Lucia, Queensland: University of Queensland Press, 1984.

Richardson, J.T.E., Mavromatis, A., Mindel, T. and Owens, A.C. Individual differences in hypnagogic and hypnopompic imagery. *J. Mental Imagery*, 1981, 5, 91-6.

Richet, C. Further experiments in hypnotic lucidity or clairvoyance. *Proc. SPR*, 1889, 6, 66-83.

Ring, K. *Heading Towards Omega.* New York: William Morrow, 1984.

Roberts, U. *Hints on Mediumistic Development.* (Private Publication: obtainable from 7, Sunny Grds. Rd., London, NW4, 1SL: 1964.)

Roberts, W.W. Rapid escape learning without avoidance learning motivated by hypothalamic stimulation in cats. *J. Comp. Physiol. Psychol.*, 1958, 51, 391-9.

Roger, H. Les secousses nerveuses de l'endormissement. *Rev. Méd. Franç.*, 1931, 12, 847-52.

Rogers, C.R. *Client-centered Therapy.* Boston: Houghton Mifflin, 1951.

Rogers, C.R. Toward a theory of creativity. In Anderson, H.H. (ed.) *Creativity and its Cultivation.* New York: Harper & Row, 1959.

Rogers, C.R. *On Becoming a Person.* Boston: Houghton Mifflin, 1961.

Roheim, G. *The Gates of the Dream.* New York: International Universities Press, 1952.

Romains, J. *Eyeless Sight: A Study of Extra-retinal Vision and the Paroptic Sense.* London and New York: Putnam's Sons, 1924.

Rose, S. *The Conscious Brain.* Harmondsworth: Penguin, 1976.

Rosett, J. *The Mechanism of Thought, Imagery, and Hallucination.* New York: Columbia University Press, 1939.

Roth, M., Shaw, J. and Green, J. The form, voltage distribution and physiological significance of the K-complex. *EEG Clin. Neurophysiol.*, 1956, 8, 385-402.

Rouquès, L. Les images prémonitoires du sommeil. *Rev. Neurol.*, 1946, 78, 371-2.

Rowland, V. Differential electroencephalographic response to conditioned auditory stimuli in arousal from sleep. *EEG Clin. Neurophysiol.*, 1957, 9, 585-94.

Rubin, F. (ed.) *Current Research in Hypnopaedia.* London: Macdonald, 1968.

Rush, J. and Jensen, A. A reciprocal distance GESP test with drawings. *J. Parapsychology*, 1949, 13, 122-34.

Russell, P. *The Brain Book.* London: Routledge & Kegan Paul, 1982.

Ryle, G. *The Concept of Mind.* Harmondsworth: Penguin, 1976.

Saint-Denys, H. de. *Dreams and How to Guide Them*. London: Duckworth, 1982. (orig. 1867).

Sanders, M., Warrington, E., Marshall, J. and Weiskrantz, L. 'Blindsight': Vision in a field defect. *Lancet*, 1974 (20 April), 707-8.

Sarbin, T.R. Contributions to role-taking theory: I. Hypnotic behavior. *Psychol. Review*, 1950, 57, 255-70.

Sartre, J.-P. *The Psychology of Imagination*. London: Methuen, 1978. (First published in French as *L'Imaginaire*, 1940.)

Saul, L.J. Dream scintillations. *Psychosom. Medicine*, 1965, 27, 286-9.

Schachtel, E.G. *Metamorphosis: On the Development of Affect, Perception, Attention and Memory*. New York: Basic Books, 1959.

Schacter, D.L. The hypnagogic state: A critical review of the literature. *Psychol. Bull.*, 1976, 83(3), 452-81.

Schacter, D.L. and Kelly, E.F. ESP in the twilight zone. *J. Parapsychol.*, 1975, 39, 27-28.

Schaefer, C.E. The importance of measuring metaphorical thinking in children. *Gifted Child Quart.*, 1975, 19, 140-8.

Schatzman, M. *The Story of Ruth*. Harmondsworth: Penguin, 1982.

Scheibel, M.L. and Scheibel, A. Structural substrates for integrative patterns in the brain stem reticular core. In *The Reticular Formation of the Brain: International Symposium*. Boston: Little Brown, 1958.

Scheibel, M. and Scheibel, A. Hallucinations and the brain stem reticular core. In West, L.J. (ed.) *Hallucinations*. New York: Grune & Stratton, 1962.

Scheibel, M., Scheibel, A., Mollica, A. and Moruzzi, G. Convergence and interaction of afferent impulses on single units of the reticular formation. *J. Neurophysiol.*, 1955, 18, 309-31.

Schilder, P. *The Image and Appearance of the Human Body: Studies in the Constructive Energies of the Psyche*. New York: International Universities Press, 1950.

Schilder, P., Pasik, P. and Pasik, T. Extrageniculostriate vision in the monkey. III. Circle vs. triangle and 'red vs. green' descrimination. *Exp. Brain Res.*, 1972, 14, 436-48.

Schiller, P. Interrelation of different senses in perception. *J. Psychol.*, 1935, 25(4), 465-9.

Schjelderup-Ebbe, T. Beiträge zur Analyse der Träume. *Z. Psychol.*, 1923, 93, 312-18.

Schlauch, R. Hypnopompic hallucinations and treatment with imipramine. *Amer. J. Psychiatry*, 1979, 136(2), 219-20.

Schlesinger, B. *Higher Cerebral Functions and Their Clinical Disorders*. New York: Grune & Stratton, 1962.

Schmeller, A. *Surrealism*. London: Methuen, 1960.

Schmoll, A. Experiments in thought-transference. *Proc. SPR*, 1887, 4, 324-37.

Schmoll, A. and Mabire, J.E. Experiments in thought transference. *Proc. SPR*, 1888, 5, 169-215.

Schneck, J.M. An evaluation of hypnagogic hallucinations. *Psychiat. Quarterly*, 1968, 42, 232-4.

Schneck, J.M. Hypnagogic hallucinations: Herman Melville's Moby Dick. *N. York State J. Medicine*, 1977, 77, 2145-7.

Schultz, G. Über hypnagoge Halluzinationen. *Msch. f. Psych.*, 1930, 75, 44-62.

Schultz, J. and Luthe, W. *Autogenic Training: A Psycho-physiologic Approach in Psychotherapy.* New York: Grune & Stratton, 1959.

Schwartz, B.A. and Fischgold, H. Introduction à l'étude polygraphique du sommeil de nuit (Mouvements oculaires et cycles de sommeil). *Vie Méd.*, 1960, 41(s1), 39-46.

Sedman, G. A clinical and phenomenological study of pseudohallucinations and related experiences. Unpublished MD thesis, Manchester University, 1964.

Sedman, G. Being an epileptic. *Psychiat. Neurol.*, 1966, 152 (Basel), 1-16.

Shaffer, L.H. Multiple attention in continuous verbal tasks. In Rabbitt, P.M. and Dornic, S. (eds) *Attention and Performance. V.* London: Academic Press, 1975.

Shallice, T. Dual functions of consciousness. *Psychol. Review*, 1972, 79, 383-93.

Shapiro, D. A perceptual understanding of color response. In Rickersman, M. (ed.) *Rorschach Psychology.* New York: John Wiley & Sons, 1960, 154-201.

Sheehan, P.W. Functional similarity of imaging to perceiving: Individual differences in vividness of imagery. *Perc. Mot. Skills*, 1966, 23, 1011-33.

Sheehan, P.W. Colour response to the TAT: An instance of eidetic imagery. *J. Psychol.*, 1968, 68, 203-9.

Sheehan, P.W. Imagery process and hypnosis: An experimental analysis of phenomena. In Sheikh, A.A. and Shaffer, J. (eds) *The Potential of Fantasy and Imagination.* New York: Brandon House, 1979.

Shepard, R.N. and Podgorny, P. Cognitive processes that resemble perceptual processes. In Estes, W. (ed.) *Handbook of Learning and Cognitive Processes.* Hillsdale, New Jersey: Erlbaum, 1978.

Sherman, S.E. Very deep hypnosis: An experimental and electroencephalographic investigation. Unpublished doctoral dissertation, Stanford University, 1971.

Sherwood, J. *The Fourfold Vision: A Study of Consciousness, Sleep and Dreams.* London: Spearman, 1965.

Short, P.L. The objective study of mental imagery. *Brit. J. Psychol.*, 1953, 44, 38-51.

Short, P.L. and Walter, W.G. The relationship between physiological variables and stereognosis. *EEG Clin. Neurophysiol.*, 1954, 6, 29-44.

Sidgwick (Mrs) H. Report on further experiments in thought-transference carried out by Professor Gilbert Murray. *Proc. SPR*, 1924, 34, 212-74.

Sidis, B. *An Experimental Study of Sleep.* Boston: Badger, 1909.

Sidis, B. The theory of the subconscious. *Proc. SPR*, 1912, 26, 319-43.

Siegel, R.K. Hallucinations. *Scient. American*, 1977, 237(4), 132-40.

Silberer, H. Report on a method of eliciting and observing certain symbolic hallucination-phenomena. In Rapaport, D. (ed.) *Organization and Pathology of Thought.* New York: Columbia University Press, 1965. (orig. 1909).

Silberer, H. *Hidden Symbolism of Alchemy and the Occult Arts.* New York: Dover Publications, 1971. (orig. 1917).

Simon, C. and Emmons, W. Learning during sleep. *Psychol. Bull.*, 1955, 52, 328-42.

Simon, C. and Emmons, W. Responses to material presented during various levels of sleep. *J. Exp. Psychol.*, 1956, 51, 89-79.

Sinclair, U. *Mental Radio: Does It Work, and How?* London: Werner Laurie, 1930.

Singer, J.L. *Daydreaming.* New York: Random House, 1966.

Singer, J.L. *Daydreaming and Fantasy.* London: Allen & Unwin, 1976.

Slap, J.W. On dreaming at sleep onset. *Psychoanal. Quart.*, 1977, 46(1), 71-81.

Slater, E., Beard, A.W. and Glithero, E. The schizophrenia-like psychoses of epilepsy. *Brit. J. Psychiatry*, 1963, 109, 95-150.

Slight, D. Hypnagogic phenomena. *J. Abn. Soc. Psychol.*, 1924, 19, 381-91.

Smythies, J.R. The stroboscopic patterns (III): Further experiments and discussion. *Brit. J. Psychol.*, 1960, 51, 247-55.

Smythies, J.R. (ed.) *Science and ESP*. London: Routledge & Kegan Paul, 1971.

Snyder, F. The new biology of dreaming. *Arch. Gen. Psychiatry*, 1963, 8, 381-91.

Snyder, F. Progress in the new biology of dreaming. *Amer. J. Psychiatry*, 1965, 122, 377-91.

Snyder, F., Hobson, J.A., Morrison, D.F. and Goldfrank, F. Changes in respiration, heart rate, and systolic blood pressure in human sleep. *J. Appl. Physiol.*, 1964, 19, 417-22.

Sparrow, F.S. *Lucid Dreaming: Dawning of the Clear Light*. Virginia Beach, Virginia: ARE Press, 1976.

Sperling, G. The information available in brief visual presentations. *Psychol. Monographs*, 1960, 74, (11, whole no. 498).

Sperry, R.W. Hemisphere deconnection and unity of conscious awareness. *Amer. Psychol.*, 1968, 23, 723-33.

Sperry, R., Gazzaniga, M. and Bogen, J. Interhemispheric relationships: The neocortical commissures: Syndromes of hemisphere disconnection. In Vinken, P. and Bruyn, G. (eds) *Handbook of Clinical Neurology*, (vol. 4). Amsterdam: North Holland Publishing Co., 1969.

Staal, F. *Exploring Mysticism*. Harmondsworth: Penguin, 1975.

Stace, W.T. *The Teachings of the Mystics*. New York: A Mentor book, 1960.

Stace, W.T. *Mysticism and Philosophy*. London: Macmillan, 1973.

Stanford, R.G. EEG alpha activity and ESP performance: A replicative study. *J. Amer. SPR*, 1971, 65, 144-54.

Stanford, R.G. Conceptual frameworks of contemporary psi research. In Wolman, B. (ed.) *Handbook of Parapsychology*. New York: Van Nostrand Reinhold, 1977.

Stanford, R.G. and Lovin, C. EEG alpha activity and ESP performance. *J. Amer. SPR*, 1970, 64, 375-84.

Starker, S. Two modes of visual imagery. *Perc. Mot. Skills*, 1974, 38, 649-50.

Stearn, J. *In Search of a Soul*. New York: Doubleday, 1973.

Steiner, R. *The Evolution of Consciousness*. London: Rudolf Steiner Press, 1979.

Sterman, M.B. The basic rest-activity cycle and sleep: Developmental considerations in man and cats. In Clemente, C.D., Purpura, D.P. and Mayer, F.E. (eds) *Sleep and the Maturing Nervous System*. New York and London: Academic Press, 1972.

Stoney, B. *Enid Blyton*. London: Hodder & Stoughton, 1974.

Storch, A. Über des archaische Denken in der Schizophrenie. *Z. Ges. Neurol. Psychiat.*, 1922, 78, 500-11.

Stoyva, J. Biofeedback techniques and the conditions for hallucinatory activity. In McGuigan, F.J. and Schoonover, R.A. (eds) *The Psychophysiology of Thinking*. New York and London: Academic Press, 1973.

Stoyva, J. and Kamiya, J. Electrophysiological studies of dreaming as the prototype of a new strategy in the study of consciousness. *Psychol. Review*, 1968, 75(3), 192-205.

Sullivan, H.S. *The Interpersonal Theory of Psychiatry*. London: Norton, 1953.

Suraci, A. Environmental stimulus reduction as a technique to effect the reactivation of crucial repressed memories. *J. Nerv. Ment. Dis.*, 1964, 138, 172-80.

Suzuki, D.T. *The Zen Doctrine of No-mind*. London: Rider, 1969.

Swedenborg, E. *The Word of the Old Testament Explained*. Bryn Athyn, Pennsylvania: Academy of the New Church, 1928-48. (orig. 1746).

Swedenborg, E. *Rational Psychology*. Philadelphia: Swedenborg Scientific Association, 1950. (orig. 1742).

Swedenborg, E. *Journal of Dreams*. New York: Swedenborg Foundation, 1977. (orig. 1859).

Szasz, T. *Ideology and Insanity*. Garden City, New York: Doubleday, 1970.

Taine, H. *Les Philosophes français du XIX siècle*. Paris: Hachette, 1857.

Taine, H. *De l'Intelligence*. Paris: Hachette, 1883.

Tanner, J.M. *Education and Physical Growth*. London: University of London Press, 1961.

Tappeiner, D.A. A psychological paradigm for the interpretation of the charismatic phenomenon of prophecy. *J. Psychol. and Theology*, 1977, 5(1), 23-9.

Tart, C. A second psychophysiological study of out of the body experience in a gifted subject. *Internat. J. Parapsychol.*, 1967, 9(1), 251-8.

Tart, C. Between waking and sleeping: The hypnagogic state. In Tart, C.T. (ed.) *Altered States of Consciousness*. New York: Wiley & Sons, 1969.

Tart, C. *On Being Stoned: A Psychological Study of Marijuana Intoxication*. Pala Alto, Cal.: Science and Behaviour Books, 1971.

Tart, C. *States of Consciousness*. New York: Dutton, 1975.

Tauber, E.S. and Green, M.R. *Prelogical Experience: An Inquiry into Dreams and Other Creative Processes*. New York: Basic Books, 1959.

Taylor, I.A. The nature of the creative process. In Smith, P. (ed.) *Creativity: An Examination of the Creative Process*. New York: Hastings House, 1959.

Teasdale, H.H. A quantitative study of eidetic imagery. *Brit. J. Ed. Psychol.*, 1934, 4, 56-74.

Tellegen, A. and Atkinson, G. Openness to absorbing and self-altering experiences ('Absorption'), a trait related to hypnotic susceptibility. *J. Abn. Psychol.*, 1974, 83(3), 268-77.

Ter Braak, J. and Van Vliet, A. Subcortical optokinetic nystagmus in the monkey. *Psychiat. Neurol. Neurochirurg.* (Amst.), 1963, 66, 277-83.

Ter Braak, J., Schenk, V. and Van Vliet, A. Visual reactions in a case of long-lasting cortical blindness. *J. Neurol. Neurosurg. Psychiat.*, 1971, 34, 140-7.

Thomas, N.W. *Thought Transference*. London: Alex Moring, 1905.

Thomson, G.N. Cerebral area essential to consciousness. *Bull. Los Angeles Neurol. Soc.*, 1951, 16, 311-34.

Thomson, G. and Nielsen, J. Area essential to consciousness; Cerebral localization of consciousness as established by neuropathological studies. *J. Amer. Med. Assn.*, 1948, 137, 285.

Timmons, B., Salamy, J., Kamiya, J. and Girton, D. Abdominal-thoracic respiratory movements and levels of arousal. *Psychon. Science*, 1972, 27(3), 173-5.

Titchener, E.B. *Lectures on the Elementary Psychology of Feeling and Attention*. New York: Macmillan, 1908.

Titchener, E.B. *Lectures on the Experimental Psychology of Thought-processes*. New York: Macmillan, 1909.

Titchener, E.B. *A Beginner's Psychology*. New York: Macmillan, 1916.

Toman, J.E., Bush, I. and Chachkes, J. Conditional features of sound-evoked responses during sleep. *Fed. Proc.*, 1958, 17, 163.

Tournay, A. Sur mes propres visions du demi-sommeil. *Rev. Neurol.*, 1941, 73, 209-24.

Trevarthen, C.B. Two mechanisms of vision in primates. *Psychol. Forsch.*, 1968, 31, 299-337.

Trömner, E. Vorgänge beim Einschlafen (Hypnagogue-Phänomene). *Journ. f. Psychol. u. Neurol.*, 1911, 17, 343-63.

Turvey, V.N. *The Beginnings of Seership*. London: Stead's Publishing House, 1911.

Tyler, D.B. Psychological changes during experimental sleep deprivation. *Dis. Nerv. Syst.*, 1955, 16, 293-9.

Tyrrell, G.N.M. Further research in extrasensory perception. *Proc. SPR*, 1936, 44, 99-168.

Tyrrell, G.N.M. *Science and Psychical Phenomena*. New York: Harpers, 1938.

Underhill, E. *Mysticism*. New York: Meridian Books, 1955.

Usher, F.L. and Burt, F.P. Thought transference. *Annals of Psychical Science*, 1909, 8, 561-600.

Van Bogaert, L. L'hallucinose pédonculaire. *Rev. Neurol.*, 1927, 1, 608-17.

Van Bogaert, L. Activité onirique et conscience. In *Rêve et conscience*. Paris: Presses Universitaires de France, 1968.

Van Dusen, W. *The Natural Depth in Man*. New York: Harper & Row, 1972.

Van Dusen, W. *The Presence of Other Worlds*. London: Wildwood House, 1975.

Van Eeden, F. A study of dreams. In Tart, C. (ed.) *Altered States of Consciousness*. New York: Wiley & Sons, 1969. (orig. 1913).

Varendonck, J. *The Psychology of Day-dreams*. New York: Macmillan, 1921.

Vernon, J.A. *Inside the Black Room*. Harmondsworth: Penguin, 1966.

Vernon, J.A., Hoffman, J. and Shiffman, H. Visual hallucinations during perceptual isolation. *Canad. J. Psychol.* 1958, 12, 31-4.

Verny, T. and Kelly, J. *The Secret Life of the Unborn Child*. London: Sphere Books, 1982.

Vihvelin, H. On the differentiation of some typical forms of hypnagogic hallucinations. *Acta Psychiat. Neurologica*, 1948, 23, 359-89.

Vivekananda (Swami). *Raja Yoga*. New York: Ramakrishna-Vivekananda Center, 1955.

Vogel, G.W. Studies in psychophysiology of dreams: III. The dream of narcolepsy. *Arch. Gen. Psychiatry*, 1960, 3, 421-8.

Vogel, G.W. A review of REM sleep deprivation. *Arch. Gen. Psychiatry*, 1975, 32, 749-61.

Vogel, G.W. Endogenous depression improvement and REM pressure. *Arch. Gen. Psychiatry*, 1977, 34, 96-7.

Vogel, G.W., Barrowclough, B. and Giesler, D.D. Limited discriminability of REM and sleep onset reports and its psychiatric implications. *Arch. Gen. Psychiatry*, 1972, 26, 449-55.

Vogel, G., Foulkes, D. and Trosman, H. Ego functions and dreaming during sleep onset. In Tart, C. (ed.) *Altered States of Consciousness*. New York: Wiley & Sons, 1969. (orig. 1966).

Von Domarus, E. The specific laws of logic in schizophrenia. In Kasanin, J. (ed.) *Language and Thought in Schizophrenia*. New York: Norton, 1964.

Von Senden, M. *Space and Sight*. Glencoe, Ill.: Free Press, 1960.

Wada, J.A. and Hamm, A.E. Paper presented at the 27th annual meeting, *Amer. EEG Soc.*, Boston, 15 and 16 June 1973.

Walker, A.E. *The Primate Thalamus*. Chicago: University of Chicago Press, 1938.

Walkup, L.E. Creativity in science through visualization. *Perc. Mot. Skills*, 1965, 21, 35-41.

Wallace, R.K. Physiological effects of transcendental meditation. *Science*, 1970, 167, 1751-4.

Wallace, R.K. and Benson, H. The physiology of meditation. In Shapiro *et al.* (eds) *Biofeedback and Self-control: 1972*. Chicago: Aldine, 1973.

Wallace, R.K., Benson, H. and Wilson, A.F. A wakeful hypometabolic state. *Amer. J. Physiol.*, 1971, 221, 795-9.

Wallas, G. The art of thought (excerpts). In Vernon, P.E. (ed.) *Creativity*. Harmondsworth: Penguin, 1978. (orig. 1926).

Walsh, W.S. *The Psychology of Dreams*. London: Kegan Paul, 1920.

Walter, W.G. Discussion on the electroencephalogram in organic cerebral disease. *Proc. Roy. Soc. Med.*, 1948, 41, 237-50.

Walter, W.G. *The Neurophysiological Aspects of Hallucinations and Illusory Experience*. London: Society for Psychical Research, 1960.

Walter, W.G. and Dovey, V.J. Electroencephalography in cases of sub-cortical tumour. *J. Neurol. Neurosurg. Psychiatry*, 1944, 7, 57-65.

Walter, W.G. and Yeager, C.L. Visual imagery and electroencephalographic changes. *Electroenceph. Clin. Neurophysiol.*, 1956, 8, 193-9.

Wambach, H. *Life Before Life*. New York: Bantam Books, 1979.

Warcollier, R. *Experimental Telepathy*. Boston: Boston Soc. for Psychic Research, 1938.

Warcollier, R. *Mind to Mind*. New York: Creative Age Press, 1948.

Ward, J. Psychology. In *Encyclopedia Britannica* (9th edn), 1883, 20, 37-85.

Warren, H.C. Some unusual visual after-effects. *Psychol. Review*, 1921, 28, 453-63.

Watkins, M.M. *Waking Dreams*. London: Gordon & Breach, 1976.

Watson, L. *Supernature*. London: Hodder & Stoughton, 1974.

Weckowicz, T.E. and Blewett, D.B. Size constancy and abstract thinking in schizophrenic patients. *J. Ment. Science*, 1959, 105, 909-34.

Weiskrantz, L. An unusual case of after-imagery following fixation of an 'imaginary' visual pattern. *Quart. J. Exp. Psychol.*, 1950, 2, 170-5.

Weiskrantz, L. Contour discrimination in a young monkey with striate cortex ablation. *Neuropsychologia*, 1963, 1, 145-64.

Weisman, A.D. Reality sense and reality testing. *Behav. Science*, 1958, 3, 228-61.

Weiss, E. *Principles of Psychodynamics*. New York: Grune & Stratton, 1950.

Weitzman, E.D. and Kremen, H. Auditory evoked responses during different stages of sleep in man. *Electroenceph. Clin. Neurophysiol.*, 1965, 18, 65-70.

Werner, H. *Comparative Psychology of Mental Development*. New York: International Universities Press, 1948.

Werner, H. and Kaplan, B. *Symbol Formation: An Organismic-developmental Approach to Language and the Expression of Thought*. New York: Wiley & Sons, 1967.

West, L.J. A general theory of hallucinations and dreams. In West, L.J. (ed.) *Hallucinations*. New York: Grune & Stratton, 1962.

Wheeler, R.H. and Cutsforth, T.D. Synaesthesia and meaning. *Amer. J. Psychol.*, 1922, 33, 361-84.

White, H.E. and Levatin, P. Floaters in the eye. *Scient. American*, 1962, 206(6), 119-27.

White, R.A. A comparison of old and new methods of response to targets in ESP experiments. *J. Amer. SPR*, 1964, 58, 21-56.

Williams, A.C. Jr. Some psychological correlates of the electroencephalogram. *Arch. Psychol.*, 1939, 34(240), 1-48.

Williams, D.H. and Cartwright, R.D. Blood pressure changes during EEG-monitored sleep. *Arch. Gen. Psychiatry*, 1969, 20, 307-14.

Williams, H.L., Tepas, D.I. and Morlock, H.E. Evoked responses to clicks and electroencephalographic stages of sleep in man. *Science*, 1962, 138, 685-6.

Williams, L. The constituents of the unconscious. *Brit. J. Psychol.* (Medical Section), 1922, 2(4), 259-72.

Williams, M.A. and Abernethy, V. Being held by a spider. *Amer. J. Psychiatry*, 1978, 135(2), 232-3.

Wilson, R.C., Guilford, J. and Christensen, P. The measurement of individual difference in originality. *Psychol. Bull.*, 1953, 50(5), 362-70.

Wilson, S. *Salvador Dali*. London: Tate Gallery Publications, 1980.

Wolstenholme, G.E.W. and Knight, J. (eds) *The Pineal Gland* (Ciba Foundation symposium). Edinburgh and London: Churchill Livingstone, 1971.

Wolters, C. (translator). *The Cloud of Unknowing*. Harmondsworth: Penguin, 1977.

Woolley, V.J. Some auto-suggested visions as illustrating dream formation. *Proc. SPR*, 1914, 27, 390-9.

Wundt, W. *Vorlesungen über die Menschen und Thierseel*. Leipzig: L. Vosz, 1863.

Wurtman, R.J. Axelrod, J. and Kelly, D.E. *The Pineal*. New York: Academic Press, 1968.

Younger, J., Adriance, W. and Berger, R. Sleep during transcendental meditation. *Perc. Mot. Skills*, 1975, 40, 953-4.

Zarcone, V., Gulevitch, G., Pivik, T. and Dement, W. Partial REM phase deprivation and schizophrenia. *Arch. Gen. Psychiatry*, 1967, 16, 297-303.

Zeig, J.K. *A Teaching Seminar with Milton H. Erickson*. New York: Brunner/Mazel, 1980.

Zikmund, V. Physiological correlates of visual imagery. In Sheehan, P. (ed.) *The Function and Nature of Imagery*. New York and London: Academic Press, 1972.

Zuckerman, M. Perceptual isolation as a stress situation. *Arch. Gen. Psychiatry*, 1964, 11, 255-76.

Zuckerman, M., Albright, R.J., Marks, C.S. and Miller, G.L. Stress and hallucinatory effects of perceptual isolation and confinement. *Psychol. Mongr.: Gen. and Applied*, 1962, 76(30), 1-15.

Zuckerman, M. and Cohen, N. Sources of reports of visual and auditory sensations in perceptual isolation experiments. *Psychol. Bull.*, 1964, 62(1), 1-20.

Zuckerman, M. and Hopkins, T.R. Hallucinations or dreams? A study of arousal levels and reported visual sensations during sensory deprivation. *Perc. Mot. Skills*, 1966, 22, 447-559.

Index